New Frontiers in Thoracic Pathology

Editor

ALAIN C. BORCZUK

SURGICAL PATHOLOGY CLINICS

www.surgpath.theclinics.com

Consulting Editor
JASON L. HORNICK

June 2024 • Volume 17 • Number 2

ELSEVIER

1600 John F. Kennedy Boulevard • Suite 1800 • Philadelphia, Pennsylvania, 19103-2899

http://www.theclinics.com

SURGICAL PATHOLOGY CLINICS Volume 17, Number 2
June 2024 ISSN 1875-9181, ISBN-13: 978-0-443-13085-4

Editor: Taylor Hayes
Developmental Editor: Saswoti Nath

Surgical Pathology Clinics (ISSN 1875-9181) is published quarterly by Elsevier Inc., 360 Park Avenue South, New York, NY 10010. Months of issue are March, June, September, and December. Business and Editorial Office: Elsevier Inc., 1600 John F. Kennedy Blvd., Ste. 1800, Philadelphia, PA 19103-2899. Accounting and Circulation Offices: Elsevier Inc., 3251 Riverport Lane, Maryland Heights, MO 63043. Periodicals postage paid at New York, NY and at additional mailing offices. Subscription prices are $253.00 per year (US individuals), $100.00 per year (US students/residents), $294.00 per year (Canadian individuals), $307.00 per year (foreign individuals), and $120.00 per year (international students/residents), $100.00 per year (Canadian students/residents). For institutional access pricing please contact Customer Service via the contact information below. Foreign air speed delivery is included in all *Clinics*' subscription prices. All prices are subject to change without notice. **POSTMASTER:** Send address changes to *Surgical Pathology Clinics*, Elsevier, 3251 Riverport Lane, Maryland Heights, MO 63043. **Customer Service: 1-800-654-2452 (US). From outside the United States, call 1-314-447-8871. Fax: 1-314-447-8029. E-mail:** JournalsCustomerServiceusa@elsevier.com **(for print support)** and JournalsOnlineSupport-usa@elsevier.com **(for online support).**

Reprints. For copies of 100 or more, of articles in this publication, please contact the Commercial Reprints Department, Elsevier Inc., 360 Park Avenue South, New York, NY 10010-1710. Tel. 212-633-3874; Fax: 212-633-3820; E-mail: reprints@elsevier.com.

Surgical Pathology Clinics of North America is covered in *MEDLINE/PubMed (Index Medicus)*.

Contributors

CONSULTING EDITOR

JASON L. HORNICK, MD, PhD
Director of Surgical Pathology and
Immunohistochemistry, Brigham and Women's
Hospital, Professor of Pathology, Harvard
Medical School, Boston, Massachusetts, USA

EDITOR

ALAIN C. BORCZUK, MD
Vice Chairperson, Anatomic Pathology,
Department of Pathology and Laboratory
Medicine, Northwell Health, Professor of
Pathology, Zucker School of Medicine at
Hofstra, Greenvale, New York, USA

AUTHORS

MARY BETH BEASLEY, MD
Professor, Department of Pathology, Icahn
School of Medicine at Mount Sinai, New York,
New York, USA

JENNIFER M. BOLAND, MD
Professor, Division of Anatomic Pathology,
Department of Laboratory Medicine and
Pathology, Mayo Clinic, Rochester, Minnesota,
USA

ALAIN C. BORCZUK, MD
Vice Chairperson, Anatomic Pathology,
Department of Pathology and Laboratory
Medicine, Northwell Health, Professor of
Pathology, Zucker School of Medicine at
Hofstra, Greenvale, New York, USA

JACKIE CHEUK KI CHAN, MD
Faculty of Medicine and Dentistry, Department
of Laboratory Medicine and Pathology, Royal
Alexandra and University of Alberta Hospitals,
Edmonton, Alberta, Canada

ANDREW CHURG, MD
Professor, Department of Pathology,
Vancouver General Hospital, University of
British Columbia, Vancouver, British Columbia,
Canada

SANJA DACIC, MD, PhD
Vice-Chair and Director of Anatomic
Pathology, Professor, Department of
Pathology, Yale School of Medicine, New
Haven, Connecticut, USA

DOUGLAS J. HARTMAN, MD
Professor of Pathology, University of
Pittsburgh Medical Center, Pittsburgh,
Pennsylvania, USA

ALIYA N. HUSAIN, MD
Professor, Department of Pathology, University
of Chicago, Chicago, Illinois, USA

DEEPALI JAIN, MD, FIAC, FRCPATH
Diagnostic Histopathologist and
Cytopathologist, Department of Pathology, All
India Institute of Medical Sciences, New Delhi,
India

SONJA KLEBE, MD, PhD
Associate Professor, Department of
Anatomical Pathology, SA Pathology

and Flinders University, Flinders Medical Centre, Bedford Park, South Australia, Australia

HUIHUA LI, MD, PhD
Assistant Professor, Department of Pathology, Duke University Medical Center, Durham, North Carolina, USA

DAVID MOFFAT, MD
Associate Professor, Department of Anatomical Pathology, SA Pathology and Flinders University, Flinders Medical Centre, Bedford Park, South Australia, Australia

ANDRE L. MOREIRA, MD, PhD
Professor, Department of Pathology, New York University Grossman School of Medicine, New York, New York, USA

SANJAY MUKHOPADHYAY, MD
Director, Pulmonary Pathology, Department of Pathology, Pathology and Laboratory Medicine Institute, Cleveland Clinic, Cleveland, Ohio, USA

NESTOR L. MULLER, MD
Professor, Department of Radiology, University of British Columbia, Vancouver, British Columbia, Canada

OANA C. ROSCA, MD
Molecular Pathologist, Cytopathologist, Assistant Professor, Donald and Barbara Zucker School of Medicine at Hofstra/Northwell, Hempstead, New York, USA; Department of Pathology and Laboratory Medicine, Greenvale, New York, USA

IRENE SANSANO, MD
Pathologist, Department of Pathology, Hospital Universitari Vall d'Hebron, Barcelona, Catalunya, Spain

RIDHI SOOD, MD, DM
Fellow Oncopathology, Department of Pathology, All India Institute of Medical Sciences, New Delhi, India

OANA E. VELE, MD
Molecular Pathologist, Assistant Professor, Donald and Barbara Zucker School of Medicine at Hofstra/Northwell, Hempstead, New York, USA; Department of Pathology and Laboratory Medicine, Lenox Hill Hospital, New York, New York, USA

AKIHIKO YOSHIDA, MD, PhD
Pathologist, Department of Diagnostic Pathology, National Cancer Center Hospital, Chuo-ku, Rare Cancer Center, National Cancer Center, Tokyo, Japan

KEN-ICHI YOSHIDA, MD, PhD
Professor of Applied Microbiology Department of Science, Technology and Innovation Graduate School of Science, Department of Diagnostic Pathology and Cytology, Osaka International Cancer Institute, Osaka, Japan

FANG ZHOU, MD
Associate Professor, Department of Pathology, New York University Grossman School of Medicine, New York, New York, USA

Contents

In the twenty- first century, there is widespread agreement that in addition to lung cancer, emphysema, and chronic bronchitis, cigarette smoking causes accumulation of pigmented macrophages, interstitial fibrosis, and Langerhans cell proliferation in various permutations. These histologic changes remain subclinical in some patients and produce clinical manifestations and imaging abnormalities in others. Debate surrounds terminology of these lesions, which are often grouped together under the umbrella of "smoking-related interstitial lung disease." This review summarizes modern concepts in our understanding of these abnormalities and explains how the recognition of smoking-related interstitial fibrosis has advanced the field.

Granulomas are frequently encountered by pathologists in all types of lung specimens and arise from diverse etiologies. They should always be reported as necrotizing or non-necrotizing, with microorganism stains performed to evaluate for infection. With attention to distribution, quality (poorly vs well-formed), associated features, and correlation with clinical, radiologic, and laboratory data, the differential diagnosis for granulomatous lung disease can usually be narrowed to a clinically helpful "short list." This review describes a practical approach to pulmonary granulomas and reviews the clinicopathological aspects of common entities, including infectious (mycobacteria, fungi) and noninfectious (hypersensitivity pneumonitis, sarcoid, and vasculitis) causes.

Although silicosis has been an established disease with a recognized cause for more than 100 years, many workers continue to be exposed to silica and new outbreaks of disease continue to occur. This article describes some of the well-established and new exposures, including denim sandblasting, artificial stone cutting, and some forms of "coal worker's pneumoconiosis." The authors review the imaging and pathology of acute silicosis (silicoproteinosis), simple silicosis, and progressive massive fibrosis and summarize known and putative associations of silica exposure, including tuberculosis, lung cancer, connective tissue disease (especially systemic sclerosis), and vasculitis.

Spindle cell lesions of the pleura and pericardium are rare. Distinction from sarcomatoid mesothelioma, which has a range of morphologic patterns, can be difficult, but accurate diagnosis matters. This article provides practical guidance for the diagnosis of primary pleural spindle cell neoplasms, focusing on primary lesions.

Lung adenocarcinoma staging and grading were recently updated to reflect the link between histologic growth patterns and outcomes. The lepidic growth pattern is regarded as "in-situ," whereas all other patterns are regarded as invasive, though with stratification. Solid, micropapillary, and complex glandular patterns are associated with worse prognosis than papillary and acinar patterns. These recent changes have improved prognostic stratification. However, multiple pitfalls exist in measuring invasive size and in classifying lung adenocarcinoma growth patterns. Awareness of these limitations and recommended practices will help the pathology community achieve consistent prognostic performance and potentially contribute to improved patient management.

Major pathologic response (MPR) and pathologic complete response (pCR) are increasingly being used in non-small cell lung carcinoma neoadjuvant clinical trials as an early endpoint of survival. MPR for all histologic types of lung cancer is $\leq 10\%$ of viable tumor, while pCR requires no viable tumor. The International Association for the Study of Lung Cancer multidisciplinary recommendation for the assessment of response in surgically resected lung carcinomas after neoadjuvant therapy was the first attempt to standardize grossing processing and microscopic evaluation.

Since US Food and Drug Administration approval of programmed death ligand 1 (PD-L1) as the first companion diagnostic for immune checkpoint inhibitors (ICIs) in non-small cell lung cancer, many patients have experienced increased overall survival. To improve selection of ICI responders versus nonresponders, microsatellite instability/mismatch repair deficiency (MSI/MMR) and tumor mutation burden (TMB) came into play. Clinical data show PD-L1, MSI/MMR, and TMB are independent predictive immunotherapy biomarkers. Harmonization of testing methodologies, optimization of assay design, and results analysis are ongoing. Future algorithms to determine immunotherapy eligibility might involve complementary use of current and novel biomarkers. Artificial intelligence could facilitate algorithm implementation to convert complex genetic data into recommendations for specific ICIs.

Adoption of molecular testing in lung cancer is increasing. Molecular testing for staging and prediction of response for targeted therapy remain the main indications, and although utilization of blood-based testing for tumor is growing, the use of the diagnostic cytology and tissue specimens is equally important. The pathologist needs to optimize reflex testing, incorporate stage-based algorithms, and understand types of tests for timely and complete assessment in the majority of cases. When tissue is limited, testing should capture the most frequent alterations to maximize the yield of what are largely mutually exclusive alterations, avoiding the need for repeat biopsy.

Artificial intelligence/machine learning tools are being created for use in pathology. Some examples related to lung pathology include acid-fast stain evaluation, programmed death ligand-1 (PDL-1) interpretation, evaluating histologic patterns of non–small-cell lung carcinoma, evaluating histologic features in mesothelioma associated with adverse outcomes, predicting response to anti-PDL-1 therapy from hematoxylin and eosin–stained slides, evaluation of tumor microenvironment, evaluating patterns of interstitial lung disease, nondestructive methods for tissue evaluation, and others. There are still some frameworks (regulatory, workflow, and payment) that need to be established for these tools to be integrated into pathology.

SURGICAL PATHOLOGY CLINICS

SERIES OF RELATED INTEREST

Clinics in Laboratory Medicine
http://www.labmed.theclinics.com/
Medical Clinics
https://www.medical.theclinics.com/

THE CLINICS ARE AVAILABLE ONLINE!
Access your subscription at:
www.theclinics.com

Preface
Thoracic Pathology—Learning from the Past to Inform the Future

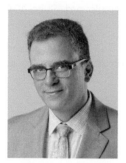

Alain C. Borczuk, MD
Editor

Thoracic pathology is a diverse combination of neoplastic and nonneoplastic diseases, and given their breadth, thoracic pathology requires frequent reexamination. Such reexamination may include incorporation of novel technologies but also conceptual changes in our interpretation of even well-established entities. This issue of *Surgical Pathology Clinics* provides a glimpse into this challenging admixture of pathologic entities.

Among the nonneoplastic diseases, this issue includes new perspectives on smoking-related diseases of the lung with suggestions on how terminology may need to change in the future. In granulomatous lung disease, what seems to be well-characterized pathology is improved upon by careful morphologic assessment of the nuances beyond necrosis. The need for pathologists to recognize historical lesions as their modern relevance becomes clearly apparent is embodied in the topic of silicosis. New frontiers include unexpected new entities, such as COVID-19 pneumonia, or in the case of interstitial lung abnormality, a clinical entity with ambiguous pathologic underpinnings. In all these topics, we see the need for change, adaptation, and further research.

Along with the neoplastic diseases, rare tumor types are being better defined by both morphology and molecular testing and as such become more readily identified. This has been especially true for the salivary gland–type lung cancers as well as for the sarcomas and spindle cell lesions of the thorax. Pathology has recognized a grading system for lung adenocarcinoma and continues to better define invasion in that entity. Increasing use of neoadjuvant therapy, including chemotherapy, radiation therapy, and immunotherapy, has required greater precision in the evaluation of the pathologic response of tumors encountered by pathologists upon tumor resection.

Beyond morphology alone, the frontiers include incorporation of new testing beyond those used in diagnosis alone. As such, pathologists need ongoing updates in the utilization of molecular

Surgical Pathology 17 (2024) xi–xii
https://doi.org/10.1016/j.path.2023.11.002
1875-9181/24/© 2023 Published by Elsevier Inc.

tests, such as microsatellite instability, mismatch repair, and tumor mutation burden, in lung cancer as well as overall utilization and incorporation of existing algorithms for predictive testing. In 2024, new frontiers must include digital pathology and artificial intelligence, as these technologies are central to the future of pathology practice across numerous subspecialties.

I thank all the authors for their insights and contributions, as well as the many colleagues who have been the source of critical thinking in the practice of thoracic pathology and pathology overall. While we learn from the past, we are constantly reinventing ourselves, and how better than with such a distinguished and enthusiastic set of peers.

Alain C. Borczuk, MD
Department of Pathology and
Laboratory Medicine
Northwell Health
Zucker School of Medicine at Hofstra
2200 Northern Boulevard, Suite 104
Greenvale, NY 11548, USA

E-mail address:
aborczuk@northwell.edu

Smoking-Related Interstitial Lung Disease
Historical Perspective and Advances in the Twenty-first Century

Sanjay Mukhopadhyay, MD[a],*, Irene Sansano, MD[b]

KEYWORDS

- Smoking • Cigarette smoking • Interstitial lung disease • Smoking-related interstitial lung disease
- Smoking-related interstitial fibrosis • Desquamative interstitial pneumonia

Key points

- The main non-neoplastic pulmonary parenchymal abnormalities caused by smoking include emphysema, interstitial fibrosis, pigmented macrophages, and Langerhans cell proliferation. Patients with these abnormalities are often asymptomatic but can present with clinical and radiologic features of interstitial lung disease.

- Smoking-related interstitial fibrosis (SRIF)—a histologically distinctive type of interstitial fibrosis that is highly specific for smoking—is usually subclinical, but may also be encountered in lung biopsies performed for evaluation of clinically evident interstitial lung disease.

- Pulmonary Langerhans cell histiocytosis in adults occurs almost exclusively in smokers and manifests as small bilateral lung nodules and/or cysts.

- The high degree of clinical and pathologic overlap between desquamative interstitial pneumonia (DIP), respiratory bronchiolitis interstitial lung disease (RBILD) and SRIF suggests that they are not discrete entities but different ways of describing various combinations of pigmented alveolar macrophages and interstitial fibrosis in smokers.

- Since macrophage accumulation within airspaces is a common and non-specific pathologic finding, so-called DIP occurs in a wide variety of clinical settings, is less specific for smoking than SRIF, and is heterogeneous in terms of prognosis and response to corticosteroids.

ABSTRACT

In the twenty-first century, there is widespread agreement that in addition to lung cancer, emphysema, and chronic bronchitis, cigarette smoking causes accumulation of pigmented macrophages, interstitial fibrosis, and Langerhans cell proliferation in various permutations. These histologic changes remain subclinical in some patients and produce clinical manifestations and imaging abnormalities in others. Debate surrounds terminology of these lesions, which are often grouped together under the umbrella of "smoking-related interstitial lung disease." This review summarizes modern concepts in our understanding of these abnormalities and explains how the recognition of smoking-related interstitial fibrosis has advanced the field.

OVERVIEW

Cigarette smoking is a well-known cause of lung cancer and obstructive lung disease, including

a Department of Pathology, Pathology and Laboratory Medicine Institute, Cleveland Clinic, 9500 Euclid Avenue, Cleveland, OH 44195, USA; b Department of Pathology, Hospital Universitari Vall d'Hebron, Passeig de la Vall d'Hebron 119-129, 08035 Barcelona, Catalunya, Spain
* Corresponding author. Department of Pathology, Cleveland Clinic, Cleveland, OH 44195.
E-mail address: mukhops@ccf.org

surgpath.theclinics.com

emphysema and chronic bronchitis. However, it has become clear over the past few decades that smoking also causes lung parenchymal abnormalities that fall under the categories of "restrictive lung disease," "interstitial lung disease," or "diffuse parenchymal lung disease," and that the pathologic hallmarks of these processes include accumulation of pigmented macrophages within respiratory bronchioles and/or alveolar lumens (airspaces), interstitial fibrosis (specifically, "ropey" collagen within alveolar septa), and Langerhans cell proliferation forming small nodules, cysts, and/or scars. The exact mix of findings and the extent and severity of each finding varies widely from patient to patient, lobe to lobe, and even from field to field within the same slide, confounding attempts at nosology. Our understanding of the clinical significance of these findings, the degree of overlap between them, and their specificity for smoking has evolved over the years. Although pulmonologists have long embraced the idea that interstitial lung disease can be caused by inhaled occupational exposures such as asbestos, silica, and coal dust, the concept that cigarette smoking can cause interstitial lung disease is relatively recent, and did not even exist in 1965 when Liebow and colleagues coined the term "desquamative interstitial pneumonia (DIP)."[1] The first major description of pulmonary Langerhans cell histiocytosis (then known as eosinophilic granuloma) in 1981 described smoking not as a cause but only as a "provocative epidemiologic factor."[2] A review in 1986 noted that 90% of the patients with pulmonary histiocytosis X were smokers but speculated that etiologic factors other than smoking might be at play.[3]

The first study introducing the paradigm that smoking can cause clinically evident interstitial lung disease appeared in 1986.[4] This, and subsequent studies,[5] led to the gradual realization that in some cases of diffuse parenchymal lung disease, smoking is the cause, not just a risk factor. The term "smoking-related interstitial lung disease" (encompassing DIP, respiratory bronchiolitis-interstitial lung disease, and pulmonary Langerhans cell histiocytosis) was introduced by Moon and colleagues in 1999[6] and subsequently adopted by others.[7]

PULMONARY LANGERHANS CELL HISTIOCYTOSIS

Langerhans cells—named after the German pathologist Paul Langerhans (1847–1888) who described them in the epidermis in 1868—are antigen-presenting dendritic cells derived from the bone marrow.[8] Between 1865 and the 1960s, various clinical syndromes that featured proliferation of histiocyte-like cells and eosinophils were described, including Letterer-Siwe syndrome, Hand–Schüller–Christian syndrome, and eosinophilic granuloma of bone.[9,10] Letterer-Siwe syndrome and Hand–Schüller–Christian syndrome typically occurred in children less than 2 years of age, while eosinophilic granuloma mainly involved bones and usually presented in children and young adults.[9–14] In 1953, these entities were grouped by Lichtenstein under the designation "histiocytosis X,"[11] a term that persisted over the next 3 decades.[12–14]

The localized pulmonary form of the disease was described in 1981 by Friedman, Liebow, and Sokoloff as "eosinophilic granuloma of lung"; the authors made the seminal observation that most patients (67 of 69) were smokers.[2] In the same year, the first immunohistochemical markers of Langerhans cells (CD1a[15] and S-100[16]) emerged. In 1987, the Writing Group of the Histiocyte Society grouped all forms of the disease under the umbrella term "Langerhans cell histiocytosis" (LCH) based on the work of French pathologist Christian Nezelof.[17–20] By 1999, the fact that nearly all patients with isolated pulmonary LCH were smokers was well documented, and pulmonary LCH was included under the umbrella of smoking-related interstitial lung disease.[6] Larger series confirmed that the vast majority of adults with pulmonary LCH are heavy cigarette smokers.[21]

CLINICAL FEATURES

Broadly speaking, LCH is extremely heterogeneous, with a clinical spectrum ranging from lethal multi-system disease requiring systemic treatment to relatively indolent single-system disease (unifocal or multifocal) that can often be managed with observation or local therapy. It encompasses LCH in children, and isolated single-system LCH of the bones, lungs, gastrointestinal tract, skin, nervous system, pituitary, oral mucosa, liver, spleen, and heart. Multisystem disease in children and young people can involve the lungs.

In contrast to extrapulmonary and systemic forms of the disease, pulmonary LCH in adults is clinically distinctive in that it occurs almost exclusively in current or former smokers[22,23] and is typically limited to the lungs.

Single-system pulmonary LCH commonly occurs in young adult smokers but can be encountered in adults of any age and affects both sexes. Although symptoms such as chronic dry cough and dyspnea are common, many patients are asymptomatic. Pneumothorax occurs in a subset, with recurrence in about half.[23] A common scenario in cases that come to lung biopsy is that a chest computed tomography (CT) performed for another reason (such as staging for newly diagnosed cancer) reveals multiple small bilateral lung nodules in an otherwise asymptomatic cigarette smoker. Like other smoking-related parenchymal lung diseases, decreased diffusing capacity for carbon monoxide (DL_{CO}) is a common pulmonary function abnormality.[23]

MICROSCOPIC FEATURES

The hallmark of pulmonary LCH is the presence of sheets (clusters) of Langerhans cells within the interstitium, forming multiple tiny (almost always <1 cm) ill-defined nodules with irregular edges.[13,24–26] These "stellate nodules" are so characteristic that the diagnosis can often be suspected at scanning magnification (**Fig. 1**). The mix of cells within the interstitium in stellate nodules is variable and includes (in proportions that vary widely from case to case) Langerhans cells, pigmented macrophages, eosinophils, and lymphocytes. Plasma cells and neutrophils are infrequent. These cells are admixed with variable amounts of collagen (fibrosis). Eosinophils can be numerous but may be absent and are not mandatory for the diagnosis. The occurrence of eosinophil-poor cases is one reason why "eosinophilic granuloma" was not an ideal term for this entity. Importantly, these lesions are not granulomas since they are collections of Langerhans cells, not epithelioid histiocytes. For this reason, the term "Langerhans cell granulomatosis"[24] is incorrect and outdated. At high magnification, Langerhans cells are similar to ordinary macrophages (histiocytes), but their nuclei are more irregular and often contain grooves, folds, or indentations,[25] resembling the kernel of a walnut. Cytoplasmic borders are poorly defined. In lung lesions, Langerhans

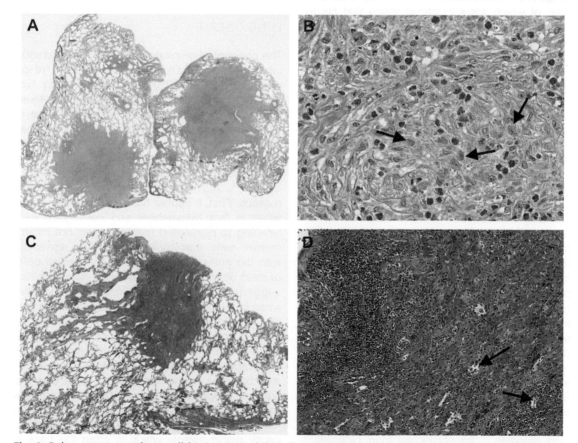

Fig. 1. Pulmonary Langerhans cell histiocytosis. (*A*) Stellate nodules (hematoxylin-eosin, original magnification ×1). (*B*) Numerous Langerhans cells (*arrows*) admixed with eosinophils and a few pigmented macrophages (hematoxylin-eosin, original magnification ×40). (*C*) Lung nodule in scarred phase of pulmonary Langerhans cell histiocytosis retains stellate shape (hematoxylin-eosin, original magnification ×1). (*D*) Scarred phase. At high magnification, there is fibrosis and a lymphoid aggregate, but Langerhans cells are absent. Note entrapped benign lung epithelium (hematoxylin-eosin, original magnification ×40).

cells are often most numerous in areas where the stroma appears slightly myxoid (mimicking organizing pneumonia). In advanced (scarred) lesions, Langerhans cells are gradually replaced by collagen, and in later stages disappear completely and cannot be demonstrated by immunohistochemistry. It is in these late-stage scars that the opinion of a pulmonary pathologist can be helpful, as the diagnosis can be suggested on hematoxylin-eosin (H&E) based on the size and shape of the nodules and the presence of prominent smoking-related changes in the background lung. Immunohistochemical stains are not mandatory but most pathologists do perform them to confirm that the lesional mononuclear cells are Langerhans cells. Langerhans cells are positive for S-100, CD1a, and Langerin (CD207).[24–26]

Other smoking-related changes are common in the background lung, the most common being pigmented macrophages within alveolar lumens (airspaces). This finding has been termed "respiratory bronchiolitis" or "DIP-like reaction," both of which are suboptimal terms that fail to convey the true nature of the process (accumulation of smoking-related pigmented macrophages). Other smoking-related changes that may be present in the background lung include emphysema and smoking-related interstitial fibrosis (SRIF).

Vascular changes have been described by Bois and colleagues, including intimal and medial thickening.[27] Eosinophils may occasionally be seen within vessel walls, which could potentially lead to misdiagnosis of a "true" vasculitis.

DIAGNOSIS

The diagnosis requires histopathologic confirmation, with the possible exception of cases where classic high-resolution computed tomography (HRCT) features are seen in the appropriate clinical context.[23,28] Pulmonary LCH in adults is defined by the presence of clusters or sheets of Langerhans cells within the interstitium of the lung. Isolated Langerhans cells are common in the lungs of cigarette smokers and are insufficient for the diagnosis if not clustered. The authors do not routinely perform *BRAF* V600E mutation testing as more than half of cases are negative, and BRAF-directed therapy is not indicated for most cases of pulmonary LCH.

Pulmonary LCH can be diagnosed in surgical lung biopsies,[24] transbronchial lung biopsies,[25] core needle biopsies,[26] and explanted lungs. It can also be encountered as an incidental finding in the background lung in lobectomies for cancer from smokers.[29] Immunostaining for CD1a in bronchoalveolar lavage fluid is frequently cited as

a diagnostic modality even though this method is seldom if ever diagnostic in practice. The poor sensitivity of this test and the lack of robust evidence justifying its use have been recently highlighted by Vehar and colleagues[30]

PROGNOSIS

Most cases of pulmonary LCH remain stable on follow-up. Regression upon smoking cessation alone has been reported.[31–33] In a subset of cases, the clinical course is characterized by progressive scarring with lung function impairment. Secondary pulmonary hypertension develops in some patients. Unsurprisingly, some patients are found to have smoking-related lung cancers. Unrelated malignancies such as lymphoma can also occur. Isolated pulmonary LCH does not progress to multisystem disease.[34] Median survival in a study of 102 adults was 12.5 years.[21]

RESPIRATORY BRONCHIOLITIS-INTERSTITIAL LUNG DISEASE

The concept of respiratory bronchiolitis interstitial lung disease (RBILD) is based on the term "respiratory bronchiolitis,(RB)" first introduced by Niewoehner and colleagues in 1974 in an autopsy study of young cigarette smokers who died of non-pulmonary disease. The authors described RB as "brown pigmented macrophages in the first-order and second-order respiratory bronchiole distal to the terminal membranous bronchiole."[35] The term "RB" is misleading for 2 reasons. First, it implies bronchiolar inflammation, when in fact Niewoehner and colleagues were referring to pigmented macrophages, not inflammatory cells that most pathologists associate with the suffix "itis" (lymphocytes, plasma cells, or neutrophils). Second, the word "bronchiolitis" suggests that the process is limited to bronchioles when in fact in smokers pigmented macrophages are commonly found within alveolar lumens (airspaces), often with minimal or no bronchiolar involvement. Even the broader definition used by Fraig and colleagues[36] that includes pigmented macrophages "within respiratory bronchioles *and adjacent airspaces*" does not adequately address the fact that RB is not an accurate term for *pigmented macrophages located solely or predominantly within alveoli*, which is often the case in practice. For these reasons, the authors find the term "pigmented airspace macrophages" to be a more accurate descriptor of the lesion that occurs in smokers than "RB." In most cases, pigmented airspace macrophages are an incidental and expected histologic finding in the lungs of current and ex-smokers.

RBILD is an entity in which RB is the only pathologic abnormality in a patient with symptoms and imaging suggestive of interstitial lung disease.[4–6,37–41] By definition, the lung biopsy should not reveal any other histologic features that would explain the clinical and radiologic findings.[4,5] Therefore, RBILD is not a pathologic diagnosis but a multidisciplinary one. The role of the pathologist is to identify RB and exclude other causes of interstitial lung disease.[6] The final label of RBILD requires the decision that RB is an adequate explanation for the clinical and radiologic findings, a subjective judgment call that is often made in the context of multidisciplinary discussion.

CLINICAL FEATURES

Patients with RBILD are almost invariably heavy cigarette smokers, with a mean age in the 30s or 40s.[4,5,38] The most common symptoms are cough and dyspnea.[4–6,38] Cases in never-smokers are rare.[6] Pulmonary function tests often reveal findings common to other smoking-related lung diseases such as reduced DL_{CO} and decreased forced vital capacity (FVC).[5,6,38] Findings on HRCT include bilateral ground-glass opacities[38] and centrilobular nodules, and can involve any lobe.[37] Concurrent centrilobular emphysema is often present on imaging.[6,37]

MICROSCOPIC FEATURES

The histologic hallmark of RBILD is RB, characterized by accumulation of pigmented macrophages within respiratory bronchioles and adjacent alveoli (**Fig. 2**).[4–6] These macrophages contain a light brown cytoplasmic pigment with occasional black specks derived from cigarette smoke. The pigment stains light blue with iron stains (Perls'/Prussian Blue). In contrast, hemosiderin, which also forms brown granules within the cytoplasm of macrophages, features larger and coarser granules, lacks black specks, and stains strongly with iron stains. Occasionally, it can be difficult to differentiate between these pigments. The amount of fibrosis permissible in RBILD is controversial and is the basis of much of the debate regarding terminology; some authors allow only minimal fibrosis in line with the original description of this entity[4,38] while others allow peribronchiolar fibrosis.[5,6]

Histologic features do not reliably differentiate between incidental RB in asymptomatic smokers and RB in RBILD. Contrary to the assertion[5] that in asymptomatic RB "peribronchiolar fibrosis and inflammation are minimal" whereas these features are more pronounced in RBILD, RB with significant peribronchiolar fibrosis is well documented in the lungs of asymptomatic cigarette smokers (see section on smoking-related interstitial fibrosis, later).[29] The authors are unaware of any study in which pathologists blinded to clinical findings have been able to distinguish between smoking-related macrophage accumulation in asymptomatic individuals and smoking-related macrophage accumulation in patients with clinical features of interstitial lung disease.

DIAGNOSIS

In most published series, the diagnosis of RBILD has required surgical lung biopsies since other disease processes cannot be definitively excluded without such biopsies.[4–6,38] It is important to remember that RB also occurs in the background lung in smokers with other forms of interstitial lung disease such as usual interstitial pneumonia (UIP).[6] Hence, the diagnosis of RBILD requires the pathologist not only to identify pigmented macrophages in the appropriate distribution but also to exclude a more clinically significant process in the biopsy that would relegate RB to the status of an incidental finding. In practice, a presumptive diagnosis of RBILD is often based on HRCT findings without biopsy confirmation, or only a transbronchial lung biopsy. Given the possibility of sampling error, the accuracy of this practice is debatable.

PROGNOSIS

The prognosis of RBILD is good, with stability or improvement in symptoms, long-term stability on imaging, and no deaths attributable to the disease.[5,38] In one study, improvement in symptoms occurred in 55% of the cases of RBILD treated with corticosteroids, and improvements in pulmonary function tests or imaging were noted in 64%.[38] However, these responses tended to be transient, with a return to baseline upon discontinuation of prednisone therapy. Improvements can also occur with smoking cessation alone.[38]

DESQUAMATIVE INTERSTITIAL PNEUMONIA

The problems with the entity DIP have been previously reviewed in detail.[42] Diagnostic criteria have evolved over the years, with various authors differing on the extent of macrophage accumulation, fibrosis, and inflammation that defines this entity.[42] In contrast to RBILD, which was described explicitly as a smoking-related disease, DIP was described prior to the recognition of

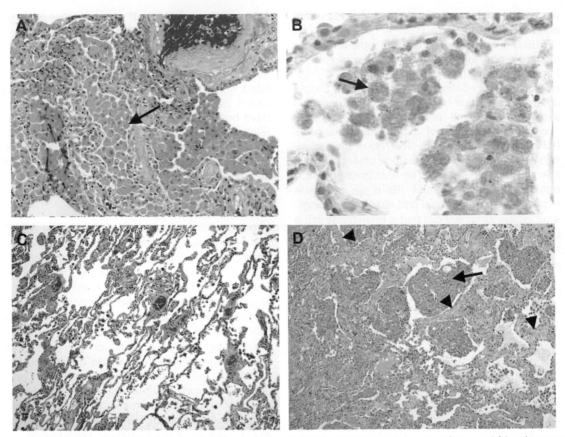

Fig. 2. Respiratory bronchiolitis interstitial lung disease (RBILD). (A) Pigmented macrophages within airspaces ("respiratory bronchiolitis") (hematoxylin-eosin, original magnification ×200). (B) Iron stain shows weak cytoplasmic staining (Perls' stain, original magnification ×400). (C) Case diagnosed at another institution as RBILD in 2007, prior to description of smoking-related interstitial fibrosis (SRIF). A few pigmented macrophages are present within airspaces but none are within "respiratory bronchioles and adjacent alveoli" (hematoxylin-eosin, original magnification ×100). (D) Another slide from the same case as C shows not peribronchiolar disease but more extensive filling of airspaces by macrophages (arrow) that some would classify as desquamative interstitial pneumonia (DIP), and ropey fibrosis (arrowhead) that we now diagnose as SRIF. This type of variability from slide to slide that defies easy classification is very common in smoking-related interstitial lung disease (hematoxylin-eosin, original magnification ×100).

smoking as a cause of interstitial lung disease. The key difference between RBILD and DIP lies in their defining histologic features. Since RBILD is defined by the presence of *pigmented* macrophages within respiratory bronchioles and adjacent airspaces—a finding strongly associated with smoking—essentially all patients are smokers, making this a *bona fide* smoking-related disease. In contrast, DIP is defined by extensive macrophage accumulation within alveoli *regardless of whether the macrophages are pigmented*, reducing its specificity for smoking. Once this fact is appreciated, it is easy to understand why some cases of DIP (those characterized by pigmented macrophages) occur in smokers while others (featuring non-pigmented macrophages) occur in never-smokers. The latter subset is not caused by smoking, is driven by a hodge-podge of unrelated causes such as connective tissue disease, drugs and exposures, and does not belong under the heading of smoking-related interstitial lung disease. This also explains why DIP is a mixed bag in terms of etiology, clinical features, response to corticosteroids, and prognosis.

The second—and widely acknowledged—problem with DIP is that it is a misnomer.[42] Since 1969, several investigators have demonstrated that the cells in the alveoli are macrophages, not desquamated pneumocytes.[43–47]

The third problem with the way DIP is defined is that its occasional occurrence in never-smokers perpetuates the misconception that DIP is a form of "idiopathic interstitial pneumonia."[38,40] DIP is thus an odd mix of cases that are clearly histologically smoking-related, and cases that lack smoking-related histologic findings (some of which may indeed be idiopathic), leading to the oxymoron "smoking-related idiopathic interstitial pneumonia."[48] Because of these problems with DIP, which are a direct consequence of its definition, the authors do not use this term in their practice.

CLINICAL FEATURES

Most patients with DIP present with cough and shortness of breath.[5,38] Approximately 80% are smokers. Clinical overlap with RBILD is significant.[5,38]

MICROSCOPIC FEATURES

The diagnosis of DIP requires alveolar filling by macrophages (**Fig. 3**), although various series

differ regarding the exact defining features.[5,38,42] Some state that the macrophages may be pigmented or non-pigmented,[5] while others require "the presence of *pigmented* macrophages diffusely involving alveolar spaces…."[38] Some authors require "diffuse alveolar septal thickening due to alveolar septal inflammation with or without fibrosis,"while others state that DIP is characterized by "diffuse interstitial fibrous thickening of the alveolar septa and a mild mononuclear cell interstitial infiltrate."[5]

DIAGNOSIS

Definitive diagnosis requires surgical lung biopsy. Radiologists often include DIP in their differential

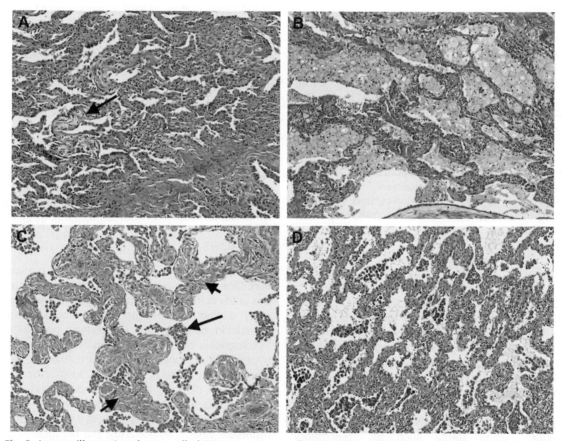

Fig. 3. Images illustrating that so-called DIP are a non-specific mixed bag. (*A*) This case was diagnosed elsewhere as DIP, but the appearance of the expanded alveolar septa suggests that the correct diagnosis is organizing acute lung injury in a smoker with pigmented airspace macrophages (hematoxylin-eosin, original magnification ×10). (*B*) The degree of alveolar filling by foamy macrophages in this case would qualify as "DIP," but this is actually the lung adjacent to a bulla from a case of Niemann–Pick disease. Non-pigmented macrophages are not smoking-related (hematoxylin-eosin, original magnification ×10). (*C*) Accumulation of pigmented macrophages within airspaces (long *arrow*) in this case is truly smoking-related, and some would classify this as DIP. However, the authors prefer the term "SRIF" because there is also ropey alveolar septal fibrosis (short *arrows*) (hematoxylin-eosin, original magnification ×10). (*D*) This type of extensive filling by macrophages can be misinterpreted as DIP. This focus was seen in a case of UIP with superimposed organizing pneumonia (not shown here) and probably represents accumulation of hemosiderin-laden macrophages secondary to congestive heart failure (hematoxylin-eosin, original magnification ×10).

diagnosis when they encounter bilateral ground-glass infiltrates on HRCT in cases that lack features of UIP or other named forms of interstitial lung disease, but the accuracy of this approach has not been validated.

PROGNOSIS

Similar to RBILD, most cases of DIP improve or remain stable on follow-up.[5] Worsening or death has been reported in a small subset.[5] Published series have not clarified whether the histologic features of the poor-prognosis subset differ in any way from the majority of patients who do well.[5] In the authors' anecdotal experience, subtle features of early UIP (such as scarring and fibroblast foci) may account for the cases that develop progressive fibrosis.

The notion that RBILD needs to be differentiated from DIP because DIP responds to corticosteroids while RBILD does not was debunked in 2005 by Ryu and colleagues, who showed that symptomatic improvement with prednisone therapy occurs more often in RBILD (55% of patients) than in DIP (24% of patients).[38] Similarly, objective improvements in pulmonary function tests and imaging were more common in RBILD (64%) than in DIP (33%). In both groups, improvements were transient, with worsening of the condition to baseline after discontinuation of treatment.[38] These findings suggest that in smoking-related interstitial lung disease (whether RBILD or DIP), responses to prednisone occur only in a subset of patients and are at best transient.

SMOKING-RELATED INTERSTITIAL FIBROSIS

SRIF is a histologically distinctive form of interstitial fibrosis characterized by thickening of alveolar septa by "ropey" collagen. The term was introduced in 2010 after a review of extensively sampled lobectomy specimens from smokers.[29] Subsequently, the existence of SRIF and its occurrence exclusively in smokers was validated by other investigators.[49–54] Interstitial fibrosis identical to SRIF has also been described by others, using terms such as "respiratory bronchiolitis-associated interstitial lung disease (RBILD) with fibrosis,"[55] "respiratory bronchiolitis with fibrosis,"[56] and "airspace enlargement with fibrosis."[57]

CLINICAL FEATURES

SRIF occurs exclusively in adult smokers of both sexes.[29,30,49–53,58] Most cases are seen in lungs resected or biopsied for other reasons, where SRIF represents an incidental smoking-related finding of no further clinical significance.[29] In this group, symptoms attributable to SRIF are absent, and SRIF is either not seen on HRCT or correlates only with minimal ground-glass opacities. However, SRIF can also be encountered in surgical lung biopsies performed for patients who present with clinical and radiologic features of interstitial lung disease.[53] In this subset of patients, common symptoms are cough and dyspnea, and the most common pulmonary function test abnormalities are decreased DL_{CO} and FVC. HRCT invariably shows bilateral ground-glass opacities without reticulation, traction bronchiectasis, or honeycombing.

MICROSCOPIC FEATURES

The defining feature of SRIF is expansion of alveolar septa by eosinophilic, paucicellular fibrosis composed of dense "ropey-appearing" collagen (**Fig. 4**).[29,59,60] This type of fibrosis typically occurs in combination with 2 other smoking-related findings: emphysema and pigmented airspace macrophages.[29] The fibrosis is commonly subpleural and patchy, but it also occurs in peribronchiolar parenchyma, and can occasionally be diffuse, closely mimicking the fibrosing variant of non-specific interstitial pneumonia (NSIP).[53] Other nonspecific findings commonly seen in SRIF include wisps of hyperplastic smooth muscle bundles within thickened alveolar septa, and scattered lymphoid follicles.[53]

DIAGNOSIS

The diagnosis of SRIF requires histologic examination. One of the greatest practical applications of this entity is that it allows pathologists to histologically distinguish smoking-related fibrosis from fibrosis in other entities, preventing pathologic misdiagnosis of UIP,[53] fibrosing NSIP,[53] fibrotic hypersensitivity pneumonitis, and connective tissue disease-related interstitial lung disease. Further, as demonstrated by Bledsoe and colleagues, it is likely that many cases formerly diagnosed as "mild asbestosis" in heavy smokers also represent SRIF.[61] Importantly, the recognition of SRIF has created a paradigm shift in the terminology of smoking-related interstitial lung disease, as it provides pathologists with a more accurate alternative term for cases of interstitial lung disease in smokers in which the only choices in the past would have been DIP or RBILD.[42,53,59,60]

PROGNOSIS

The prognosis of pure SRIF is excellent, whether encountered as an incidental finding in lung

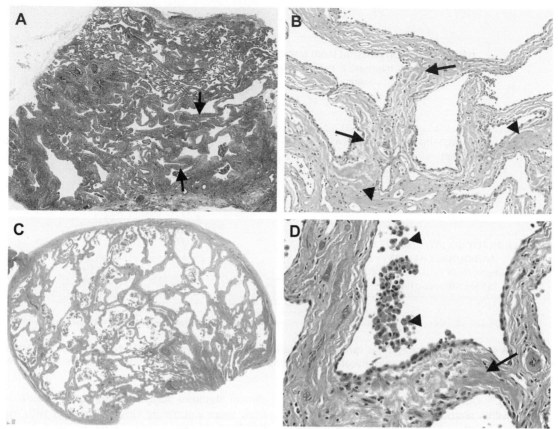

Fig. 4. Smoking-related interstitial fibrosis (SRIF). (*A*) Background lung in a lobectomy specimen shows striking interstitial fibrosis (*arrows*) in emphysematous lung (hematoxylin-eosin, original magnification × 1). (*B*) Ropey collagen (*arrows*) and admixed smooth muscle bundles (*arrowheads*) (hematoxylin-eosin, original magnification ×40). (*C*) SRIF in a patient with clinical and radiologic features of interstitial lung disease. The stiff, boxy appearance that results from alveolar septal fibrosis in emphysematous lung is typical of SRIF (hematoxylin-eosin, original magnification ×1). D (hematoxylin-eosin, original magnification × 100). (*D*) High magnification from the same case as part C shows interstitial expansion by paucicellular ropey collagen (*arrow*). Note pigmented macrophages in adjacent airspace (*arrowheads*) (hematoxylin-eosin, original magnification ×40).

resections or in patients presenting with clinical evidence of interstitial lung disease. When SRIF occurs as an incidental finding in the background lung of another entity (such as UIP or diffuse alveolar damage), the outcome is driven by the prognosis of the main entity.

COMBINED PULMONARY FIBROSIS AND EMPHYSEMA

Combined pulmonary fibrosis and emphysema (CPFE) is defined as the coexistence of emphysema and parenchymal fibrosis (most commonly UIP) in the same lung.[62–65] It is important to distinguish this entity from SRIF (which also features a combination of emphysema and fibrosis) because the prognosis of SRIF is excellent whereas the prognosis of CPFE is poor.

CLINICAL FEATURES

Most patients with CPFE are men (male: female ratio = 9:1) with a mean age of 65 to 70 years,[65]; nearly all are current or ex-smokers.[62,64] Cough and exertional dyspnea are common presenting symptoms. Finger clubbing is seen in 43%.[64] Pulmonary function tests reflect the superimposition of 2 entities that cause counterbalancing physiologic effects.[62] Common features include hypoxemia, relative preservation of spirometric values and lung volumes,[62,64] and disproportionate impairment of gas exchange characterized by decreased DL_{CO}.[62,63]

MICROSCOPIC FEATURES

The most common microscopic finding in CPFE is the coexistence of UIP and emphysema in the

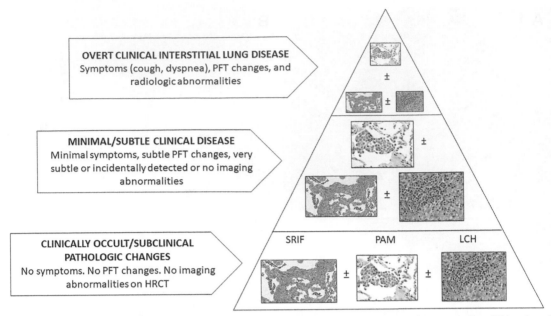

PFT: pulmonary function test, HRCT: high-resolution computed tomography, SRIF: smoking-related interstitial fibrosis, PAM: pigmented airspace macrophages, LCH: Langerhans cell histiocytosis

Fig. 5. This schematic illustrates those various combinations of the same smoking-related pathologic abnormalities (pigmented macrophages, ropey alveolar septal fibrosis, and/or Langerhans cell nodules) can be encountered in different clinical contexts.

same lung.[65] Concurrent RB (pigmented macrophages within airspaces) is common.[65] The co-existence of UIP and emphysema often complicates recognition of UIP because emphysema often further distorts the architecture of fibrotic lung (sometimes forming "thick-walled cysts")[65] or is so prominent that it overshadows the fibrosis. This complicating effect of concurrent emphysema has also been noted on imaging.[64] For prognostic purposes, it is important to distinguish between the 2 major types of histologic fibrosis that occur in emphysematous lungs (SRIF and CPFE/UIP), a distinction that can be challenging in some cases because both types of fibrosis may occasionally coexist. Features that favor CPFE over pure SRIF include evidence of reticulation or honeycombing on imaging, and microscopic evidence of fibroblast foci, significant scarring, or honeycomb change.

DIAGNOSIS

CPFE is usually diagnosed by HRCT[65] but it can also be suggested on the basis of pathologic findings. Some authors accept combinations of emphysema with interstitial pneumonias other than UIP[62,64,65] while others only include UIP.[63] It is likely that patients whose HRCTs feature emphysema and ground-glass opacities/ground-glass attenuation without reticulation or honeycombing have SRIF, not CPFE; a perusal of the

clinical literature suggests that such cases have likely been incorrectly lumped together with true CPFE; this may explain why some cases of "CPFE" have a favorable survival.[62]

PROGNOSIS

Like UIP, CPFE is associated with poor survival.[65] Potential complications include pulmonary hypertension (which, if present, worsens the prognosis), acute lung injury, and lung cancer.[62,65]

SUMMARY

Much progress has been made since the 1980s, when pathologists first recognized that smoking can cause interstitial lung disease.[4–6] In the twenty-first century, it has become clear that interstitial lung abnormalities on HRCT are common in smokers,[66] that emphysema and UIP can occur in the same lung (this entity is known as CPFE),[65] and that smoking also causes a morphologically distinctive type of interstitial fibrosis in emphysematous lungs characterized by alveolar septal expansion by "ropey" collagen that differs from UIP (this entity is termed SRIF)[29,55]; the latter observation has been acknowledged as a milestone in our understanding of coexistent pulmonary fibrosis and emphysema.[65] Despite these advances, nomenclature of the overlapping entities RBILD, DIP, and SRIF remains confusing,[67] with persistent use of outdated misnomers. Despite terminological problems, it is well-established that smoking-related histologic abnormalities such as pigmented airspace macrophages and ropey interstitial fibrosis most commonly occur as incidental subclinical findings in the lungs of asymptomatic smokers without radiologic abnormalities (Fig. 5). They are also most likely the basis of ground-glass opacities in smokers with subtle or no symptoms and minimal pulmonary function abnormalities. Finally, these same changes occasionally account for symptoms *and* radiologic features of interstitial lung disease in heavy smokers.[53,55] It is time to definitively classify cases with clinical and radiologic features of interstitial lung disease and smoking-related histologic findings as *smoking-related interstitial lung disease* and stop labeling them as "idiopathic interstitial pneumonias."

CLINICS CARE POINTS

- Cigarette smoking causes emphysema, interstitial fibrosis (characterized by "ropey" collagen within alveolar septa), accumulation of pigmented macrophages within airspaces, and proliferations of Langerhans cells in the interstitium.

- Patients with smoking-related pathologic abnormalities may be asymptomatic (with or without radiologic abnormalities) or symptomatic, with clinical and radiologic features of interstitial lung disease.

- The recognition of SRIF as a histologically distinctive type of interstitial fibrosis that is highly specific for smoking is a milestone not just because it describes a previously overlooked type of fibrosis in emphysematous lungs but also because it provides pathologists with a means of distinguishing smoking-related fibrosis from interstitial fibrosis caused by other etiologies.

- Pulmonary Langerhans cell histiocytosis in adults is almost invariably smoking-related and is isolated to the lungs.

- DIP, RBILD, and SRIF are different ways of defining various combinations of pigmented alveolar macrophages and interstitial fibrosis in smokers.

- DIP is an outdated misnomer. Since its definition is based on a common non-specific finding (macrophage accumulation within alveoli), it is a heterogeneous mixed bag, and is less specific for smoking than SRIF.

SOURCES OF SUPPORT AND FUNDING

None.

CONFLICT OF INTEREST DECLARATION:

The authors have nothing to disclose.

DISCLOSURES

The authors have no conflicts pertinent to this manuscript.

REFERENCES

1. Liebow AA, Steer A, Billingsley JG. Desquamative interstitial pneumonia. Am J Med 1965;39:369–404.
2. Friedman P, Liebow AA, Sokoloff J. Eosinophilic granuloma of lung. Clinical aspects of primary pulmonary histiocytosis in the adult. Medicine 1981;60:385–92.
3. Hance AJ, Basset F, Saumon G, et al. Smoking and interstitial lung disease. The effect of cigarette smoking on the incidence of pulmonary histiocytosis X and sarcoidosis. Ann NY Acad Sci 1986;465:643–56.
4. Myers JL, Veal C, Shin M, et al. Respiratory bronchiolitis causing interstitial lung disease. A clinicopathologic study of six cases. Am Rev Respir Dis 1987;135:880–4.
5. Yousem SA, Colby TV, Gaensler EA. Respiratory bronchiolitis-associated interstitial lung disease and its relationship to desquamative interstitial pneumonia. Mayo Clin Proc 1989;64:1373–80.
6. Moon J, du Bois RM, Colby TV, et al. Clinical significance of respiratory bronchiolitis on open lung biopsy and its relationship to smoking related interstitial lung disease. Thorax 1999;54:1009–14.
7. Ryu JH, Colby TV, Hartman TE, et al. Smoking-related interstitial lung diseases. A concise review. Eur Respir J 2001;17:122–32.
8. Merad M, Ginhoux F, Collins M. Origin, homeostasis and function of Langerhans cells and other langerin-expressing dendritic cells. Nat Rev Immunol 2008;8:935–47.
9. Greenberger JS, Crocker AC, Vawter G, et al. Results of treatment of 127 patients with systemic histiocytosis (Letterer-Siwe syndrome, Schuller-Christian syndrome and multifocal eosinophilic granuloma). Medicine 1981;60:311–38.
10. Lichtenstein L, Jaffe HL. Eosinophilic granuloma of bone. With report of a case. Am J Pathol 1940;16:595–604.
11. Lichtenstein L. Histiocytosis X, integration of eosinophilic granuloma of bone, Letterer-Siwe disease and Schuller-Christian disease as related manifestations

of a single nosologic entity. Arch Pathol 1953;56: 84–102.

12. Favara BE, McCarthy RC, Mierau GW. Histiocytosis X. Hum Pathol 1983;14:663–76.

13. Colby TV, Lombard C. Histiocytosis X in the lung. Hum Pathol 1983;14:847–56.

14. Basset F, Corrin B, Spencer H, et al. Pulmonary histiocytosis X. Am Rev Respir Dis 1978;118:811–20.

15. Murphy GF, Bhan AK, Sato S, et al. Characterization of Langerhans cells by the use of monoclonal antibodies. Lab Invest 1981;465–8.

16. Cocchia D, Michetti F, Donato R. Immunohistochemical and immunocytochemical localization of S-100 antigen in normal human skin. Nature 1981;294: 85–7.

17. Kobayashi M, Tojo A. Langerhans cell histiocytosis in adults: advances in pathophysiology and treatment. Cancer Sci 2018;109:3707–13.

18. No authors listed. Histiocytosis syndromes in children. Lancet 1987;1:208–9.

19. Nezelof C, Basset F, Rousseau MF. Histiocytosis X. Histogenetic arguments for a Langerhans cell origin. Biomedicine 1973;18:365–71.

20. Nezelof C, Basset F. From histiocytosis X to Langerhans cell histiocytosis: a personal account. Int J Surg Pathol 2001;9:137–46.

21. Vassallo R, Ryu JH, Colby TV, et al. Pulmonary Langerhans'-cell histiocytosis. N Engl J Med 2000;342: 1969–78.

22. Suri HS, Yi ES, Nowakowski GS, et al. Pulmonary Langerhans cell histiocytosis. Orphanet J Rare Dis 2012;7:16.

23. Amarilys-Calderon A, Vassallo R, Yi ES, et al. Smoking-related interstitial lung diseases. Immunol Allergy Clin North Am 2023;43:273–87.

24. Travis WD, Borok Z, Roum JH, et al. Pulmonary Langerhans cell granulomatosis (histiocytosis X). A clinicopathologic study of 48 cases. Am J Surg Pathol 1993;17:971–86.

25. Baqir M, Vassallo R, Maldonado F, et al. Utility of bronchoscopy in pulmonary Langerhans cell histiocytosis. J Bronchology Interv Pulmonol 2013;20: 309–12.

26. Mukhopadhyay S, Eckardt S, Scalzetti EM. Diagnosis of pulmonary Langerhans cell histiocytosis by CT-guided core biopsy of lung: a report of 3 cases. Thorax 2010;65:833–5.

27. Bois MC, May AM, Vassallo R, et al. Morphometric study of pulmonary arterial changes in pulmonary Langerhans cell histiocytosis. Arch Pathol Lab Med 2018;142:929–37.

28. Goyal G, Tazi A, Go RS, et al. International expert consensus recommendations for the diagnosis and treatment of Langerhans cell histiocytosis in adults. Blood 2022;139:2601–21.

29. Katzenstein AL, Mukhopadhyay S, Zanardi C, et al. Clinically occult interstitial fibrosis in smokers: classification and significance of a surprisingly common finding in lobectomy specimens. Hum Pathol 2010;41:316–25.

30. Vehar SJ, Ribeiro Neto ML, Culver DA, et al. CD1a staining in bronchoalveolar lavage in pulmonary Langerhans cell histiocytosis. Barking up the wrong tree!". J Bronchology Interv Pulmonol 2022;29: e33–5.

31. Mogulkoc N, Veral A, Bishop PW, et al. Pulmonary Langerhans' cell histiocytosis: radiologic resolution following smoking cessation. Chest 1999;115: 1452–5.

32. Von Essen S, West W, Sitorius M, et al. Complete resolution of roentgenographic changes in a patient with pulmonary histiocytosis X. Chest 1990;98:765–7.

33. Negrin-Dastis S, Butenda D, Dorzee J, et al. Complete disappearance of lung abnormalities on high-resolution computed tomography: a case of histiocytosis X. Can Respir J 2007;14:235–7.

34. Tazi A, de Margerie C, Naccache JM, et al. The natural history of adult pulmonary Langerhans cell histiocytosis: a prospective multicentre study. Orphanet J Rare Dis 2015;10:30.

35. Niewoehner DE, Kleinerman J, Rice DB. Pathologic changes in the peripheral airways of young cigarette smokers. N Engl J Med 1974;291:755–8.

36. Fraig M, Shreesha U, Savici D, et al. Respiratory bronchiolitis: a clinicopathologic study in current smokers, ex-smokers, and never-smokers. Am J Surg Pathol 2002;26:647–53.

37. Park JS, Brown KK, Tuder R, et al. Respiratory bronchiolitis-associated interstitial lung disease: radiologic features with clinical and pathologic correlation. J Comput Assist Tomogr 2002;26:13–20.

38. Ryu JH, Myers JL, Capizzi SA, et al. Desquamative interstitial pneumonia and respiratory bronchiolitis-associated interstitial lung disease. Chest 2005; 127:178–84.

39. Heyneman LE, Ward S, Lynch DA, et al. Respiratory bronchiolitis, respiratory bronchiolitis-associated interstitial lung disease, and desquamative interstitial pneumonia: different entities or part of the spectrum of the same disease process? Am J Roentgenol 1999;173:1617–22.

40. American Thoracic Society, European Respiratory Society. American Thoracic Society/European Respiratory Society international multidisciplinary consensus classification of the idiopathic interstitial pneumonias. Am J Respir Crit Care Med 2002;165: 277–304.

41. Craig PJ, Wells AU, Doffman S, et al. Desquamative interstitial pneumonia, respiratory bronchiolitis and their relationship to smoking. Histopathology 2004; 45:275–82.

42. Mukhopadhyay S, Aesif SW, Sansano I. Five simple reasons to discard DIP, or why we should stop calling dolphins big fish. J Clin Pathol 2020;73:762–8.

43. Shortland JR, Darke CS, Crane WAJ. Electron microscopy of desquamative interstitial pneumonia. Thorax 1969;24:192–208.

44. Farr GH, Harley RA, Hennigar GR. Desquamative interstitial pneumonia. An electron microscopic study. Am J Pathol 1970;60:347–70.

45. Tubbs RR, Benjamin SP, Reich NE, et al. Desquamative interstitial pneumonitis. Chest 1977;72:159–65.

46. Valdivia E, Hensley G, Leory EP, et al. Morphology and pathogenesis of desquamative interstitial pneumonitis. Thorax 1977;32:7–18.

47. Mutton AE, Hasleton PS, Curry A, et al. Differentiation of desquamative interstitial pneumonia (DIP) from pulmonary adenocarcinoma by immunocytochemistry. Histopathology 1998;33:129–35.

48. Flaherty KR, Fell C, Aubry MC, et al. Smoking-related idiopathic interstitial pneumonia. Eur Respir J 2014;44:594–602.

49. Fabre A, Treacy A, Lavelle LP, et al. Smoking-related interstitial fibrosis: evidence of radiologic regression with advancing age and smoking cessation. COPD 2017;14:603–9.

50. Primiani A, Dias-Santagata D, Iafrate AJ, et al. Pulmonary adenocarcinoma mutation profile in smokers with smoking-related interstitial fibrosis. Int J Chronic Obstr Pulm Dis 2014;9:525–31.

51. Wick MR. Pathologic features of smoking-related lung diseases, with emphasis on smoking-related interstitial fibrosis, and a consideration of differential diagnoses. Semin Diagn Pathol 2018;35:315–23.

52. El-Kersh K, Perez RL, Smith JS, et al. Smoking-related interstitial fibrosis and pulmonary hypertension. BMJ Case Rep 2013. https://doi.org/10.1136/bcr-2013-008970, bcr2013008970.

53. Vehar SJ, Yadav R, Mukhopadhyay S, et al. Smoking-related interstitial fibrosis in patients presenting with diffuse parenchymal lung disease. Am J Clin Pathol 2023;159:146–57.

54. Otani H, Tanaka T, Murata K, et al. Smoking-related interstitial fibrosis combined with pulmonary emphysema: computed tomography-pathologic correlative study using lobectomy specimens. Int J Chronic Obstr Pulm Dis 2016;11:1521–32.

55. Yousem SA. Respiratory bronchiolitis-associated interstitial lung disease with fibrosis is a lesion distinct from fibrotic nonspecific interstitial pneumonia: a proposal. Mod Pathol 2006;19:1474–9.

56. Reddy TL, Mayo J, Churg A. Respiratory bronchiolitis with fibrosis. High-resolution computed tomography findings and correlation with pathology. Ann Am Thorac Soc 2013;10:590–601.

57. Kawabata Y, Hoshi E, Murai K, et al. Smoking-related changes in the background lung of specimens resected for lung cancer: a semiquantitative study with correlation to postoperative course. Histopathology 2008;53:707–14.

58. Pannunzio A, Mukhopadhyay S. Are respiratory bronchiolitis, emphysema and smoking-related interstitial fibrosis (SRIF) accurate markers of smoking status? A histologic study of 119 surgically resected lung specimens. Mod Pathol 2017;30(Suppl 2):488A, [abstract].

59. Katzenstein AL. Smoking-related interstitial fibrosis (SRIF): pathologic findings and distinction from other chronic fibrosing lung diseases. J Clin Pathol 2013;66:882–7.

60. Katzenstein AL. Smoking-related interstitial fibrosis (SRIF), pathogenesis and treatment of usual interstitial pneumonia (UIP), and transbronchial biopsy in UIP. Mod Pathol 2012;25(Suppl 1):S68–78.

61. Bledsoe JR, Christiani DC, Kradin RL. Smoking-associated fibrosis and pulmonary asbestosis. Int J Chronic Obstr Pulm Dis 2015;10:31–7.

62. Jankowich MD, Rounds SIS. Combined pulmonary fibrosis and emphysema syndrome. Chest 2012;141:222–31.

63. Ryerson CJ, Hartman T, Elicker BM, et al. Clinical features and outcomes in combined pulmonary fibrosis and emphysema in idiopathic pulmonary fibrosis. Chest 2013;144:234–40.

64. Cottin V, Nunes H, Brillet P-Y, et al. Combined pulmonary fibrosis and emphysema: a distinct underrecognized entity. Eur Respir J 2005;26:586–93.

65. Cottin V, Selman M, Inoue Y, et al. Syndrome of combined pulmonary fibrosis and emphysema. An official ATS/ERS/ALAT research statement. Am J Respir Crit Care Med 2022;4:e7–41.

66. Washko GR, Hunninghake GM, Fernandez IE, et al. Lung volumes and emphysema in smokers with interstitial lung abnormalities. N Engl J Med 2011;364:897–906.

67. Konopka KE, Myers JL. A review of smoking-related interstitial fibrosis, respiratory bronchiolitis, and desquamative interstitial pneumonia: overlapping histology and confusing terminology. Arch Pathol Lab Med 2018;142:1177–81.

Granulomatous Lung Diseases
A Practical Approach and Review of Common Entities

Jackie Cheuk Ki Chan, MD[a], Jennifer M. Boland, MD[b,c],*

KEYWORDS

• Granuloma • Necrotizing • Pulmonary • Lung • Infection

Key points

- Granulomas are frequently encountered in needle core biopsies, transbronchial biopsies, resections for a mass, and medical wedge biopsies.
- Granulomas should always be reported as necrotizing or non-necrotizing.
- Acid-fast bacilli stain, fungal stain, and polarized light examination should be performed on all granulomas.
- The differential diagnosis can be narrowed by attention to distribution, quality (poorly vs well-formed), and associated features.

ABSTRACT

Granulomas are frequently encountered by pathologists in all types of lung specimens and arise from diverse etiologies. They should always be reported as necrotizing or non-necrotizing, with microorganism stains performed to evaluate for infection. With attention to distribution, quality (poorly vs well-formed), associated features, and correlation with clinical, radiologic, and laboratory data, the differential diagnosis for granulomatous lung disease can usually be narrowed to a clinically helpful "short list." This review describes a practical approach to pulmonary granulomas and reviews the clinicopathological aspects of common entities, including infectious (mycobacteria, fungi) and noninfectious (hypersensitivity pneumonitis, sarcoid, and vasculitis) causes.

OVERVIEW

Granulomas are defined as a collection of epithelioid histiocytes, with or without the presence of multinucleated giant cells.[1,2] Epithelioid histiocytes are activated macrophages with morphologic features reminiscent of epithelial cells (polygonal shape, abundant cytoplasm), often forming tight interdigitated junctions with each other, lending a cohesive appearance.[3,4] Histologically, epithelioid histiocytes typically show indistinct cell borders and elongated, curved nuclei.[2]

Granulomas are the most common specific non-neoplastic diagnosis in pulmonary core needle biopsies[5,6] and are also frequently seen in transbronchial biopsies, excisional and wedge biopsies, and lobectomies. They carry a broad differential diagnosis regarding etiology (Box 1). As

---

[a] Department of Laboratory Medicine and Pathology, Royal Alexandra and University of Alberta Hospitals, 10240 Kingsway NW, Edmonton, Alberta, Canada, T5H 3V9; [b] Department of Laboratory Medicine and Pathology, Mayo Clinic, Rochester, MN, USA; [c] Division of Anatomic Pathology, Mayo Clinic, 200 First Street SW, Rochester, MN 55905, USA
* Corresponding author.
E-mail address: boland.jennifer@mayo.edu

Surgical Pathology 17 (2024) 173–192
https://doi.org/10.1016/j.path.2023.11.004
1875-9181/24/

Box 1
Common etiologies of pulmonary granulomas

- Infectious
  - Mycobacteria
    - *Mycobacterium tuberculosis*
    - Nontuberculous mycobacteria
  - Fungi
    - *Histoplasma*
    - *Blastomyces*
    - *Cryptococcus*
    - *Coccidioides*
    - *Pneumocystis*
  - Parasites
    - *Paragonimus*
    - *Dirofilaria*
    - *Schistosoma*
    - *Strongyloides*
- Noninfectious
  - Hypersensitivity pneumonitis
  - Sarcoidosis
  - Berylliosis
  - Hot tub lung
  - Lymphoid interstitial pneumonia
  - Granulomatous-lymphocytic interstitial lung disease
  - Granulomatosis with polyangiitis
  - Eosinophilic granulomatosis with polyangiitis
  - Aspiration
  - Talc granulomatosis
  - Rheumatoid nodule
  - Adverse drug reaction

such, this review aims to summarize the various entities in the differential of granulomatous lung disease and to provide an approach to narrow the differential based on specific features. Admittedly, not all cases can be given a confident and specific diagnosis despite careful clinical, pathologic, and radiologic review. Occasional cases of granulomatous inflammation may also be attributed to multiple concurrent processes, which can lead to diagnostic confusion.[7] However, by assessing for certain key morphologic features, the pathologist can often render a specific

diagnosis or provide a targeted, clinically useful differential diagnosis.

GENERAL APPROACH TO PULMONARY GRANULOMAS

Whenever possible, pulmonary granulomas should be evaluated for the presence of necrosis, anatomic distribution, and quality (tight and well-formed vs loose and poorly formed or somewhere in between). The presence of critical associated features such as vasculitis, foreign body material, and infectious organisms should always be evaluated. In addition, clinical, microbiological, laboratory, and radiographic data should also be reviewed to help establish the diagnosis. These key features are summarized in **Box 2**, and each discussed briefly in the following sections.

First, the presence and quality of necrosis should be assessed. The differential diagnosis of

Box 2
Important features in evaluation of pulmonary granulomas

- Presence of necrosis
- Well-formed vs poorly formed granulomas
- Distribution of disease
  - Lymphatic
  - Peribronchiolar
  - Vascular
- Associated features:
  - Vasculitis
  - Foreign material
  - Microorganisms
- Clinical history
  - Infectious history (travel, sick contacts)
  - Environmental/occupational exposure history
  - Birds, mold, farming, hot tub, beryllium, intravenous drug use
  - Immune status
  - Autoimmune disease history
  - Medication history
- Radiographic features
  - Focality and location
  - Size
  - Cavitation

(Continued)

necrotizing granulomas is fairly short and primarily includes infection, granulomatosis with polyangiitis (GPA), and aspiration. Rheumatoid nodule could also be considered in the correct clinical context. The quality of necrosis is important: rheumatoid nodules and aspiration are often associated with eosinophilic necrotic debris (**Fig. 1**), whereas GPA classically has basophilic necrosis (**Fig. 2**). Infectious necrosis may be eosinophilic or basophilic, but the former is more common. The presence of non-necrotizing and necrotizing granulomas is also worth noting, as this is common in infection, but not in GPA or rheumatoid nodule. If all granulomas are non-necrotizing, the differential is broader and includes infection, hypersensitivity pneumonitis (HP), sarcoid, and adverse drug reaction, among others.

Second, the anatomic distribution of the granulomas is also diagnostically useful. An exquisite lymphatic distribution—involving the pleura, interlobular septa, and bronchovascular bundles—is characteristic of sarcoidosis. If the granulomas are only seen in a peribronchiolar distribution, HP and aspiration should be considered. Perivascular distribution should trigger concern for vasculitis, intravascular drug injection, and sarcoidosis. Infectious granulomas can show nearly any distribution, and therefore, infection must be included in the differential diagnosis of essentially all cases of granulomatous lung disease.

Third, the quality of the granulomas—well-formed or poorly formed—should be assessed. "Well-formed" granulomas refer to tightly compacted collections of epithelioid histiocytes which are discrete and well-circumscribed, and more

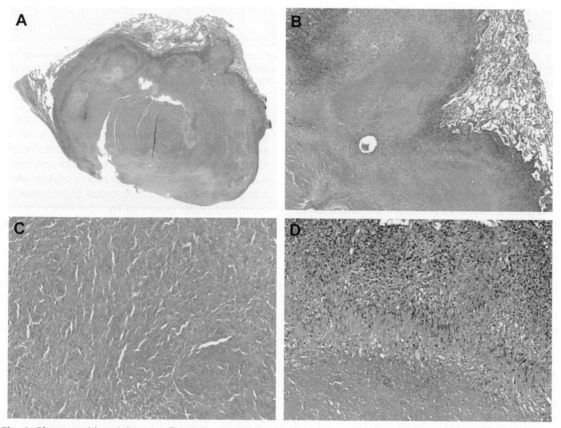

Fig. 1. Rheumatoid nodules are often (*A*) peripheral/subpleural in distribution, showing (*B*) central necrosis surrounded by lymphohistiocytic inflammation. (*C*) The necrosis is often bland, and (*D*) the histiocytes show a palisading configuration.

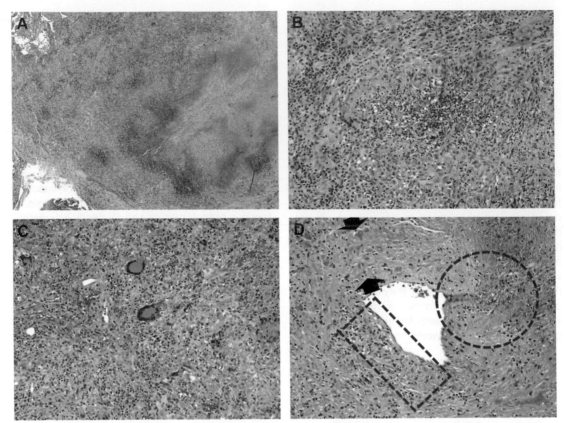

Fig. 2. Granulomatosis with polyangiitis (GPA) shows (*A*) geographic, basophilic necrosis rimmed by granulomas, (*B*) neutrophilic microabscesses, (*C*) hyperchromatic giant cells, and (*D*) necrotizing vasculitis, where the vessel wall is involved by suppurative necrosis (circle), karyorrhectic neutrophils (rectangle), and fibrinoid necrosis (between *arrows*).

often associated with sarcoidosis and infection (**Fig. 3**). In contrast, "poorly-formed" granulomas show poorly circumscribed, loose aggregates of epithelioid histiocytes and giant cells, often with intervening lymphocytes such that the histiocytes and giant cells are not in contact with one another. Poorly formed granulomas are associated with HP, infection, and adverse drug reactions (**Fig. 4**). Some granulomas will show morphology somewhere in between classic well-formed and poorly formed granulomas; although these "moderately formed" granulomas are not specific, they are most common in infection, adverse drug reaction, and hot tub lung.

Notable features that may be observed in granulomatous lung disease include vasculitis, polarizable or foreign material, and microorganisms. The character of vascular inflammation should always be carefully considered: true necrotizing vasculitis with fibrinoid necrosis of the vascular wall is likely related to GPA. However, simple vascular wall inflammation without fibrinoid necrosis may be due to infection, and prominent vascular wall

granulomas without necrosis may be seen in sarcoidosis. Familiarity with the typical histologic features of aspirated vegetable matter will make a definitive diagnosis of aspiration possible when it is present (**Fig. 5**). Granulomas should also be examined under polarized light for foreign material, especially talc particles which may indicate aspirated or injected pill material (**Fig. 6**). It should also be noted that multinucleated giant cells can produce endogenous cytoplasmic calcifications that are weakly polarizable; these needle-like endogenous calcification should not be confused with polarizable foreign material.

For all pulmonary granulomas, infection must be excluded. Therefore, special stains for fungi (Grocott methenamine silver [GMS] or periodic acid Schiff) and acid-fast bacilli (AFB) (eg, Ziehl–Neelsen) should be ordered for all such cases. To maximize sensitivity on resected necrotizing granulomas, it is recommended to perform these stains on at least two blocks, and the necrotic areas should be carefully examined for microorganisms.[8] It should be noted that tissue stains

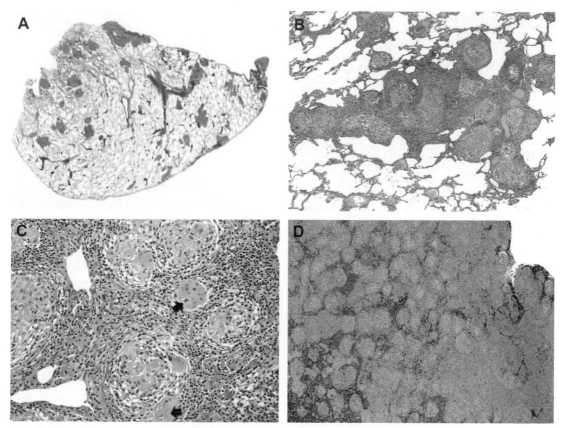

Fig. 3. (*A*) Pulmonary sarcoidosis showing multiple well-defined nodules in a lymphatic distribution. (*B*) The nodules comprise multiple well-formed, non-necrotizing granulomas, often surrounded by lamellar fibrosis. (*C*) Eosinophilic, star-shaped asteroid bodies within giant cells (*arrows*) are a frequent but nonspecific feature. (*D*) The hilar lymph nodes are commonly involved, also showing well-formed, non-necrotizing granulomas and fibrosis.

for microorganisms have inferior sensitivity compared with culture, so correlation with culture results should always be performed.

Despite these techniques, the etiology of many granulomas remains uncertain using histologic examination alone. However, by incorporating clinical, microbiological, laboratory, and radiographic data, a specific cause can often be established.[9–11] To evaluate for infection, an infectious history—for example, travel and sick contacts—should be carefully reviewed, along with culture, serology, and other microbiological testing results. Environmental and occupational exposure histories are also important. Birds/bird feathers, agricultural grains, hot tubs, chemical exposures, and many more organic antigen exposures are linked with HP.[12,13] Occupational exposures (eg, beryllium) may be relevant. A history of intravenous drug use may be a clue to pulmonary talcosis. Other important considerations in the medical history include any known inherited or acquired immunodeficiency (eg, common variable immunodeficiency [CVID], human immunodeficiency virus [HIV], and organ

transplant) or autoimmunity (eg, rheumatoid arthritis), along with autoimmune serologies. Antineutrophil cytoplasmic antibody (ANCA) studies may be very helpful in cases of suspected GPA. Medication review may reveal drugs commonly associated with granulomas (eg, methotrexate) or may indicate unmentioned medical conditions (eg, proton-pump inhibitors suggesting acid reflux, a risk factor for aspiration). Any condition leading to impaired swallowing or airway compromise should also be noted as a risk factor for aspiration.

Radiology review can be very helpful to determine the anatomic distribution (focal/diffuse) and thus narrow the differential diagnosis: for example, a focal nodular infiltrate would be more typical for infection, aspiration, or GPA, but would render HP very unlikely.[7]

By using a similar approach of comprehensive histologic and medical data review, previous studies of pulmonary granulomas reached specific diagnoses in 58% to 77% of cases.[5,7–11] To aid pathologists in this task, the common infectious and noninfectious etiologies for pulmonary

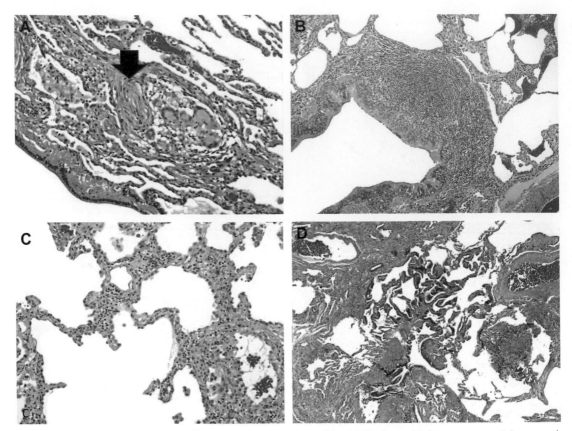

Fig. 4. The key histologic features of hypersensitivity pneumonitis. (*A*) Peribronchiolar, non-necrotizing, poorly-formed granulomas. Organizing pneumonia (*arrow*) is sometimes present. (*B*) Chronic bronchiolitis. (*C*) Interstitial chronic inflammation. (*D*) Peribronchiolar metaplasia, where the bronchiolar epithelium extends along the alveolar septal surface, is sometimes seen.

granulomas will be discussed in more detail in the following sections.

INFECTIOUS CAUSES OF GRANULOMATOUS LUNG DISEASE

Mycobacteria and fungi are the most important infectious causes of pulmonary granulomas.[2,9,11] Parasites such as *Paragonimus* spp may also cause granulomatous inflammation.[14] Viral infections generally do not produce granulomas; however, infections by HIV, Epstein–Barr virus or human T-lymphotropic virus type 1 may result in lymphoid interstitial pneumonia (LIP), which sometimes has non-necrotizing granulomas.[15] There is also a single case report of granulomatous inflammation in an immunocompromised patient with COVID-19 pneumonia and active leukemia.[16]

MYCOBACTERIA

Mycobacteria are the most frequently identified organisms in pulmonary granulomas outside the United States.[11] Mycobacterial infection should

always be considered in the differential diagnosis of pulmonary granulomas due to the wide range of possible morphologic features; often a mix of both necrotizing and non-necrotizing granulomas are present, and they can range from poorly to well-formed. The granulomas are often peribronchiolar in distribution (**Fig. 7**), but can be lymphatic. Although special stains can highlight AFB, a negative AFB stain does not exclude mycobacterial infection, which can be culture positive and AFB stain negative.[17] Histologic features cannot reliably distinguish between tuberculous and nontuberculous (atypical) mycobacteria; speciation requires cultures or polymerase chain reaction (PCR) methods, which are higher yield when necrosis is present.[17–19] Ultimately, the diagnosis of tuberculosis relies on the synthesis of clinical presentation, infectious history, radiologic findings, immunologic assays, biopsy, and microbiology results.[17]

In contrast to cases of active tuberculosis, where organisms are often abundant, organisms can be rare and difficult to identify in chronic atypical mycobacterial infection. Therefore, diagnosis

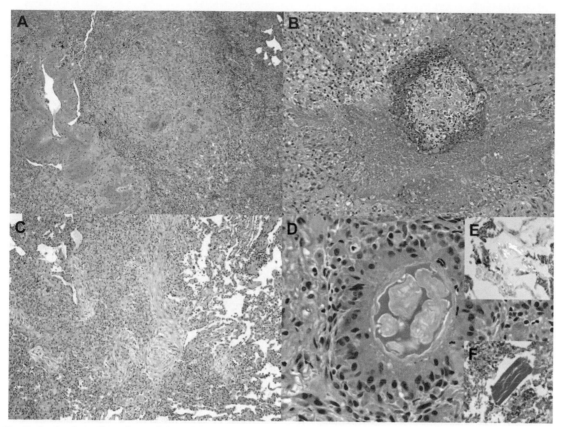

Fig. 5. Aspiration often shows (*A*) well-formed granulomas with giant cells, (*B*) neutrophilic microabscesses, and (*C*) organizing pneumonia. The granulomas are frequently associated with the aspirated material, which may include (*D*) vegetable matter, (*E*) pill fillers (polarizable talc), and (*F*) skeletal muscle (meat).

often relies on clinical context in conjunction with microbiological testing. Atypical mycobacterial infection may show prominent middle lobe/lingula involvement by bronchiectasis or chronic bronchiolitis, a condition commonly known as "Middle Lobe Syndrome," which classically occurs in elderly, nonsmoking, white women.[20–22] The bronchiectasis in this setting may be a primary or secondary issue, as ectatic bronchi are prone to atypical mycobacterial infection, but chronic infection may also lead to bronchiectasis. On high-resolution computed tomography (HRCT) images, patients with atypical mycobacterial infection can also show a "tree-in-bud" pattern, with predominantly peripheral, small bronchiolocentric nodules (see **Fig. 7**D), corresponding to inflammatory bronchiolitis.[22]

FUNGI

In the United States, fungi are more commonly identified in pulmonary granulomas than mycobacteria.[11] In pulmonary granulomas with suspected fungal infection, the patient's immune status, geographic location, travel history, and social history often suggest the responsible fungus.[23] Cultures are useful, though certain species such as *Pneumocystis jirovecii* do not grow in culture, requiring PCR. In contract to mycobacteria, in many instances, the morphologic features of the fungus in tissue can be used to identify it or at least give a narrow differential diagnosis. **Table 1** summarizes the key distinguishing features of common pulmonary fungi.

HISTOPLASMOSIS

Histoplasmosis (Histo) is endemic to many regions worldwide. In the United States, it is found in the Mississippi and Ohio River valleys and many Mid-eastern states.[23,24] The etiologic agent is *Histoplasma capsulatum,* a dimorphic fungus often found in damp soil rich in bird or bat excrement. Risk factors include occupational exposures such as construction, demolition, chicken coop cleaning, and pest waste removal, as well as adventure sports such as cave exploration.[24] In the human body, *H capsulatum* exists mainly as

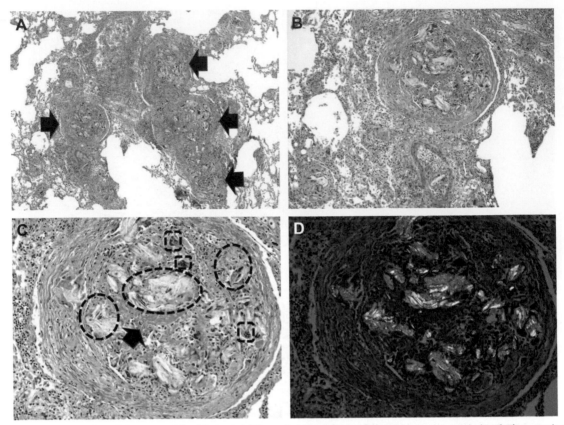

Fig. 6. Talc granulomatosis showing (*A*) lumenal filling of multiple pulmonary arteries (*arrows*). (*B, C*) The arteries contain refractile, transparent-to-brown exogenous pill material (*circles*), fibrinous thrombus (*arrow*), and foreign body giant cells (*rectangles*). (*D*) The talc from the pill material is polarizable.

yeast. Cultures for pulmonary histoplasmosis are often negative, and morphologically, the granulomas are difficult to distinguish from those of coccidioidomycosis or tuberculosis.[25] Morphologic evaluation with fungal stains can therefore be a key to the diagnosis, in addition to serologic testing.

Histologically, *Histoplasma* yeasts are oval and often have a tapering end (slightly tear-drop shaped), uniformly small (2–4 μm) in size, and show narrow-based budding (**Fig. 8**). They are typically associated with large necrotizing granulomas, especially those that are hyalinized or calcified. The organisms can be found both inside and outside of macrophages. In acute or disseminated disease, the yeasts are predominantly located in macrophages, and the alveoli and/or interstitium may be diffusely involved by a lymphohistiocytic infiltrate, in addition to geographic necrosis and/or necrotizing granulomas. In the setting of diffuse alveolar involvement, the yeasts of *H capsulatum* may mimic those of *P jirovecii*, which do not bud, can show frequent crescent shapes, and are often seen in severely immunocompromised patients.

BLASTOMYCOSIS

Blastomycosis is caused by *Blastomyces dermatitidis*, a dimorphic fungus found in warm, moist soil, rotting wood, beaver dams, and watershed areas worldwide.[23,26,27] In North America, endemic areas include the Mississippi and Ohio river valleys; the South, Southeast, and North Central states in the United States; and US and Canadian territories adjacent to the Great Lakes.[27] The diagnosis can be made on histology, culture, or serology.[23,26] Of note, several culture-confirmed blastomycosis cases have had negative microscopic tissue examination.[27]

Morphologically, pulmonary blastomycosis manifests in immunocompetent patients as necrotizing granulomas containing large (8–15 μm) round yeasts of relatively uniform size, showing thick and refractile double-contour walls and broad-based budding (**Fig. 9**). These granulomas are often associated with neutrophilic infiltrates. The organisms may also be present in alveolar spaces.[26] Although often visible on hematoxylin and eosin (H&E) stains, the morphology is best

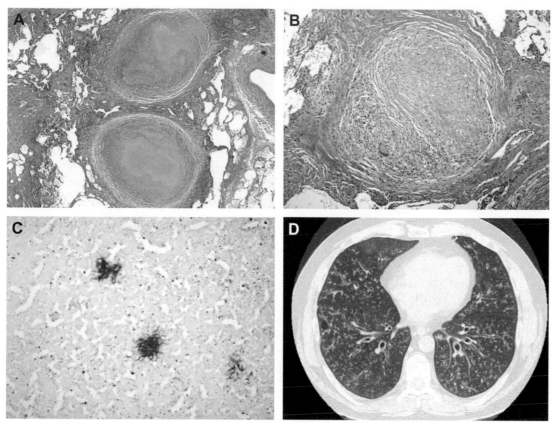

Fig. 7. (*A, B*) Peribronchiolar necrotizing granulomas in mycobacteria infection, with occasional multinucleated giant cells. (*C*) AFB stain highlights acid-fast bacilli. (*D*) "Tree-in-bud" pattern on chest CT, showing centrilobular nodules with linear branching, caused by non-tuberculous mycobacteria infection.

exemplified on fungal stains. The morphologic differential for *Blastomyces* includes *Cryptococcus neoformans*, which differs in having variable yeast sizes, frequent mucin capsule, and narrow-based budding.

COCCIDIOIDOMYCOSIS

Coccidioides spp is responsible for coccidioidomycosis, with *C immitis and C posadasii* being the main pathogenic species. These organisms are dimorphic fungi that dwell in arid, alkaline soil, and are limited to the Western Hemisphere.[28] The disease is endemic to the southwestern United States (primarily Arizona and California), parts of Mexico, and Central and South America.[29] It has recently been described to have an expanded range, including Washington, Oregon, Utah, Nevada, and Texas, potentially due to climate change.[28,30] Most infections are asymptomatic and are often incidentally identified as solitary pulmonary nodules or thin-walled cavities on imaging.[28] Dissemination typically occurs in immunocompromised hosts but has also been

Table 1
Distinguishing features of fungi commonly associated with pulmonary granulomas

Fungus	Size (μm)	Variability	Buds	Additional Features
Histoplasma	2–4	No	Yes (narrow-based)	Pointed end (teardrop-shaped)
Blastomyces	8–15	No	Yes (broad-based)	Neutrophils
Cryptococcus	4–15	Yes	Yes (narrow-based)	Capsule
Coccidioides	2–5/30–200	Yes	No	Eosinophils
Pneumocystis	3.5–7	No	No	Crescent shapes

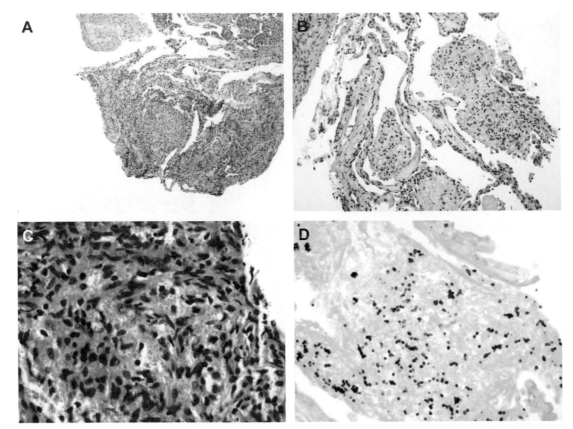

Fig. 8. Histoplasmosis can show pulmonary granulomas (*A*) or, less commonly, alveolar exudates (*B*). (*C*) The granular "dots" in the histiocytes correspond to *Histoplasma* organisms highlighted on GMS stain (*D*), showing uniformly small yeasts with narrow-based budding.

reported in immunocompetent individuals with remote exposures.[31,32] The organism can be identified on histology, cultures, or serology.

Coccidioides spp exist predominantly as round spherules in the human body, causing necrotizing granulomas in the lungs. It is the largest routinely encountered fungal organism, showing spherules of variable sizes (30–200 μm). These thick-walled spherules contain many small, non-budding endospores (2–5 μm), which are eventually expelled, leaving behind empty or collapsed spherules (**Fig. 10**). The nearby tissue often shows an eosinophilic infiltrate. The large spherules are often found on H&E but are best visualized on fungal stains. Morphologically, the endospores may resemble small yeasts like *Histoplasma*. However, unlike *Histoplasma*, *Coccidioides* spp do not bud and often grow in culture from infected tissue.[23]

CRYPTOCOCCOSIS

Pulmonary cryptococcosis is usually caused by *C neoformans or C gattii,* often in immunocompromised hosts.[33] *Cryptococcus spp* are encapsulated

yeasts typically found in soil, bird (particularly pigeon) feces, and tree hollows.[23,33] It has a worldwide distribution.[34] Cryptococcosis may also present with meningitis and can disseminate.[33] As respiratory tract colonization is not uncommon, positive cultures should be interpreted in context of clinical presentation, radiographic findings, and histologic results.[33,35] Serologic studies and molecular methods may also help establish the diagnosis.[33] Of note, occasional histologically confirmed cases may be culture-negative.[11,23]

On microscopy, *Cryptococcus* can show both non-necrotizing and necrotizing granulomas, though granuloma formation might be hindered in immunocompromised patients. The granulomas often contain many giant cells with foamy cytoplasm containing numerous organisms. The organisms are large (4–15 μm), rounded yeasts of variable sizes (**Fig. 11**). They show narrow-based budding and typically are surrounded by a mucin-rich capsule, which can be highlighted by mucicarmine stain, but capsule-deficient forms exist. The cell wall of *Cryptococcus* is often positive with Fontana-Masson stain. The main

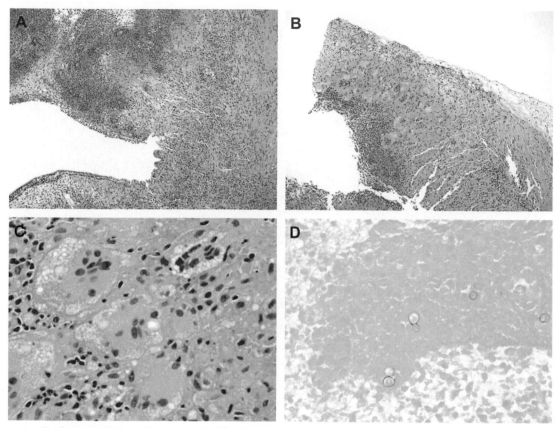

Fig. 9. (*A, B*) Blastomycosis showing necrotizing peribronchiolar granulomatous inflammation, often associated with neutrophilic infiltrate. (*C*) Yeast-form organisms may reside within multinucleated giant cells. (*D*) GMS stain highlights large yeasts with relatively uniform size, broad-based budding, and a thick, refractile, double-contour wall.

histologic differential diagnosis includes *Histoplasma* and *Blastomyces spp*, but both lack the capsule and size variability of *Cryptococcus*, and *Blastomyces* demonstrates broad-based budding.

PNEUMOCYSTIS

P jirovecii is a fungus pathogenic almost exclusively in immunocompromised individuals, including those with a history of HIV, malignancy, or transplant. Its natural reservoir remains unknown. In the lung, the organism exists as cysts (highlighted by GMS or toluidine blue) and trophozoites (highlighted by Giemsa and Diff-Quik).[36] Radiographically, a "crazy paving" pattern may be observed, along with nodules and cavitary lesions.[23] As *P jirovecii* does not grow in culture, diagnosis relies on tissue examination or molecular methods such as PCR.[36]

Microscopically, *P jirovecii* usually manifests as eosinophilic frothy alveolar exudates in profoundly immunosuppressed patients. However, especially in patients with less severe immunosuppression,

occasional necrotizing or non-necrotizing granulomas may be identified.[23] The organisms are non-budding yeast-like cysts of relatively uniform size (3.5–7 μm). These cysts range from round/oval to crushed/crescent shapes, and sometimes show central intracystic dots of enhanced staining (**Fig. 12**). The morphologic differential for *P jirovecii* includes *H capsulatum* (which buds and lacks the central dot and crescent shape) and the endospores of *Coccidioides* spp (which show size variation and are accompanied by large thick-walled spherules). In small biopsies where neither spherules nor budding are identified, definitive classification may not be possible, and the reported differential diagnosis may include all three organisms.[23]

PARASITES

Increased global travel has led to parasitic infections being seen more outside their endemic regions. Thus, surgical pathologists have a valuable role in identifying parasitic infections,

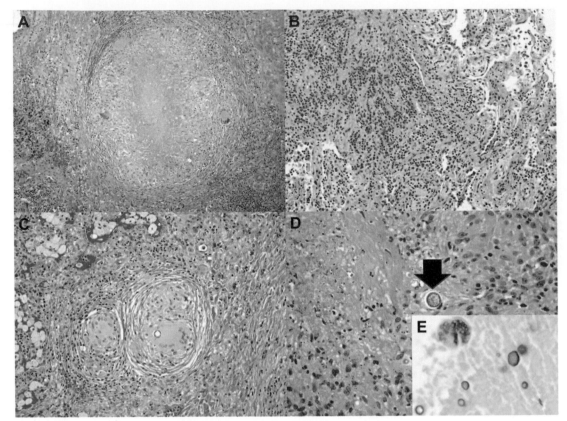

Fig. 10. (*A, B*) *Coccidioides* granulomas are often associated with an eosinophilic infiltrate. (*C*) The large spherules, which may be empty, can often be seen on H&E, within giant cells. (*D*) A spherule (*arrow*) still contains endospores. (*E*) GMS stain highlights the variably-sized spherules, including one still containing numerous non-budding endospores.

especially when they are not suspected clinically. Although parasitic infections vary greatly in microscopic manifestations—including eosinophilic pneumonia/abscess, vasculitis, pleuritis, fibrosis, empyema, and acute lung injury—many can also cause granulomatous inflammation, including paragonimiasis, dirofilariasis, schistosomiasis, and strongyloidiasis.[14,37–39] Identification and careful examination of the organisms and/or eggs in tissue can lead to identification in many cases, which is covered in detail elsewhere.[14]

NONINFECTIOUS CAUSES OF GRANULOMATOUS LUNG DISEASE

For many cases in which an infectious etiology cannot be proven, the noninfectious causes of granulomatous lung disease must also be considered, which are a broad and varied group of diseases. Correlation with clinical, radiographic, and laboratory data is optimally performed to aid in the differential diagnosis of these cases.

HYPERSENSITIVITY PNEUMONITIS

HP is an inflammatory and sometimes fibrotic disease of the interstitium and small airways, typically due to an immune-mediated reaction triggered by an inhaled antigen in susceptible individuals.[13] The inciting agents are numerous. They may be organic (eg, fungi, avian proteins, thermophilic actinomyces associated with agricultural grain) or inorganic (eg, polyurethane products, antibiotics) and include many occupational and environmental exposures (hence names such as farmer's lung, bird fancier's disease, and hot tub lung).[12,13] HP can present acutely or chronically, with symptoms including dyspnea and cough and HRCT findings classically including ground-glass opacities, mosaic attenuation, expiratory air trapping, and frequent upper lobe predilection. A variable amount of interstitial fibrosis may be present, as the disease can become fibrotic in later stages.

Non-fibrotic HP requires three histologic features for confident diagnosis (see **Fig. 4**)[13].

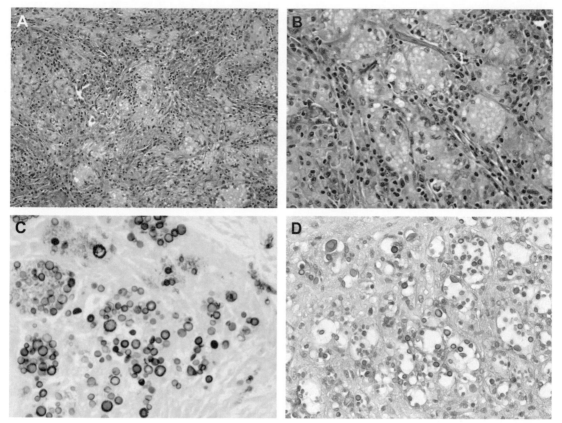

Fig. 11. (*A*) *Cryptococcus* may cause granulomas with many giant cells containing foamy cytoplasm. (*B*) On higher power, the organisms can be seen within the giant cells. (*C*) GMS shows large yeasts of variable sizes, with narrow-based budding. (*D*) Mucicarmine highlights the mucin-rich capsule.

1. Poorly formed, non-necrotizing granulomas: often small, typically within the interstitium of the peribronchiolar regions and alveolar walls. Within the giant cells, cholesterol clefts and Schaumann bodies are common but not specific. Granulomas may spill into peribronchiolar air spaces and be associated with organizing pneumonia, but the interstitial granulomas are more specific for HP.
2. Chronic bronchiolitis: lymphocytic infiltrates in the small airways which may be accompanied by peribronchiolar metaplasia (extension of bronchiolar epithelium onto adjacent alveolar septa), bronchiolectasis, and mucostasis.
3. Interstitial chronic inflammation: mainly consisting of lymphocytes and plasma cells, often bronchiolocentric but may extend more diffusely into the alveolar walls.

Fibrotic HP should show the features above (often more prominent in the less fibrotic areas), accompanied by subpleural and centriacinar fibrosis. The pattern of fibrosis often resembles usual interstitial pneumonia, with patchy fibrosis, fibroblastic foci, and subpleural honeycombing. However, some cases of fibrotic HP show a more diffuse and uniform fibrosis, without honeycombing, reminiscent of nonspecific interstitial pneumonia (NSIP).

The differential diagnosis includes infection (especially atypical mycobacteria), LIP, hot tub lung, and adverse drug reaction. Exclusion of these conditions typically requires clinical, radiographic, and microbiological correlation.[12,13]

HOT TUB LUNG

Hot tub lung is a diffuse lung disease associated with aerosolized exposure to *Mycobacterium avium* complex (MAC), with clinical, radiological, and histologic findings that overlap with typical HP. The patients are often immunocompetent and usually are exposed to hot tub water contaminated with MAC. Generally considered a hypersensitivity reaction and not a true infection, some uncertainty remains as to whether a component of infection is involved.[12,13,40]

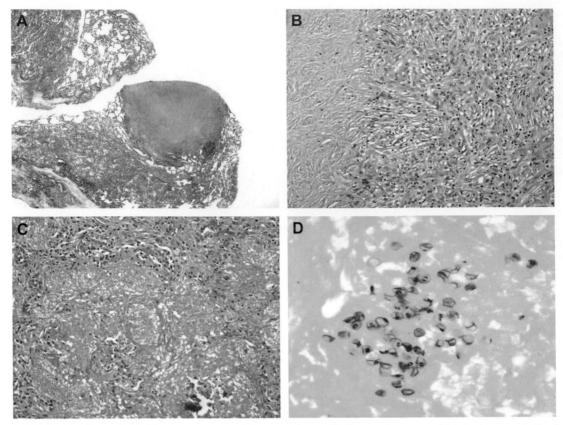

Fig. 12. (A, B) *P jirovecii* manifesting as a necrotizing granuloma. (C) The most common histologic presentation is eosinophilic, frothy intra-alveolar infiltrates. (D) On GMS stain, they appear as non-budding yeast-like cysts of relatively uniform size, some ovoid with central dots, and others with crescent shapes.

Histologically, although the patchy chronic interstitial pneumonia, bronchiolocentric granulomas, and occasional organizing pneumonia may resemble HP, the granulomas of hot tub lung tend to be more cohesive and a bit larger, and are often in the airspaces of distal bronchioles and alveoli. MAC organisms are not usually identifiable on AFB stains.[13,40] Definitive diagnosis requires a history of hot tub use or exposure to water aerosol contaminated with MAC.[41]

SARCOIDOSIS

Sarcoidosis is a multisystemic disease characterized by non-necrotizing granulomas in various organs, most often the lungs and/or mediastinal lymph nodes. The incidence is highest in Scandinavian countries and among African Americans.[42–44] Pulmonary sarcoidosis is diagnosed based on clinical presentation (cough, dyspnea, wheeze), radiologic findings (bilateral hilar lymphadenopathy, nodules in lymphatic distribution), non-necrotizing granulomas on biopsy, and exclusion of other granulomatous conditions,

particularly infection.[42,44] Although spontaneous regression is common, more than 10% of patients show progression of lung disease, and the overall mortality rate is about 7% at 5 years.[45]

On histologic examination, sarcoidosis shows well-formed, non-necrotizing granulomas that are often surrounded by concentric lamellar rings of fibrosis (see **Fig. 3**). The granulomas are described as "naked"—showing a relative lack of lymphoid cuff compared with other granulomas, particularly those of infection and hypersensitivity pneumonia. The granulomas are characteristically distributed along lymphatic routes (bronchovascular bundles, pleura, and interlobular septa)—making transbronchial biopsies high-yield. Some histiocytes or multinucleated giant cells may contain Schaumann bodies or asteroid bodies, but these findings are nonspecific. Lymph node involvement is typical and may be a helpful diagnostic clue. If the disease progresses, the granulomas may be replaced by dense fibrosis.[44]

Sarcoidosis is a diagnosis of exclusion. The most important differential diagnosis is infection, which must be excluded clinically before a diagnosis of sarcoid is rendered. Other less common entities in the differential diagnosis include berylliosis, adverse drug reaction, and foreign body reaction. Interestingly, sarcoid-like reaction can also be observed in the setting of malignancy (eg, seminoma, lymphoma) and may abate with treatment of the malignancy.

CHRONIC BERYLLIUM DISEASE

Chronic beryllium disease (CBD) is an occupational lung disease caused by inhaled beryllium. At-risk occupations include beryllium extraction/processing, metal machining, and computer, aerospace, ceramics, and electronic industries.[41] The symptoms, imaging, and biopsy findings may be identical to sarcoidosis.[41,46] Therefore, the diagnosis is based on beryllium exposure history, documented beryllium sensitivity via lymphocyte proliferation test, and non-necrotizing granulomas on lung biopsy.[46] Similar to sarcoidosis, CBD shows non-necrotizing granulomas in a lymphatic distribution and hilar lymph node involvement. However, unlike sarcoidosis, CBD can also show poorly formed granulomas and interstitial chronic inflammation.[47]

LYMPHOID INTERSTITIAL PNEUMONIA AND GRANULOMATOUS–LYMPHOCYTIC INTERSTITIAL LUNG DISEASE

LIP is a rare interstitial lung disease usually associated with autoimmune disorders (eg, Sjogren syndrome and lupus) or immunodeficiencies (eg, CVID, selective IgA deficiency [IgAD], HIV).[15] Interestingly, radiographic features of LIP are often noted to include prominent cyst formation, but a recent study noted that radiologically suspected LIP (often based on striking cyst formation) does not translate into a pathologic LIP diagnosis in many cases.[15] On histopathology, LIP should show dense, diffuse expansion of the alveolar septa by inflammatory cells consisting of mainly T lymphocytes, plasma cells, and macrophages, with frequent lymphoid aggregates and scattered germinal centers.[48] Small, loosely formed, non-necrotizing granulomas are sometimes identified.[15] The main differential diagnosis includes HP (which shows less intense alveolar septal inflammation, few germinal centers, but more peribronchiolar inflammation and presence of organizing pneumonia) and low-grade B-cell lymphomas (which shows a predominance of monoclonal B cells, often in lymphatic distribution).[2]

LIP shows significant clinicopathological overlap with the entity "granulomatous-lymphocytic interstitial lung disease" (GLILD). Although the most common pulmonary manifestation of CVID and IgAD is recurrent infections, interstitial lung disease is not uncommon.[49] GLILD is a term that has been used to describe the combination of non-necrotizing granulomas and benign interstitial lymphoid infiltrates in a patient with primary antibody deficiency due to CVID or IgAD. The lymphoid infiltrates may encompass many different pathologic patterns, including follicular bronchiolitis, peribronchiolar lymphoid aggregates without germinal centers, LIP, and NSIP (**Fig. 13**). Organizing pneumonia is a common finding, and fibrosis may be present. There are no well-established diagnostic criteria for GLILD nor is there consensus regarding its clinical significance.[49–51] Because of this, a recent study suggests GLILD may not be a useful concept and suggests that more descriptive pathologic diagnoses could be rendered in the setting of CVID and IgAD.[49]

VASCULITIS: GRANULOMATOSIS WITH POLYANGIITIS AND EOSINOPHILIC GRANULOMATOSIS WITH POLYANGIITIS

GPA is the most important vasculitic process that involves the lung. GPA belongs to the group of systemic necrotizing ANCA-associated vasculitides, which involve predominantly small vessels, show few to no immune deposits, and are often associated with myeloperoxidase ANCA or proteinase 3 (PR3) ANCA.[52,53] GPA is characterized by necrotizing vasculitis of small to medium vessels and necrotizing granulomas of the upper and lower respiratory tract. Sinonasal disease and necrotizing glomerulonephritis are also common features; eyes, skin, and peripheral nervous system can also be affected.[52] Lung involvement can be the only presenting feature.[41] GPA typically shows strong association with PR3-ANCA.[53] Diagnosis is based on clinical presentation, detection of ANCA by immunoassays or immunofluorescence, CT findings (multiple lung nodules, often with thick-walled cavities), and sometimes surgical biopsy.[41,54,55]

Histologically, GPA shows geographic areas of necrosis surrounded by palisading granulomas (see **Fig. 2**). The necrosis contains abundant neutrophils and nuclear debris, lending a "dirty" blue appearance. Neutrophilic microabscesses and multinucleated giant cells with characteristic darkly hyperchromatic nuclei are frequent. Because the presence of necrosis, granulomas, and microabscesses can also be observed in infection, the presence of necrotizing vasculitis should always be assessed. Necrotizing vasculitis

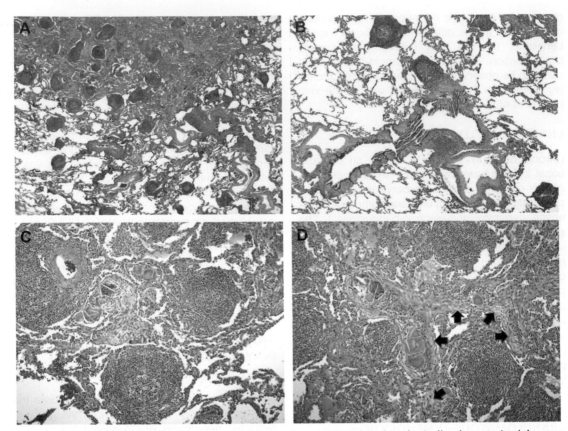

Fig. 13. Granulomatous-lymphocytic interstitial lung disease (GLILD) is histologically characterized by non-necrotizing granulomas and various forms of lymphocytic infiltrates, including (*A*) follicular bronchiolitis, featuring numerous peribronchiolar lymphoid aggregates and (*B*) some with germinal centers. (*C*) There may be lymphoid interstitial pneumonia-like alveolar interstitial chronic inflammation. Small, loose, non-necrotizing granulomas are also seen. (*D*) Additionally, organizing pneumonia (*arrows*) may be present.

may be focal or transmural, and should show fibrinoid necrosis of the vessel wall; it may or may not have associated granulomas and/or suppuration.[41] Capillaritis—karyorrhectic neutrophils and fibrinoid necrosis in the capillary walls—is not specific for GPA but can be the only finding in small biopsies.[41] Airway inflammation and organizing pneumonia may be present. Compact, non-necrotizing granulomas and hilar lymph node involvement are unusual for GPA and should raise concern for infection.[41] Prominent eosinophils are also rare. Although ANCA results may be helpful, false positives are seen in some infections, so special stains for microorganisms and clinical microbiological testing should always be performed.[54]

Eosinophilic GPA (EGPA) is another ANCA-associated, multisystemic vasculitis that often involves the respiratory tract. However, unlike GPA, the histologic features observed in lung biopsies from EGPA are often not very specific, and the diagnosis requires correlation with the required clinical features. EGPA is almost universally associated with asthma and eosinophilia in blood and tissue.[52,56] The most common radiologic finding in the lung is peripheral, bilateral, migratory opacities.[55] The diagnosis is often based on clinical findings and/or biopsy of extrapulmonary sites.[56] This is because the classical histologic triad for EGPA in the lung, including eosinophilic pneumonia, necrotizing granulomas, and necrotizing vasculitis, is uncommonly seen.[41,56] Eosinophilic pneumonia alone is the most common pattern observed in lung biopsies from patients with EGPA, in which case the diagnosis strongly relies on the clinical factors mentioned above.

ASPIRATION

Aspiration is one of the most underrecognized granulomatous conditions, both clinically and histologically.[7,57] It often occurs in those with impaired gag, cough, and swallowing reflexes (ie, neuromuscular disease, prior stroke, heavy drug or alcohol abuse, and recent sedation/intubation), and may also be asymptomatic, especially in younger individuals.[41,58] The aspirated material is usually food remnants, some of which persist for longer periods and are therefore more likely to be recognized histologically, especially vegetable matter and pill filler fragments.[41,57] Aspiration pneumonitis or pneumonia may occur as an inflammatory reaction to the aspirated material and the accompanying gastric acid/bacteria.

Histologically, aspiration is characterized by bronchiolocentric inflammation and well-formed intraluminal granulomas with giant cells, often with small foci of central necrosis, and associated with neutrophilic microabscesses (see Fig. 5).[13,58,59] The granulomas are most often closely related to the aspirated material. Organizing pneumonia is also a common feature.[57,59] Vegetable/plant matter like seeds, lentils, legumes, starch granules, and nuts can persist for a long time in the lungs and are recognized by their thick cell walls and internal septations. Material seen under plane-polarized light typically represents pill fillers such as talc. The presence of confidently identified foreign material in the airspaces allows for a definitive diagnosis of aspiration pneumonia and effectively excludes important differential diagnostic considerations. The location of the foreign material in the airspace is important, because foreign material can also be introduced into the lung through the vasculature (see the following section).

TALC GRANULOMATOSIS

Talc granulomatosis, also known as intravenous talcosis and Drug Abuser's Lung, refers to granulomatous lung disease resulting from the intravenous injection of crushed pills, most often opioids, amphetamines, barbiturates, or methylphenidate.[41,60] The pill fragments then get lodged in the pulmonary vascular system. Histologically, there are diffuse perivascular granulomas containing plate- or needle-shaped crystals of talc or other pill fillers (methylcellulose, crospovidone), which are at least partially birefringent under polarized light (see Fig. 6).[60,61] Talc granulomatosis may cause interstitial fibrosis and pulmonary hypertension with organizing thrombosis and arterial remodeling.[61] The typical histologic features allow a definitive diagnosis, so long as the foreign material is confidently located in the vascular structures and not the airspaces, because pill material can also be aspirated into the lung.

RHEUMATOID NODULE

Pulmonary rheumatoid nodules are usually associated with active rheumatoid arthritis requiring systemic therapy. Their presence is correlated with elevated disease severity and increased mortality.[62] Patients that develop pulmonary rheumatoid nodules usually also have cutaneous rheumatoid nodules and high titers of rheumatoid factor. The nodules tend to be multiple and are often subpleural. Histologically, pulmonary rheumatoid nodules show identical morphology to the more common cutaneous nodules, characterized by necrotizing ("necrobiotic") granulomas with palisading histiocytes and central bland necrosis (see Fig. 1). If abundant neutrophils or eosinophils are present, alternate diagnoses should be considered. The diagnosis of pulmonary rheumatoid nodule requires clinical and microbiological correlation; infection is the prime differential diagnosis based on morphologic features, and rheumatoid arthritis patients are often on immunosuppressant treatments, making them more prone to pulmonary infections.[41]

ADVERSE DRUG REACTION

Adverse drug reaction can cause granulomatous reaction in the lungs, and the granulomas are most commonly poorly to moderately formed. In some cases, the granulomas might be accompanied by bronchiolitis and interstitial inflammation, making the pattern of adverse drug reaction indistinguishable from HP.[63] The prototypic drug for granulomatous pneumonitis is methotrexate, for which there can be acute lung injury associated with focal organizing pneumonia, predominantly non-necrotizing granulomas, perivascular inflammation, and eosinophils.[64] A large number of other medications have been implicated in pulmonary granulomatous reactions, with the most common categories being tumor necrosis factor (TNF)-alpha antagonists (eg, infliximab, etanercept), interferon or peg-interferon therapeutics, and immune checkpoint inhibitors (eg, pembrolizumab, nivolumab).[65] Other implicated drugs include Bacillus Calmette-Guerin vaccine, sulfasalazine, isoniazid, fluoxetine, and mesalamine.[41,65] Drug databases such as Pneumotox (https://www.pneumotox.com) may be helpful to further evaluate a specific drug in question, as there is an ever-expanding list of granuloma-inducing medications.

SUMMARY

In summary, granulomas are frequently observed in all types of lung specimens, including core biopsies, transbronchial biopsies, wedge biopsies, and lobectomies, and arise from diverse causes. Granulomas should always be reported as necrotizing or non-necrotizing, which helps to refine the differential diagnosis. The possibility of infection should always be evaluated using special stains and/or microbiologic methods. The differential diagnosis of granulomatous lung disease can be narrowed by paying attention to granuloma distribution, quality, and associated features, which can lead to a more focused and clinically helpful pathology report.

CLINICS CARE POINTS

- Granulomas should always be reported as necrotizing or non-necrotizing.

- All pulmonary granuomas should have microorganism stains performed.

- The differnetial diagnosis for necrotizing pulmonary granuolomas primarily includes infection, aspiration, and granulomatosis with polyangiits.

- The differential diagnosis for non-necrotizing pulmonary granulomas is broad, but can be narrowed to a "short list" by paying attention to distriubtion and quality of the granuolomas, along with associated features.

DISCLOSURE

No disclosures or conflicts of interest.

REFERENCES

1. Adams DO. The granulomatous inflammatory response. A review. Am J Pathol 1976;84(1):164–92.
2. Mukhopadhyay S, Gal AA. Granulomatous lung disease: an approach to the differential diagnosis. Arch Pathol Lab Med 2010;134(5):667–90.
3. McClean CM, Tobin DM. Macrophage form, function, and phenotype in mycobacterial infection: lessons from tuberculosis and other diseases. Pathog Dis 2016;74(7). https://doi.org/10.1093/femspd/ftw068.
4. Ramakrishnan L. Revisiting the role of the granuloma in tuberculosis. Nat Rev Immunol 2012;12(5):352–66.
5. Doxtader EE, Mukhopadhyay S, Katzenstein AL. Core needle biopsy in benign lung lesions: pathologic findings in 159 cases. Hum Pathol 2010;41(11):1530–5.
6. Gong Y, Sneige N, Guo M, et al. Transthoracic fine-needle aspiration vs concurrent core needle biopsy in diagnosis of intrathoracic lesions: a retrospective comparison of diagnostic accuracy. Am J Clin Pathol 2006;125(3):438–44.
7. Hutton Klein JR, Tazelaar HD, Leslie KO, et al. One hundred consecutive granulomas in a pulmonary pathology consultation practice. Am J Surg Pathol 2010;34(10):1456–64.
8. Ulbright TM, Katzenstein AL. Solitary necrotizing granulomas of the lung: differentiating features and etiology. Am J Surg Pathol 1980;4(1):13–28.
9. Mukhopadhyay S, Wilcox BE, Myers JL, et al. Pulmonary necrotizing granulomas of unknown cause: clinical and pathologic analysis of 131 patients with completely resected nodules. Chest 2013;144(3):813–24.
10. Aubry MC. Necrotizing granulomatous inflammation: what does it mean if your special stains are negative? Mod Pathol 2012;25(Suppl 1):S31–8.
11. Mukhopadhyay S, Farver CF, Vaszar LT, et al. Causes of pulmonary granulomas: a retrospective study of 500 cases from seven countries. J Clin Pathol 2012;65(1):51–7.
12. Miller R, Allen TC, Barrios RJ, et al. Hypersensitivity pneumonitis a perspective from members of the pulmonary pathology society. Arch Pathol Lab Med 2018;142(1):120–6.
13. Raghu G, Remy-Jardin M, Ryerson CJ, et al. Diagnosis of hypersensitivity pneumonitis in adults. an official ATS/JRS/ALAT clinical practice guideline. Am J Respir Crit Care Med 2020;202(3):e36–69.
14. Boland JM, Pritt BS. Histopathology of parasitic infections of the lung. Semin Diagn Pathol 2017;34(6):550–9.
15. Fraune C, Churg A, Yi ES, et al. Lymphoid interstitial pneumonia (LIP) revisited: a critical reappraisal of the histologic spectrum of "radiologic" and "pathologic" lip in the context of diffuse benign lymphoid proliferations of the lung. Am J Surg Pathol 2023;47(3):281–95.
16. Usturalı Keskin E, Tastekin E, Can N, et al. Granulomatous inflammation in pulmonary pathology of 2019 novel coronavirus pneumonia: case report with a literature review. Surgical and Experimental Pathology 2020;3(1). https://doi.org/10.1186/s42047-020-00071-2.
17. Jain D, Ghosh S, Teixeira L, et al. Pathology of pulmonary tuberculosis and non-tuberculous mycobacterial lung disease: Facts, misconceptions, and practical tips for pathologists. Semin Diagn Pathol 2017;34(6):518–29.
18. Corpe RF, Stergus I. Is the histopathology of non-photochromogenic mycobacterial infections distinguishable from that caused by Mycobacterium tuberculosis? Am Rev Respir Dis 1963;87:289–91.
19. Tang YW, Procop GW, Zheng X, et al. Histologic parameters predictive of mycobacterial infection. Am J Clin Pathol 1998;109(3):331–4.
20. Einarsson JT, Einarsson JG, Isaksson H, et al. Middle lobe syndrome: a nationwide study on clinico-pathological features and surgical treatment. Clin Respir J 2009;3(2):77–81.

21. Kwon KY, Myers JL, Swensen SJ, et al. Middle lobe syndrome: a clinicopathological study of 21 patients. Hum Pathol 1995;26(3):302–7.

22. Griffith DE, Aksamit T, Brown-Elliott BA, et al. An official ATS/IDSA statement: diagnosis, treatment, and prevention of nontuberculous mycobacterial diseases. Am J Respir Crit Care Med 2007;175(4):367–416.

23. Roden AC, Schuetz AN. Histopathology of fungal diseases of the lung. Semin Diagn Pathol 2017; 34(6):530–49.

24. Arauz AB, Papineni P. Histoplasmosis. Infect Dis Clin North Am 2021;35(2):471–91.

25. Zimmerman LE. Demonstration of Histoplasma and Coccidioides in so-called tuberculomas of lung: preliminary report on thirty-five cases. AMA Arch Intern Med 1954;94(5):690–9.

26. Taxy JB. Blastomycosis: contributions of morphology to diagnosis: a surgical pathology, cytopathology, and autopsy pathology study. Am J Surg Pathol 2007;31(4):615–23.

27. Patel AJ, Gattuso P, Reddy VB. Diagnosis of blastomycosis in surgical pathology and cytopathology: correlation with microbiologic culture. Am J Surg Pathol 2010;34(2):256–61.

28. Crum NF. Coccidioidomycosis: a contemporary review. Infect Dis Ther 2022;11(2):713–42.

29. McCotter OZ, Benedict K, Engelthaler DM, et al. Update on the epidemiology of coccidioidomycosis in the United States. Med Mycol 2019; 57(Supplement_1):S30–40.

30. Chow NA, Kangiser D, Gade L, et al. Factors influencing distribution of coccidioides immitis in soil, Washington State, 2016. mSphere 2021;6(6): e0059821.

31. Agarwal P, Gami R, Osman AF, et al. Disseminated coccidioidomycosis in an immunocompetent male who lived in an endemic region in the remote past: a case report. Cureus 2022;14(5):e25249.

32. Ashizawa H, Iwanaga N, Kurohama H, et al. Pulmonary coccidioidomycosis complicated by nontuberculous mycobacterial pulmonary diseases with a literature review. Jpn J Infect Dis 2023. https://doi.org/10.7883/yoken.JJID.2023.073.

33. Setianingrum F, Rautemaa-Richardson R, Denning DW. Pulmonary cryptococcosis: A review of pathobiology and clinical aspects. Med Mycol 2019;57(2):133–50.

34. Diaz JH. The disease ecology, epidemiology, clinical manifestations, and management of emerging Cryptococcus gattii complex infections. Wilderness Environ Med 2020;31(1):101–9.

35. Duperval R, Hermans PE, Brewer NS, et al. Cryptococcosis, with emphasis on the significance of isolation of Cryptococcus neoformans from the respiratory tract. Chest 1977;72(1):13–9.

36. Apostolopoulou A, Fishman JA. The pathogenesis and diagnosis of pneumocystis jiroveci pneumonia.

J Fungi (Basel) 2022;8(11). https://doi.org/10.3390/jof8111167.

37. Boland JM, Vaszar LT, Jones JL, et al. Pleuropulmonary infection by Paragonimus westermani in the United States: a rare cause of Eosinophilic pneumonia after ingestion of live crabs. Am J Surg Pathol 2011;35(5):707–13.

38. Flieder DB, Moran CA. Pulmonary dirofilariasis: a clinicopathologic study of 41 lesions in 39 patients. Hum Pathol 1999;30(3):251–6.

39. Lin AL, Kessimian N, Benditt JO. Restrictive pulmonary disease due to interlobular septal fibrosis associated with disseminated infection by Strongyloides stercoralis. Am J Respir Crit Care Med 1995; 151(1):205–9.

40. Khoor A, Leslie KO, Tazelaar HD, et al. Diffuse pulmonary disease caused by nontuberculous mycobacteria in immunocompetent people (hot tub lung). Am J Clin Pathol 2001;115(5):755–62.

41. Rosen Y. Pathology of granulomatous pulmonary diseases. Arch Pathol Lab Med 2022;146(2): 233–51.

42. Grunewald J, Grutters JC, Arkema EV, et al. Sarcoidosis. Nat Rev Dis Primers 2019;5(1):45.

43. Hena KM. Sarcoidosis epidemiology: race matters. Front Immunol 2020;11:537382.

44. Tana C, Donatiello I, Caputo A, et al. Clinical features, histopathology and differential diagnosis of sarcoidosis. Cells 2021;11(1). https://doi.org/10.3390/cells11010059.

45. Belperio JA, Shaikh F, Abtin FG, et al. Diagnosis and treatment of pulmonary sarcoidosis: a review. JAMA 2022;327(9):856–67.

46. MacMurdo MG, Mroz MM, Culver DA, et al. Chronic beryllium disease: update on a moving target. Chest 2020;158(6):2458–66.

47. Freiman DG, Hardy HL. Beryllium disease. The relation of pulmonary pathology to clinical course and prognosis based on a study of 130 cases from the U.S. beryllium case registry. Hum Pathol 1970;1(1): 25–44.

48. Travis WD, Costabel U, Hansell DM, et al. An official American Thoracic Society/European Respiratory Society statement: Update of the international multidisciplinary classification of the idiopathic interstitial pneumonias. Am J Respir Crit Care Med 2013; 188(6):733–48.

49. Larsen BT, Smith ML, Tazelaar HD, et al. GLILD Revisited: pulmonary pathology of common variable and selective IgA immunodeficiency. Am J Surg Pathol 2020;44(8):1073–81.

50. Bates CA, Ellison MC, Lynch DA, et al. Granulomatous-lymphocytic lung disease shortens survival in common variable immunodeficiency. J Allergy Clin Immunol 2004;114(2):415–21.

51. Rao N, Mackinnon AC, Routes JM. Granulomatous and lymphocytic interstitial lung disease: a spectrum

of pulmonary histopathologic lesions in common variable immunodeficiency–histologic and immunohistochemical analyses of 16 cases. Hum Pathol 2015;46(9):1306–14.

52. Jennette JC, Falk RJ, Bacon PA, et al. 2012 revised International Chapel Hill Consensus Conference Nomenclature of Vasculitides. Arthritis Rheum 2013;65(1):1–11.

53. Kitching AR, Anders HJ, Basu N, et al. ANCA-associated vasculitis. Nat Rev Dis Primers 2020;6(1):71.

54. Bossuyt X, Cohen Tervaert JW, Arimura Y, et al. Position paper: Revised 2017 international consensus on testing of ANCAs in granulomatosis with polyangiitis and microscopic polyangiitis. Nat Rev Rheumatol 2017;13(11):683–92.

55. Feragalli B, Mantini C, Sperandeo M, et al. The lung in systemic vasculitis: radiological patterns and differential diagnosis. Br J Radiol 2016;89(1061):20150992.

56. Katzenstein AL. Diagnostic features and differential diagnosis of churg-strauss syndrome in the lung. a review. Am J Clin Pathol 2000;114(5):767–72.

57. Mukhopadhyay S, Katzenstein AL. Pulmonary disease due to aspiration of food and other particulate matter: a clinicopathologic study of 59 cases diagnosed on biopsy or resection specimens. Am J Surg Pathol 2007;31(5):752–9.

58. Barnes TW, Vassallo R, Tazelaar HD, et al. Diffuse bronchiolar disease due to chronic occult aspiration. Mayo Clin Proc 2006;81(2):172–6.

59. Yousem SA, Faber C. Histopathology of aspiration pneumonia not associated with food or other particulate matter: a clinicopathologic study of 10 cases diagnosed on biopsy. Am J Surg Pathol 2011;35(3):426–31.

60. Krause ML, Boland JM, Maleszewski JJ, et al. An unusual cause of diffuse pulmonary infiltrates. Arthritis Care Res 2013;65(3):487–90.

61. Griffith CC, Raval JS, Nichols L. Intravascular talcosis due to intravenous drug use is an underrecognized cause of pulmonary hypertension. Pulm Med 2012;2012:617531.

62. Esposito AJ, Chu SG, Madan R, et al. Thoracic manifestations of rheumatoid arthritis. Clin Chest Med 2019;40(3):545–60.

63. Flieder DB, Travis WD. Pathologic characteristics of drug-induced lung disease. Clin Chest Med 2004;25(1):37–45.

64. Imokawa S, Colby TV, Leslie KO, et al. Methotrexate pneumonitis: review of the literature and histopathological findings in nine patients. Eur Respir J 2000;15(2):373–81.

65. Cohen Aubart F, Lhote R, Amoura A, et al. Drug-induced sarcoidosis: an overview of the WHO pharmacovigilance database. J Intern Med 2020;288(3):356–62.

Update on Silicosis

Andrew Churg, MD[a],*, Nestor L. Muller, MD[b]

KEYWORDS

- Silicosis • Lung cancer • Connective tissue disease • Acute silicosis

---

Key points

- Silicosis has not disappeared, and there is a resurgence in some industries.
- Pathologically, silicosis can appear as alveolar proteinosis (acute silicosis), simple silicosis, or progressive massive fibrosis.
- Silicosis increases the risk of lung cancer; the data are less strong for silica exposure without silicosis.
- Silica exposure increases the risk of tuberculosis.
- Silica exposure increases the risk of connective tissue disease, particularly systemic sclerosis.

ABSTRACT

Although silicosis has been an established disease with a recognized cause for more than 100 years, many workers continue to be exposed to silica and new outbreaks of disease continue to occur. This article describes some of the well-established and new exposures, including denim sandblasting, artificial stone cutting, and some forms of "coal worker's pneumoconiosis." The authors review the imaging and pathology of acute silicosis (silicoproteinosis), simple silicosis, and progressive massive fibrosis and summarize known and putative associations of silica exposure, including tuberculosis, lung cancer, connective tissue disease (especially systemic sclerosis), and vasculitis.

OVERVIEW

Silicosis is an ancient disease, but one that, despite long-standing recognition of the dangers associated with silica inhalation, has never disappeared, and is even increasing in frequency in some contemporary populations. For the pathologist, silicosis is important to recognize, both in terms of accurate diagnosis and in terms of potential compensation for affected workers, but recognition is sometimes confounded by a lack of familiarity with the various morphologic appearances of silicosis as well as by the complexities of radiologic (chest radiograph) classification schemes. The pathologist may also be asked to comment on whether another process, for example, lung cancer, can be linked with silica exposure in a given case. In this brief review, the authors cover these topics and provide practical advice for the diagnosis of silicosis and its complications.

Silica refers to silicon dioxide, chemical formula SiO_2. Silica occurs either naturally or as a result of human activity, in crystalline and amorphous forms, and this distinction is important, because amorphous forms of silicon dioxide, such as diatomaceous earth, glass, or fiberglass, are not fibrogenic. Silicosis is a result of exposure to some type of crystalline silica. The common crystalline forms are quartz, tridymite, and cristobalite. Many rocks have high concentrations of quartz; for example, sandstone is typically up to 67% quartz and granite 25% to 40% quartz. Tridymite and cristobalite are much less frequently encountered but can be created by heating amorphous

---

Funding: There was no specific funding for this project.
[a] Department of Pathology, Vancouver General Hospital and University of British Columbia, JPPN 1401 Vancouver General Hospital 910 West 10th Avenue, Vancouver, British Columbia V5Z 1M9, Canada;
[b] Department of Radiology, Vancouver General Hospital, 910 W 10th Avenue, Vancouver, BC, V5Z 1M9 Canada
* Corresponding author.
E-mail address: achurg@mail.ubc.ca

silica, such as diatomaceous earth, to high temperatures, and are also found in silica refractory bricks.[1,2]

One important distinction that is frequently misunderstood is between silica and silicates. Silicates are minerals with a cation such as magnesium or aluminum and silica groups. For example, talc is a magnesium silicate with the chemical formula $Mg_3Si_4O_{10}(OH)_2$, and mica (muscovite) is an aluminum potassium silicate with formula $Al_2K_2O_6Si$. Asbestos fibers are also silicates. The potential pulmonary toxicity of silicate minerals varies enormously. Some, such as talc or asbestos, are fibrogenic at high doses, but the associated pathologic picture is quite different from silicosis, and these exposures do not predispose to mycobacterial infections, a well-recognized complication of silica exposure. Some forms of asbestos are also potent mesothelial carcinogens, a property not seen with either silica or most silicates.

CURRENT POPULATIONS AT RISK

It has been recognized since the beginning of the twentieth century that exposure to silica causes the specific disease, silicosis (for a detailed historical review see Rosenthal[3]). Nonetheless, one hundred years later, silica exposure is still common in many countries, and although there are notional permitted exposure levels to silica, these vary enormously from country to country, may be insufficient to prevent silicosis, and may be ignored, leading to new outbreaks of disease. Currently, it is estimated that there are 23 million workers in China, 11 million in India, 3 million in the European Union, 2 million in Brazil, and 2 million in the United States with exposure to respirable crystalline silica.[1,4-7] Leung and colleagues[1] reported that in China more than 500,000 new cases of silicosis were diagnosed between 1991 and 1995 and that there are still 6000 new cases and 24,000 silicosis-related deaths per year. Where strict dust control measures have been implemented and followed, silicosis rates have plummeted. For example, with an estimated 600,000 workers exposed to crystalline silica in the United Kingdom from 1990 to 1993, there were 28 silicosis-related deaths in 1993 and 10 in 2008.[7]

A wide variety of occupations in which stone is mined, quarried, crushed, or cut, or in which silica-containing materials are used for grinding and sandblasting, or in the manufacture of ceramics and refractories, have the potential for significant silica exposure. **Box 1** shows an abbreviated list of potential silica exposures;

Box 1
Occupations at risk of silicosis and silica-related diseases
Traditional Sources of Exposure
Mining
Quarrying
Stone cutting
Manufacture/use of silica abrasives and fillers
Foundry work
Ceramic and refractory manufacture
Sandblasting and grinding
Construction work (concrete cutting/drilling)
New Sources of Exposure
Hydraulic fracking
Denim sandblasting
Fabrication/installation of artificial (engineered) stone countertops
Coal mine in parts of Appalachia where the mines are excavating small coal seams

---

greater detail can be found in Leung and colleagues[1] and Weill and colleagues.[2]

Despite the well-recognized dangers of silica exposure, new outbreaks associated with high incidences of disease continue to be reported from occupational settings where dust control standards are lacking or not enforced. Contemporary data on sandstone miners in India show a radiologic prevalence of 37% to 52% simple silicosis and 7.5% progressive massive fibrosis (PMF, see Clinical and radiologic classification of silicosis section for definitions of these terms).[8,9] Similarly, Govindagoudar and colleagues[10] reported in 2021 that 465 of 729 (64%) stone crushing workers in the Indian state of Haryana were found to have silicosis, with 23% having PMF.

Another small but lethal epidemic of silicosis has been described in workers using sandblasting to create "distressed" denim jeans in Turkey. In a cohort of 145 such workers, 9 died over a 4-year period, with a mean age at death of 24 years.[11,12] Radiologic reassessment of 74 of these workers between 2007 and 2011 showed that the prevalence of silicosis increased from 55% to 96%.

Rapidly progressive and severe silicosis has been seen worldwide in workers who manufacture and cut artificial (engineered) stone kitchen and bathroom countertops.[13] Artificial stone is typically made of around 90% silica mixed with binders and coloring agents. Dry cutting releases dust that is nearly pure silica, and such exposures have led to high incidences of both simple silicosis and PMF with extremely short latencies (7–20 years) and the appearance of disease at a young age (reviewed in Leso and colleagues[13]).

Hydraulic fracking has been a cause of concern for silicosis risk because of the widespread use of silica sand in the fracking process,[6,14] but thus far there do not seem to be actual reported cases of silicosis in fracking workers.

It is also important to remember that the notional name of an occupation can hide significant silica exposure. What was at first thought to be an (unexplained) resurgence of severe coal workers' pneumoconiosis with disease appearing at a young age and leading to death or lung transplantation has recently been described in contemporary US Central Appalachian coal miners.[15] However, detailed pathologic examination showed that in fact this process was actually silicosis[16] and the silica exposure arose from the newer practice of mining small coal seams, as opposed to historic very large seams, with high silica exposure from cutting through the rock overburden around the seams.

CLINICAL AND RADIOLOGIC CLASSIFICATION OF SILICOSIS

Silicosis can be classified by clinical findings, especially latency (time from first exposure to the appearance of disease), imaging findings, and pathologic findings (**Table 1**). Acute silicosis, also called silicoproteinosis, is typically seen with high levels of exposure to finely divided dust. The latency is short, ranging from a few weeks to a few years. Currently, silicoproteinosis is fairly uncommon but has been reported in sandblasters, including denim sandblasters, brick masons, and artificial stone workers, and we found small amounts of silicoproteinosis in coal miners with accelerated silicosis.[16]

Accelerated and chronic silicosis are also sometimes referred to as forms of nodular silicosis.[17] The clinical distinction is based on latency: accelerated silicosis manifests within 5 to 10 years of initial exposure and chronic silicosis with latencies greater than 10 years, and patients with accelerated silicosis have more rapid disease progression than those with chronic silicosis.

On imaging, the CT manifestations of silicoproteinosis consist of centrilobular nodules, bilateral ground-glass opacities and dependent areas of consolidation with calcification, or bilateral ground-glass opacities with superimposed interlobular septal thickening resulting in the so-called crazy paving pattern[18,19] (**Fig. 1A**). This latter pattern is indistinguishable from autoimmune alveolar proteinosis.

The radiographic and CT findings of accelerated and chronic silicosis consist of multiple small nodules involving mainly the upper lobes. Nodules up to 1 cm are referred to as simple silicosis. On CT, the nodules typically measure 2 to 5 mm in diameter, are usually sharply defined, may be calcified, and have a centrilobular and subpleural predominance[19,20] (**Fig. 1B**). Bilateral hilar and mediastinal enlargement and calcification are commonly present.

PMF is characterized by the development of large irregular nodular opacities greater than 1 cm or mass-like areas of dense consolidation and scarring in the upper lobes, usually bilateral and symmetric[21] (**Fig. 1C**). Calcification is commonly evident within these conglomerate masses.

The functional and prognostic consequences of these various forms of silicosis are covered in Functional effects, treatment, and prognosis section.

PATHOLOGIC FEATURES OF SILICOSIS

On biopsy (**Fig. 2A**), acute silicosis resembles alveolar proteinosis of other causes, but in our

---

Table 1
Clinical, radiologic, and pathologic classification of silicosis

Clinical Term	Latency	Imaging Findings	Pathologic Findings
Acute silicosis (silicoproteinosis)	Weeks to years	Crazy paving pattern	Alveolar proteinosis but may also have silicotic nodules
Accelerated silicosis	5–10 y	Usually upper zone nodules <1 cm and/or progressive massive fibrosis	Simple silicotic nodules, but silicoproteinosis and/or progressive massive fibrosis may be present
Chronic silicosis	>10 y	Upper zone nodules <1 cm and/or progressive massive fibrosis. Interstitial fibrosis may be present	Simple silicotic nodules and/or progressive massive fibrosis. Interstitial fibrosis may be present

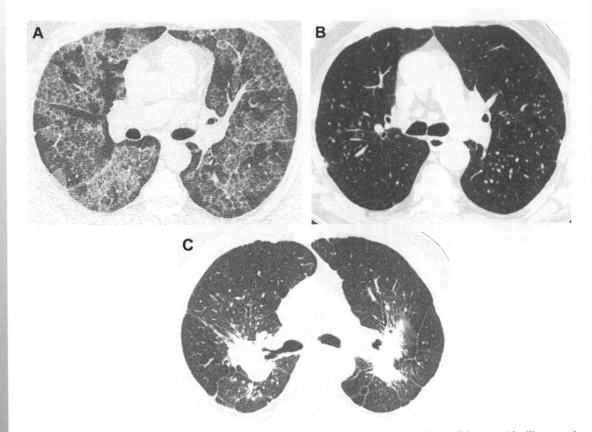

Fig. 1. Imaging of silicosis. (*A*) Silicoproteinosis. High-resolution CT in a 48-year-old sandblaster with silicoproteinosis demonstrates bilateral ground-glass with superimposed linear opacities representing interlobular septa, resulting in a crazy-paving pattern. (*B*) Chronic silicosis. High-resolution CT in a 78-year-old man shows multiple bilateral well-defined small centrilobular nodules. Also noted are a few subpleural nodules. (*C*) PMF. High-resolution CT in a 67-year-old man demonstrates irregular bilateral upper lobe masses with adjacent scarring. Also noted are scattered centrilobular nodules.

experience, there is always a mild chronic interstitial inflammatory infiltrate in silicoproteinosis, a finding that is often absent in other forms of alveolar proteinosis. On polarization (**Fig. 2**B), very small, weakly birefringent, silica particles are usually present. Cases of acute silicosis can also have more typical silicotic nodules (described as follows).

In accelerated and chronic silicosis, nodules are visible to the naked eye on gross examination of lung specimens. With exposures to fairly pure silica, the silicotic nodules are typically pale blue or pale green, but if the exposure is to silica with another dust, then the nodules may be colored. For example, in coal miners, silicotic nodules are often black on gross examination, and in hematite (iron ore) miners, red.

Microscopically, in simple silicosis, established silicotic nodules have a center of whorled collagen with a variable surrounding collar of dust and dust-laden macrophages. In workers with current or recent dust exposure, the surrounding macrophage collar is frequently prominent (**Fig. 3**A) but

if exposure is remote, then the nodule may be almost "bare" (**Fig. 3**B). Pathologically, the same size-based distinction used in imaging between simple silicosis and PMF applies: PMF lesions are greater than 1 cm in diameter and are formed by conglomeration of simple silicotic nodules (**Fig. 3**C). Sometimes, very early silicotic nodules are encountered in which there is disorganized collagen in the midst of dust-laden macrophages (**Fig. 3**D); these are difficult to recognize as manifestations of silicosis unless there is a dust exposure history. Old simple silicotic and PMF lesions can be calcified.

Silica itself is invisible on H&E stain. Polarization can be helpful but also misleading in diagnosing silicosis. Crystalline silica is poorly birefringent, is usually round to polygonal, and is very pale orange or red (**Fig. 4**A), but depending on the nature of the exposure, more or less white, brightly birefringent silicate needle-like particles may be found (see **Fig. 4**A). The latter are not diagnostic of silicosis.

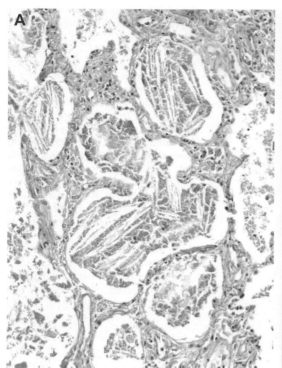
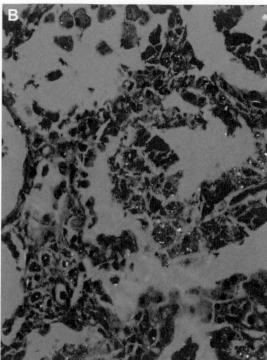

Fig. 2. Silicoproteinosis (acute silicosis). (*A*) Typical appearance of alveolar proteinosis. Note that the interstitial inflammatory infiltrate, something that is often lacking in primary (autoimmune) proteinosis but is invariably present in silicoproteinosis. (*B*) Polarized light image. The silica particles appear as weakly birefringent-rounded structures with a red to orange color.

Silicotic nodules can also be found in some cases in the pleura and in hilar and mediastinal lymph nodes. By definition, at least one silicotic nodule must be present in the lung parenchyma or pleura to permit a diagnosis of silicosis; if nodules are only present in lymph nodes, silicosis cannot be diagnosed.

Diffuse interstitial fibrosis is sometimes present in patients with silica exposure, and the question then arises as to whether this process is a manifestation of silicosis or is interstitial fibrosis of some other etiology, for example, idiopathic pulmonary fibrosis. Pathologically, a somewhat arbitrary but practical rule of thumb is that if silicotic nodules are present (**Fig. 4**B), then the fibrosis is probably also a manifestation of silicosis.

Additional illustrations of the pathologic features of silicosis can be found in Ref.[22]

PATHOLOGIC DIFFERENTIAL DIAGNOSIS

Important morphologic differentials for silicotic nodules include old infectious granulomas and mixed dust pneumoconiosis. Old infectious granulomas (**Fig. 5**A) typically have dense but unorganized collagen, as opposed to the whorled collagen of silicotic nodules and do not have the peripheral dust-laden macrophages of silicotic nodules. Nodules of mixed dust pneumoconiosis (ie, nodules caused by exposure to silica plus another dust) can be harder to differentiate because they often have a collar of dust-laden macrophages similar to those in silicotic nodules, but the central collagen is disorganized and not whorled (**Fig. 5**B).

SILICA EXPOSURE AND TUBERCULOSIS

Historically, silicosis and tuberculosis were often confused, and in the nineteenth century, this problem delayed recognition of silica as a specific disease. It is now clear that there is an increased risk of tuberculosis even without radiologic evidence of silicosis, and the increased risk applies to both pulmonary and extrapulmonary TB.[23] Some idea of the magnitude of the effect can be seen in the report of Cowie and colleagues.[24] They followed 1153 South African gold miners who initially did not have evidence of TB. More than 7 years, the relative risk for developing TB was 2.8 (95% confidence interval [CI] 1.9–4.1) for those with radiologic silicosis compared with those without and

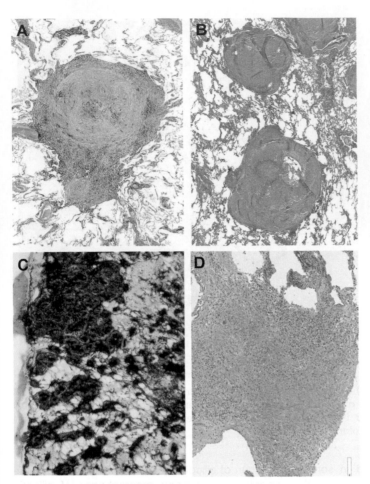

Fig. 3. Appearances of chronic silicosis. Simple silicosis: (*A*) Silicotic nodule with whorled collagen in the center and a prominent collar of dust-laden pigmented macrophages. This appearance is usually seen with current or recent dust exposure. (*B*) Simple silicosis. Three older silicotic nodules without dust collars. This appearance is usually seen when exposure is fairly remote. (*C*) Simple silicosis and PMF. A Gough (1-mm paper) section showing individual simple silicotic nodules which agglomerate to form the PMF lesion. (*D*) Simple silicosis. A very early silicotic lesion with extensive dust-laden macrophages and beginning formation of the collagenous center. This lesion does not look like a typical silicotic nodule and a history of exposure is crucial to making the correct diagnosis. (Image courtesy Dr Carlyne Cool, Denver, CO.)

the risk increased with increasing radiologic severity of silicosis. TB was also diagnosed in 23 of 335 men without radiologic silicosis.

There is dispute about the risks associated with radiologically visible silicosis versus just silica exposure. In a meta-analysis, Erhlich and colleagues[25] calculated a pooled relative risk across eight studies of 4.01 (95% CI 2.28–5.88) for TB in workers with silicosis, with consistent increases in risk with increasing profusion of silicotic nodules on imaging. Controlling for the presence of radiologic silicosis, there was also an increasing risk with increasing amounts and duration of silica exposure, with an overall risk of around 2.0. However, chest radiographs miss some cases of pathologically proven silicosis,[26] so the actual risk numbers may be smaller.

SILICA EXPOSURE AND LUNG CANCER

There are more than 60 studies and several meta-analyses examining the relationship between silica exposure and lung cancer, with not entirely consistent results. Kurihara and Wada[27] performed a meta-analysis using reports from 1966 to 2001. They found that for silicotics, the relative risk was 2.37 (95% CI 1.98–2.84) but for those without silicosis, there was no increased risk (relative risk 0.96; 95% CI 0.81–1.15). Only a few studies allowed them to evaluate silicotics who were smokers versus nonsmokers, and here, the risk was 4.47 (95% CI 3.17–6.30) for smokers; exposure to silica and cigarette smoke was not multiplicative.

More recently, Liu and colleagues[28] published an analysis of more than 34,000 workers with silica exposure and a 34.5 year mean follow-up time. Exposures were reconstructed and broken down into increasing exposure quartiles, with relative risks of 1.26, 1.54, 1.68, and 1.70 by increasing exposure. Overall, after adjustment for potential confounders including smoking, workers with silica exposure had a 61% increase in lung cancer risk compared with those without silica exposure, and the risks were similar in those with or without silicosis. Smokers exposed to the highest cumulative amounts of silica had a 5.07 risk that seemed to be multiplicative with silica exposure. Similarly, Wang and colleagues[29] studied 17,000 workers

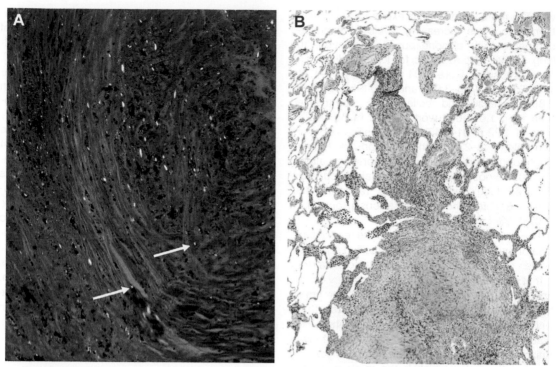

Fig. 4. (*A*) Polarized light examination of a silicotic nodule showing brightly birefringent elongated particles. These are silicates and not silica; the silica particles are weakly birefringent and rounded (*arrows*). (*B*) A silicotic nodule with early interstitial fibrosis.

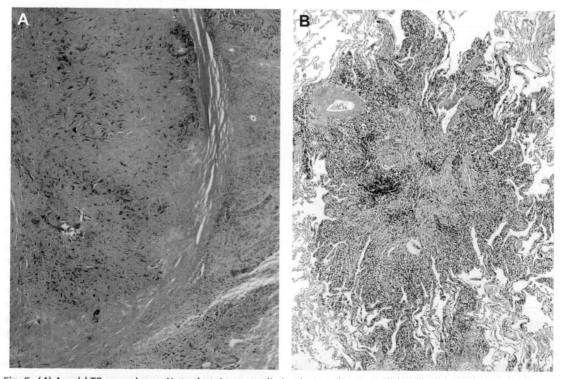

Fig. 5. (*A*) An old TB granuloma. Note that, in contradistinction to silicotic nodules which have whorled collagen, there is no organization to the collagen. (*B*) A mixed dust (here silica and hematite) nodule. In mixed dust nodules, there typically is a prominent peripheral collection of dust-laden macrophages but the collagenous core is composed of disorganized collagen.

with 1 or more years of silica exposure and divided them into three increasing levels of exposure; compared with a nonexposed population, the lung cancer hazard ratios for low, medium, and high exposures were 0.94 (95% CI 0.52–1.71), 1.86 (95% CI 1.15–3.00), and 1.65 (95% CI 0.95–2.86). Lacasse and colleagues[30] summarized data from 1,615,000 workers and found relative risks of 1.22 (1.01–1.47) with low silica exposure and 1.84 (1.48–2.28) with high exposure. Poinen-Rughooputh and colleagues[31] reported on almost 127,000 exposed workers and calculated standardized lung cancer mortality ratios of 2.32 (1.91–2.81) for those with silicosis and 1.78 (1.07–2.96) for those without.

The above data are cited to give the reader some idea of the problem. IARC has classified silica as a human carcinogen,[32] but the conclusion, we draw is that silica is, relatively, a weak pulmonary carcinogen, with the greatest (and still not very strong) effect in those with silicosis and lesser effects in those without. Also, as pointed out by Kurihara and Wada[27] and confirmed by the pathology study of Hnizdo and colleagues,[26] detection of silicosis by chest radiographs, which is the method used in these studies, misses some fraction of cases and thus misclassifies some silicotics as non-silicotics, so that the apparent effects in non-silicotics are actually smaller than the published numbers would suggest. To the extent there is an interaction with smoking, it would seem to be weak.

SILICA EXPOSURE AND CONNECTIVE TISSUE DISEASE

Current evidence indicates that silica exposure is associated with an increased prevalence of auto-antibodies and an increased risk of various types of connective tissue disease. Freire and colleagues[33] reviewed the literature on scleroderma and silica. They found 32 published series encompassing 254 silica-exposed patients, of whom 96% were males. Conversely, taking reports of patients with scleroderma, silica exposure was reported in 38% to 86% of men but only 0% to 2.7% of women. Whether this difference is caused by a gender-specific biologic effect is uncertain, but more likely reflects differences in occupational exposures between men and women. Of particular importance, diffuse forms of scleroderma were more prevalent than localized forms in both sexes with silica exposure, and there was a very high incidence (81%) of interstitial lung disease. The important conclusion to draw from these data is that a history of silica exposure should be sought in men who are diagnosed with scleroderma.

Less information, perhaps reflecting weaker associations, has been published for other forms of connective tissue disease. Yahya and colleagues[34] reported a 2.4 fold (95% CI 1.0–5.6) risk of anti-citrullinated antibody-positive rheumatoid arthritis in men with silica exposure, and an even higher risk for ever-smokers with silica exposure (7.5 [95% CI 2.3–24.2]) compared with never-smokers not exposed to silica. Similarly, Stolt and colleagues[35] found a silica-exposure risk of 2.34 (95% CI 1.17–4.68) for anti-citrullinated rheumatoid arthritis in a series of 577 rheumatoid arthritis patients compared with 659 controls without rheumatoid arthritis; in exposed current smokers, the risk increased to 7.36 (95% CI 3.31–16.38) and there seemed to be a multiplicative interaction between silica exposure and smoking.

There are also a small number of cases of lupus described in patients with silica exposure.[36] Again, there is a male predominance, as opposed to the usual female predominance in lupus patients that probably reflects occupational differences.

SILICA AND VASCULITIS

A few studies have examined the question of whether silica exposure is associated with ANCA-positive vasculitis. Gomez-Puerta and colleagues[37] carried out a meta-analysis of published data and found six useable reports with an overall risk of 2.56 (95% CI 1.51–4.36) for all ANCA-associated vasculitides comparing silica-exposed to non-exposed populations. For microscopic polyangiitis, specifically, the relative risk was 3.95 (95% CI 1.89–8.24) and for granulomatosis with polyangiitis (Wegener's) the risk was 3.56 (95% CI 1.85–6.82).

FUNCTIONAL EFFECTS, TREATMENT, AND PROGNOSIS

Acute silicosis (silicoproteinosis) typically presents with shortness of breath and may be indistinguishable from the much more common primary (autoimmune) alveolar proteinosis on clinical and radiologic grounds if a history of dust exposure is not evident. Assay for GM-CSF antibodies can be useful, because these are not found in acute silicosis. The prognosis of acute silicosis is poor; both steroids and whole lung lavage have been tried, but without clear benefit, and such patients tend to have progressive disease leading to death or transplantation.[4]

Patients with accelerated and chronic silicosis may present with shortness of breath, but can be asymptomatic with disease first detected on imaging. Pulmonary function testing can show obstructive and/or restrictive abnormalities, which in general correlate with the severity of radiologic findings. Patients with low profusion simple silicosis may have essentially normal pulmonary function, whereas those with PMF typically have significant and often increasing impairment that may lead to death or lung transplantation. Because silica is poorly cleared from lung, disease progression after cessation of exposure is common. Control of dust exposure is crucial to preventing disease, because there is no treatment, beyond lung transplantation, for functionally impairing accelerated and chronic silicosis. OHSA[38] has recently reduced the permitted exposure level for crystalline silica to an 8 hour time weighted average of 50 $\mu g/m^3$ in an attempt to further reduce the incidence of disease.

DISCLOSURE

The authors have nothing to disclose.

REFERENCES

1. Leung CC, Yu IT, Chen W. Silicosis. Lancet 2012; 379:2008–18.
2. Weill H, Jones RN, Parkes RW. Silicosis and related diseases. In: Parkes WR, editor. Occupational lung disorders. 3rd Edition. Oxford: Butterworth-Heineman; 1994. p. 285–339.
3. Rosenthal P-A. Silicosis: a world history. Baltimore: Johns Hopkins University Press; 2017.
4. Krefft S, Wolff J, Rose C. Silicosis: an update and guide for clinicians. Clin Chest Med 2020;41: 709–22.
5. The Lancet Respiratory Medicine. The world is failing on silicosis. Lancet Respir Med 2019;7:283.
6. Silica, crystalline. Occupational Safety and Health Administration. Safety and health Topics Web site. Available at: https://www.osha.gov/dsg/topics/silica-crystalline/.
7. Sauve JF. Historical and emerging workplaces affected by silica exposure since the 1930 Johannesburg conference on Silicosis, with special reference to construction. Am J Ind Med 2015;58(Suppl 1):S67–571.
8. Dhoonia 54, Nandi SS, Dhatrak SV, Sarkar K. Silicosis, progressive massive fibrosis and silico-tuberculosis among workers with occupational exposure to silica dusts in sandstone mines of Rajasthan state: an urgent need for initiating national silicosis control programme in India. J Family Med Prim Care 2021;10:686–91.
9. Dhooria Rajavel S, Raghav P, Gupta MK, et al. Silico-tuberculosis, silicosis and other respiratory morbidities among sandstone mine workers in Rajasthan: a cross-sectional study. PLoS One 2020;15:e0230574.
10. Govindagoudar MB, Singh PK, Chaudhry D, et al. Burden of Silicosis among stone crushing workers in India. Occup Med (Lond) 2022;72:366–71.
11. Akgun M, Araz O, Ucar EY, et al. Silicosis Appears Inevitable Among Former Denim Sandblasters: A 4-Year Follow-up Study. Chest 2015;148:647–54.
12. Albez FS, Araz Ö, Yılmazel Uçar E, et al. Long-term follow-up of young denim sandblasters in Turkey. Occup Med (Lond) 2022;72:403–10.
13. Leso V, Fontana L, Romano R, et al. Artificial Stone Associated Silicosis: A Systematic Review. Int J Environ Res Public Health 2019;16:568–73.
14. OSHA-NIOSH Hazard Alert: Worker Exposure to Silica during Hydraulic Fracturing. www.OSHA.gov DTSEM 6/2012.
15. Wade WA, Petsonk EL, Young B, et al. Severe occupational pneumoconiosis among West Virginian coal miners: one hundred thirty-eight cases of progressive massive fibrosis compensated between 2000 and 2009. Chest 2011;139:1458–62.
16. Cohen RA, Petsonk EL, Rose C, et al. Lung pathology in U.S. coal workers with rapidly progressive pneumoconiosis implicates silica and silicates. Am J Respir Crit Care Med 2016;193:673–80.
17. Silicosis 2010 case definition. Centers for Disease Control and Prevention. Surveillance case definitions Web site. 2010. Available at: https://wwwn. cdc.gov/nndss/conditions/silicosis/case-definition/2010/.
18. Souza CA, Marchiori E, Goncalves LP, et al. Comparative study of clinical, pathological and HRCT findings of primary alveolar proteinosis and silicoproteinosis. Eur J Radiol 2012;81:371–8.
19. Akira M, Suganuma N. Imaging diagnosis of pneumoconiosis with predominant nodular pattern: HRCT and pathologic findings. Clin Imaging 2023; 97:28–33.
20. Antao VC, Pinheiro GA, Terra-Filho M, et al. High-resolution CT in silicosis: correlation with radiographic findings and functional impairment. J Comput Assist Tomogr 2005;29:350–6.
21. Walkoff L, Hobbs S. Chest imaging in the diagnosis of occupational lung diseases. Clin Chest Med 2020;41:581–603.
22. Gibbs AR, Wagner JC. Diseases due to silica. In: Churg A, Green FHY, editors. Pathology of occupational lung disease. 2nd Edition. Baltimore: Williams and Wilkins; 1998. p. 209–33.
23. Lanzafame M, Vento S. Mini-review: Silico-tuberculosis. J Clin Tuberc Other Mycobact Dis 2021;23: 100218.
24. Cowie RL. The epidemiology of tuberculosis in gold miners with silicosis. Am J Respir Crit Care Med 1994;150:1460–2.
25. Ehrlich R, Akugizibwe P, Siegfried N, et al. The association between silica exposure, silicosis and tuberculosis: a systematic review and meta-analysis. BMC Publ Health 2021;21:953.

26. Hnizdo E, Murray J, Sluis-Cremer GK, et al. Correlation between radiological and pathological diagnosis of silicosis: an autopsy population based study. Am J Ind Med 1993;24:427–45.

27. Kurihara N, Wada O. Silicosis and smoking strongly increase lung cancer risk in silica-exposed workers. Ind Health 2004;42:303–14.

28. Liu Y, Steenland K, Rong Y, et al. Exposure-response analysis and risk assessment for lung cancer in relationship to silica exposure: a 44-year cohort study of 34,018 workers. Am J Epidemiol 2013;178:1424–33.

29. Wang D, Yang M, Ma J, et al. Association of silica dust exposure with mortality among never smokers: A 44-year cohort study. Int J Hyg Environ Health 2021;236:113793.

30. Lacasse Y, Martin S, Gagné D, et al. Dose-response meta-analysis of silica and lung cancer. Cancer Causes Control 2009;20:925–33.

31. Poinen-Rughooputh S, Rughooputh MS, Guo Y, et al. Occupational exposure to silica dust and risk of lung cancer: an updated meta-analysis of epidemiological studies. BMC Publ Health 2016;16:1137.

32. Silica, some silicates, coal dust, and para-aramid fibers. IARC monograph evaluating carcinogenic risks to humans. Lyon: IARC; 1997.

33. Freire M, Alonso M, Rivera A, et al. Clinical peculiarities of patients with scleroderma exposed to silica: A systematic review of the literature. Semin Arthritis Rheum 2015;45:294–300.

34. Yahya A, Bengtsson C, Larsson P, et al. Silica exposure is associated with an increased risk of developing ACPA-positive rheumatoid arthritis in an Asian population: evidence from the Malaysian MyEIRA case-control study. Mod Rheumatol 2014;24:271–4.

35. Stolt P, Yahya A, Bengtsson CEIRA Study Group, Rönnelid J, Lundberg I, Klareskog L, Alfredsson L, EIRA Study Group. Silica exposure among male current smokers is associated with a high risk of developing ACPA-positive rheumatoid arthritis. Ann Rheum Dis 2010;69:1072–6.

36. Fukushima K, Uchida HA, Fuchimoto Y, et al. Silica-associated systemic lupus erythematosus with lupus nephritis and lupus pneumonitis: A case report and a systematic review of the literature. Medicine (Baltim) 2022;101:e28872.

37. Gómez-Puerta JA, Gedmintas L, Costenbader KH. The association between silica exposure and development of ANCA-associated vasculitis: systematic review and meta-analysis. Autoimmun Rev 2013;12:1129–35.

38. Occupational Exposure to Crystalline Silica: Final Rule https://www.osha.gov/laws-regs/federalregister/2016-03-25-1.

Pathology of COVID-19 Lung Disease

Alain C. Borczuk, MD

KEYWORDS

- Long COVID-19 • Diffuse alveolar damage • Persistent COVID-19

Key points

- Severe COVID-19 lung pathology is diffuse alveolar damage at different stages.
- Thrombosis, characteristic of severe cases early in the pandemic, is less frequently reported.
- Pathogenesis of severe lung disease includes disturbed interferon responses, complement activation, delayed adaptive immune response, and neutrophil extracellular trap formation.
- Long COVID remains pathologically poorly defined, with patterns that include persistent lung injury beyond 30 days and eventual lung fibrosis.

ABSTRACT

The pathology of severe COVID-19 lung injury is predominantly diffuse alveolar damage, with other reported patterns including acute fibrinous organizing pneumonia, organizing pneumonia, and bronchiolitis. Lung injury was caused by primary viral injury, exaggerated immune responses, and superinfection with bacteria and fungi. Although fatality rates have decreased from the early phases of the pandemic, persistent pulmonary dysfunction occurs and its pathogenesis remains to be fully elucidated.

OVERVIEW

At the end of 2019, a new pulmonary infection was noted in the Hubei province of China. Within several months of early 2020, this infection became a widespread pandemic. As per the WHO coronavirus dashboard, there have been more than 770 million cases worldwide with reported nearly 7 million deaths, which is a calculated fatality rate of just under 1%.[1,2]

Early in the pandemic it was found that the causal agent of this infection was a coronavirus, named the severe acute respiratory syndrome associated coronavirus 2 (SARS-CoV-2), and the disease was referred to as COVID-19.[2] Although COVID-19-related illnesses involved multiple organ systems, the fatal cases were largely the result of pulmonary disease and the inflammatory consequences of infection.[3] This review focuses on the pathology of COVID-19 pneumonia.

CLINICAL FEATURES OF COVID-19 DISEASE

The initial symptoms of COVID-19 included fever, cough, fatigue, loss of appetite, and, in some instances, loss of the sense of olfaction. Some patients may have experienced mild symptoms before more severe ones, and it is likely that there was an incubation period of roughly 5 days before symptom onset. Severe illness occurred in about 15% of patients, with critical illness in about 5%.[4] Patient presentations included cough, fever, as well as dyspnea and shortness of breath, an indication of the frequency of pulmonary disease. A subset of patients developed severe disease with hypoxemia but without significant dyspnea.

In a series of more than 174,000 adult patients with SARS-Cov-2 infection in the initial phase of the pandemic, severe disease is seen in about 20% with an overall mortality of 11.6%.[5] In this series, the mortality rate decreased substantially in

Department of Pathology, Northwell Health, 2200 Northern Boulevard Suite 104, Greenvale, NY 11548, USA
E-mail address: aborczuk@northwell.edu

Surgical Pathology 17 (2024) 203–214
https://doi.org/10.1016/j.path.2023.11.006
1875-9181/24/© 2023 Elsevier Inc. All rights reserved.

surgpath.theclinics.com

the latter portions of 2020, indicating that efforts to treat and mitigate the injury associated with the disease were successful, even before widespread vaccination.

Although the fatality rate of COVID-19 has decreased from the initial phases of the pandemic, much of our understanding of the pathology of this disease came from autopsy studies largely performed in the pre-vaccination period. Among the underlying causes of fatal cases included risk factors that were associated with patient age, and comorbid conditions including hypertension, cardiac disease, diabetes, pulmonary disease, and preexisting malignancy.

PATHOLOGY OF ACUTE COVID-19 PNEUMONIA

A component of the COVID-19 impact on the respiratory system involved the upper airway and included the trachea and bronchi. Grossly, small mucosal ulcers were seen, spanning 2 to 3 mm. Histologically, these small ulcers showed neutrophilic inflammation (Fig. 1A). Although not every series described these lesions, they were noted in several reports and were unassociated with intubation. In addition to this acute inflammation of the upper airway, chronic inflammation has also been reported.[6–8]

One of the most prominent findings in the lungs in autopsy series were increased weights, with combined lung weights exceeding 1300 g. This increase in lung weight was associated with multifocal, diffuse, and multilobular consolidation (Fig. 1B). In addition to the consolidation, grossly visible thrombi were also seen in a subset of cases (Fig. 1C). This will be discussed further when focusing on thrombosis in COVID-19.

The main histologic pattern of disease seen in fatal COVID-19 lung injury is diffuse alveolar damage as part of the acute respiratory distress syndrome.[6,7,9–15] Although in the earliest phases this is histologically subtle in that there is pulmonary edema and congestion, later phases show exudate in the form of hyaline membranes. These hyaline membranes eventually resolve and give way to the proliferative phase with type 2 pneumocyte hyperplasia and eventual fibroblastic proliferation. Although the organizing phase develops in conjunction with duration of disease, one of the features of these autopsy series was the finding of new hyaline membranes alongside the organizing and proliferative phase of diffuse alveolar damage (Fig. 2A). This temporal heterogeneity was an indication of ongoing injury superimposed on the healing or proliferative phase of acute respiratory

distress syndrome (ARDS). Although acutely ill patients can have many causes of diffuse alveolar damage which include ventilator-associated injury and sepsis, in a subset of patients continued viral-associated lung injury as well as immune-mediated injuries was the major mechanism of the severe and diffuse lung injury. However, it is also clear that superimposed bacterial and fungal infections complicated the disease course in patients with severe lung injury (Fig. 2B). Those patients who survived the initial acute lung injury outcomes included resolution and progression to fibrotic lung disease (see Long COVID-19 section).

Viral cytopathic change was not definitively demonstrated histopathologically.[12,16] Type 2 pneumocytes showed multi-nucleation and enlargement with cytoplasmic eosinophilic and basophilic bodies. However, correlation with ultrastructure does not indicate these to be viral inclusions.

In addition to diffuse alveolar damage, organizing pneumonia was also described in a subset of cases characterized by fibroblastic tufts within alveolar spaces.[10,17] The frequency of this finding varies from study to study, although radiologic appearance supports the impression that organizing pneumonia is a feature of this disease (see Fig. 2B). With longer standing disease, airway squamous metaplasia[6,12,16–19] was identified and this likely reflects a bronchiolitis that precedes the diffuse alveolar damage (Fig. 2C). Some groups describe the presence of acute fibrinous and organizing pneumonia (Fig. 2D) as a pattern of acute lung injury which is likely a manifestation of alveolar lung injury with vascular leak.[20,21]

For patients that survived the initial injurious process the organizing phase of diffuse alveolar damage can progress to fibrosis also reported. These patients had organizing phase of diffuse alveolar damage (DAD) with progression to fibrosis.[10,11,16,22–24] This phase likely reflects inability to resolve the organizing diffuse alveolar damage and in these patients for the most part viral infection is not seen. Some of these fibrotic cases (Fig. 2E) have been described in the non-autopsy setting in lungs that were removed at the time of transplant.[25]

Another autopsy feature from the early phases of the pandemic is the presence of thrombosis. Large thrombi including pulmonary emboli were seen,[6,12,13,26] but in addition to this, smaller artery (Fig. 2F) and capillary bed microthrombi were also identified.[7,10–14,17,27] The frequency of this finding in COVID-19 lung injury seems to be higher than that described in prior series of the acute respiratory distress syndrome. In addition, thrombi were also seen in extra-pulmonary locations, including

Fig. 1. Histology of tracheal ulceration with fibrinous layer and acute inflammation and reactive and regenerative epithelium at ulcer edges (A) Gross pathology of lungs showing discoloration in parches which correspond to areas of consolidation (B) Gross pathology of lungs showing multifocal thrombosis in pulmonary artery branches of various diameter

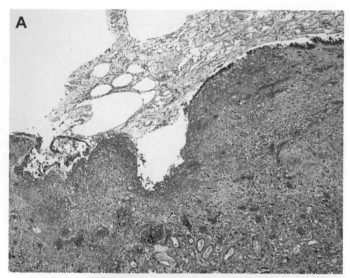

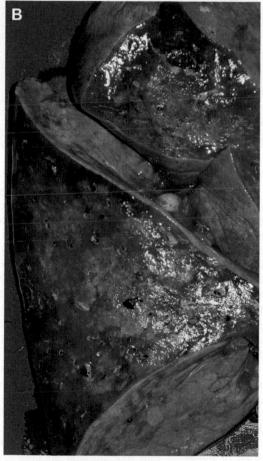

unusual sites such as prostate.[28–30] A large proportion of cases across various autopsy series demonstrated platelet/fibrin or platelet thrombi in the lung among patients who had fatal COVID-19 disease. It is notable that in later phases of the pandemic, patients with COVID-19 pneumonia with severe illness were less likely to show this hyperthrombotic state[31] and it is unclear whether this is the result of different viral variants or was the impact of vaccination.[32]

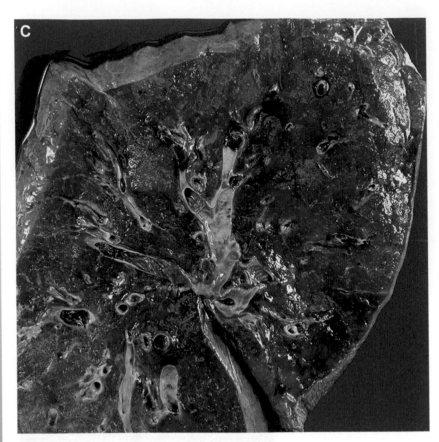

Fig. 1. (*C*).

It was also hypothesized that the vascular injury and remodeling resulted in endothelial injury and the phenomenon known as intussusceptive or sprouting angiogenesis.[33] Although this had been described previously in the acute lung injury setting, it seemed that this was a more frequent finding in COVID-19 pneumonia when compared with matched cases with influenza. This consistent finding of injury to the vascular bed has led to the hypothesis that this injury was not only pro-thrombotic in the acute setting but may impact organ function in the convalescent and post-COVID period.[34,35]

Although it is clear from autopsy studies that direct viral infection occurs in type 2 pneumocytes and macrophages in the lung,[15,36,37] it is less clear whether the ongoing lung injury is due to the persistence of viral infection or the impact of viral infection on the immune status in the lung. There are multiple lines of evidence that macrophage subsets are affected by COVID-19 pneumonia, but it is also clear that neutrophils play an important role.[36,38] Some cases demonstrate an interstitial accumulation of neutrophils. Although the suppuration of an acute bronchopneumonia[6,12,14,29,30,39] is assumed to be superinfection with bacteria or fungi, there remain cases in which neutrophilic infiltration of the lung is seen without a specific second pathogen.[6,8,40] In these cases, it has been hypothesized that the neutrophil infiltrate is a manifestation of an innate immune response to COVID-19,[41] which have been described as neutrophil extracellular traps (NETs). NETs are decondensed chromatin strands studded with citrullinated histones that can entrap and kill pathogens when neutrophils undergo apoptosis. This is a key feature of innate immunity but can become dysregulated and injurious. This can drive platelet aggregation, abnormal release of cytokines, and complement activation all of which are features of COVID-19 pneumonia.[42–44] The finding of citrullinated histone H3 supports the hypothesis that neutrophils are responding to viral infection with the formation of NETs. The connection between NETs, activation of complement, and induction of thrombosis is a potential explanation for the severe lung injury with microthrombosis that was seen in these early series of COVID-19 pneumonia.[45–47] In fact, given that NET formation is thought to be involved in the killing of pathogens, it may be that an exaggerated response of this kind before the development of an adaptive immune response contributes to the severe lung injury in COVID-19 pneumonia.

Fig. 2. Diffuse alveolar damage with organizing phase of type 2 pneumocyte hyperplasia and fibroblastic proliferation, alongside exudative phase with hyaline membranes. (*A*) Intra-alveolar suppurative inflammation in a case of organizing diffuse alveolar damage raises a secondary bacterial or fungal acute bronchopneumonia. (*B*) Small airway shows extensive squamous metaplasia. (*C*) Intra-alveolar filling with fibrinous material and some fibroblasts characteristic of acute fibrinous and organizing pneumonia.

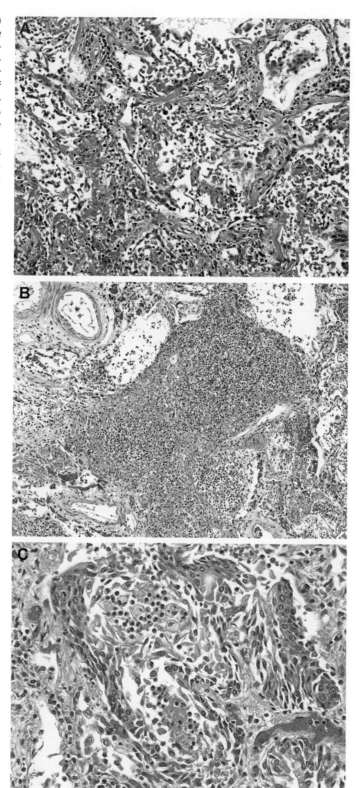

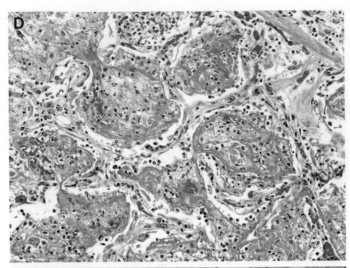

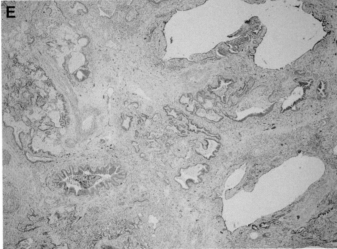

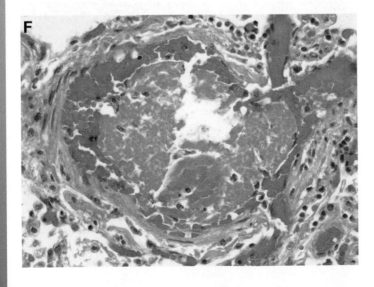

Fig. 2. (*D*) An area of pulmonary fibrosis with remodeling of the lobule with loss of alveolar architecture "microscopic honeycomb lung." (*E*) A thrombus in a small artery showing very early organization (*F*).

Fig. 3. Hematoxylin and eosin area of exudative diffuse alveolar damage corresponding to the field of view in *B* and *C* (*A*). Immunohistochemistry for COVID-19 spike protein shows intense reactivity in denuded cells and in hyaline membranes (*B*). RNA in situ hybridization for spike mRNA shows intense cellular staining as well as staining in hyaline membranes (*C*).

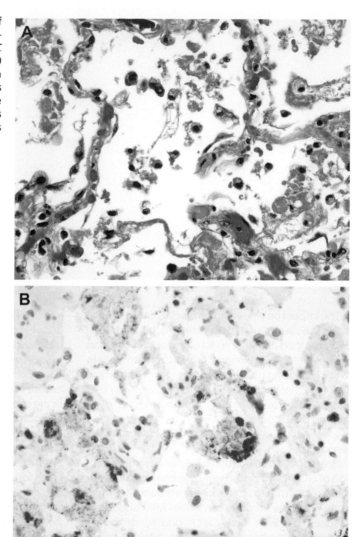

Viral presence has been demonstrated in the large airway epithelium and in lung tissue in alveolar zones in the acute setting. Using immunohistochemistry for spike protein and in situ hybridization for viral RNA, tissue sections of lung show reactivity in hyaline membranes, type 2 pneumocytes and macrophages (**Fig. 3**A–C). Some series showed viral presence only in the first 10 days after illness initiation, but others showed evidence of virus in the lung well beyond 2 weeks,[24] albeit in a smaller number of cases. Overall, in fatal cases, the median days of illness in which lung tissue was shown to be positive was 14 days[48] and overall by 30 days, virus is not identified in the majority of cases. Interestingly, when hyaline membranes are present, there is a higher rate of identification of viral protein and RNA within these areas of acute lung injury,[6] even when in the background of the proliferative phase of diffuse alveolar damage.

PATHOGENESIS

The underlying pathogenesis of tissue injury and COVID-19 disease in the lung includes aberrant interferon-related responses, recruitment of inflammatory and immune cells that are either functionally altered or excessively recruited by the cytokine milieu, and complement activation.[49] Interferon-related responses are critical to the control of viral infections. The subtypes of interferon response are also important in creating a balance between the control of disease and inducing tissue injury. Reduced interferon responses are associated with severe COVID-19 disease and may be the result of inherited interferon mutations, neutralizing autoantibodies, or depleted plasmacytoid dendritic cells. It may be that successful interferon responses result in viral clearance, but in severe COVID-19 cases, successful clearance does not occur.[50,51]

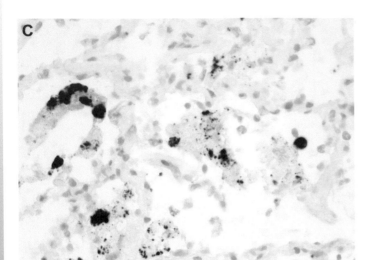

Fig. 3.

The impact on viral infection on cytokine response is also notable in that the degree of neutrophil degranulation and the impact on cytokine activation could lead to a prolonged pro-inflammatory state which some had coined cytokine storm[52] and which would be manifested by the severe tissue injury that was seen. Pro-inflammatory states may also be favored by the persistence of M1 type macrophage responses in lieu of a transition to M2 macrophage response.[53]

Given these observations, the successful resolution of COVID-19 pneumonia depends on an eventual switch from the initial innate immune response to an adaptive immune response. Mild disease is associated with an appropriate antibody-mediated anti-viral response. The cytokine milieu of severe disease seems to indicate a predominance of innate immune responses.[51,54] In addition, the neutrophilic response itself may be maladaptive in enriching for dysfunctional granulocytes[55] that are more likely to respond by NET formation. The damage to the epithelial cell may also result in a persistent secretion of cytokines that recruit macrophages that are pro-inflammatory and the combination of the type 2 pneumocyte hyperplasia and abnormal recruitment of these pro-inflammatory macrophages may generate a persistent cycle of tissue injury.[36,56] Some of this pro-inflammatory cycle may be driven by the propensity of the type 2 pneumocytes and macrophages to viral reinfection or by proposed delayed maturation of these cells to as compared with their normal counterparts.

Eventually, the adaptive immune response should allow for viral clearance. However, in severe cases, changes in the CD4 positive T-cell population as well as reduced CD8 positive T-cell cytotoxic effects demonstrate an insufficient shift toward adaptive immunity.[57] This was also manifested by a decrease in B-cell evolution with an increased proportion of naïve B cells, including those without a specific antibody response.[51] This suggests that severe COVID-19 disease is associated with a delay in the production of active antiviral antibodies.

Examination of lung tissue from COVID-19 pneumonia showed that complement activation was a key injurious factor and that this complement activation drives thrombosis as well as NET formation.[58] This increase in complement activation associated with COVID-19 respiratory failure was notably greater than that previously reported in other viral infections such as influenza.[59] Here, again interferon responses can activate complement factors and these may be favored by the presence of altered lung with increase numbers of type 2 pneumocytes. The association of complement activation, thrombosis, and NETs were supported by tissue-based studies demonstrating the presence of microthrombi and C5B-9 deposits in the vascular bed of the lung.[60] This complement activation also contributes to the abnormal cytokine environment within the damaged tissue.

LONG COVID-19

The precise definition of long COVID remains elusive. The current definitional framework for three phases of COVID produced by the National Institute for Health and Care Excellence from the United Kingdom defines acute COVID-19 in cases with symptomatology up to 4 weeks with ongoing symptomatic COVID-19 lasting a period of 4 to 12 weeks and post-COVID-19 an illness greater than 12 weeks without an alternative diagnosis.[61] Although long COVID was not a definition established in this series, it is likely that this entity reflects cases beyond 4 weeks of illness.

The clinical manifestations of long COVID-19 in the lung have also been difficult to precisely correlate with pathologic findings. In part, this is due to limited situations with tissue sampling. However, series that have examined COVID-19 disease beyond 4 weeks indicate fatigue, dyspnea, chest pain, and cough as the main symptoms with a significant rate of readmission and even a significant rate of ultimate mortality.[62] Decreased exercise capacity and abnormalities in pulmonary function tests have been reported[31,63] as well as persistent abnormalities on imaging which include both subacute type findings such as ground glass opacities, as well as features that associate with the development of lung fibrosis. Of note as months' progress, reductions in diffusion capacity and the establishment of restrictive physiology indicate a progression to fibrosis. On the optimistic side, a significant number of patients followed 6 and 12 months after disease onset showed resolution of respiratory symptoms. It was noted that diffusion impairment can persist at 1 year, perhaps related to the severity of the original disease.[64]

It is possible that a subset of patients with ongoing symptomatic COVID-19 have persistent viral infection without viral clearance. Such cases are not well described, but may be associated with immunodeficiency, such as that induced by rituximab therapy. Such patients seem to have persistent imaging findings of organizing pneumonia but with ultimate progression to diffuse alveolar damage in a period greater than 4 weeks after their initial COVID-19 infection and with persistent evidence of viral infection by nasal swab. These cases overall remain anecdotal and it is unclear to what proportion these cases contribute to what is observed as long COVID.

In patients requiring lung transplantation, which is generally after a period after viral clearance (which is required for transplant eligibility), the pattern has been reported as organizing diffuse alveolar damage with fibrosis as well as acute bronchopneumonia and exudative diffuse alveolar damage.[65] In patients who receive single lung transplantation, there may be ongoing improvement in the non-transplanted native lung after transplantation indicating some degree of reversibility even at that phase.[66]

The pathology of pulmonary COVID-19 persisting more than 12 weeks is also not well-defined. Some patients do develop diffuse interstitial fibrosis (see **Fig. 2E**). The persistent lung injury in this phase has been studied to a degree and the themes of immune dysfunction and incomplete cellular maturation resulting in persistent dysfunctional immune and epithelial responses remain.[67–69] The cause of this persistent immune dysfunction and type 2 pneumocyte immaturity is unclear, but studies that have examined populations of cells in the respiratory tract indicate abnormal monocyte and dendritic cell populations that contribute to abnormal interferon responses.[68] Although these would be pro-inflammatory responses despite viral clearance because of this persistent pro-inflammatory state and ongoing lung injury that occurs in a subset of patients is of unknown cause. There is also a hypothesis that there is persistent autoimmunity in patients with long COVID-19 and that such autoantibodies may target particular organ systems with symptoms typical of that organ dysfunction manifested.[70] In this hypothesis, autoantibodies to central nervous system may contribute to neurologic dysfunction, and those targeting lung may be contributing to persistent pulmonary dysfunction.

SUMMARY

The pathology of acute COVID-19 lung disease may vary based on disease severity. Although bronchiolitis and organizing pneumonia may be features of this disease, severe cases may be most commonly associated with diffuse alveolar damage. Thrombosis, a feature of the early phases of the pandemic, seems to have decreased over time. The pathology of long COVID-19 lung disease is still being defined, and persistent lung injury as diffuse alveolar damage and ultimately fibrosis are features seen in tissues sampled, such a lung explants.

CLINICS CARE POINTS

- Severe COVID-19 cases are characterized by diffuse alveolar damage of acute respiratory distress syndrome.

- Thrombosis, characteristic of severe cases early in the pandemic, is now less commonly seen.

- Some patients with ongoing symptomatic COVID-19 have immunosuppression, including treatment with rituximab.

- Lung injury may persist and result in organ failure requiring transplantation.

DISCLOSURE

The author has nothing to disclose.

REFERENCES

1. Dong E, Du H, Gardner L. An interactive web-based dashboard to track COVID-19 in real time. Lancet Infect Dis 2020;20:533–4.
2. Zhu N, Zhang D, Wang W, et al. A Novel Coronavirus from Patients with Pneumonia in China, 2019. N Engl J Med 2020;382:727–33.
3. Borczuk AC. Pulmonary pathology of COVID-19: a review of autopsy studies. Curr Opin Pulm Med 2021;27:184–92.
4. Berlin DA, Gulick RM, Martinez FJ. Severe Covid-19. N Engl J Med 2020;383:2451–60.
5. Bennett TD, Moffitt RA, Hajagos JG, et al. Clinical Characterization and Prediction of Clinical Severity of SARS-CoV-2 Infection Among US Adults Using Data From the US National COVID Cohort Collaborative. JAMA Netw Open 2021;4:e2116901.
6. Borczuk AC, Salvatore SP, Seshan SV, et al. COVID-19 pulmonary pathology: a multi-institutional autopsy cohort from Italy and New York City. Mod Pathol 2020;33:2156–68.
7. Bradley BT, Maioli H, Johnston R, et al. Histopathology and ultrastructural findings of fatal COVID-19 infections in Washington State: a case series. Lancet 2020;396:320–32.
8. Menter T, Haslbauer JD, Nienhold R, et al. Postmortem examination of COVID-19 patients reveals diffuse alveolar damage with severe capillary congestion and variegated findings in lungs and other organs suggesting vascular dysfunction. Histopathology 2020;77:198–209.
9. De Michele S, Sun Y, Yilmaz MM, et al. Forty Postmortem Examinations in COVID-19 Patients. Am J Clin Pathol 2020;154:748–60.
10. Falasca L, Nardacci R, Colombo D, et al. Postmortem Findings in Italian Patients With COVID-19: A Descriptive Full Autopsy Study of Cases With and Without Comorbidities. J Infect Dis 2020;222:1807–15.
11. Valdivia-Mazeyra MF, Salas C, Nieves-Alonso JM, et al. Increased number of pulmonary megakaryocytes in COVID-19 patients with diffuse alveolar damage: an autopsy study with clinical correlation and review of the literature. Virchows Arch 2021;478:487–96.
12. Grosse C, Grosse A, Salzer HJF, et al. Analysis of cardiopulmonary findings in COVID-19 fatalities: High incidence of pulmonary artery thrombi and acute suppurative bronchopneumonia. Cardiovasc Pathol 2020;49:107263.
13. Hanley B, Naresh KN, Roufosse C, et al. Histopathological findings and viral tropism in UK patients with severe fatal COVID-19: a post-mortem study. Lancet Microbe 2020;1:e245–53.
14. Remmelink M, De Mendonca R, D'Haene N, et al. Unspecific post-mortem findings despite multiorgan viral spread in COVID-19 patients. Crit Care 2020;24:495.
15. Sauter JL, Baine MK, Butnor KJ, et al. Insights into pathogenesis of fatal COVID-19 pneumonia from histopathology with immunohistochemical and viral RNA studies. Histopathology 2020;77:915–25.
16. Kommoss FKF, Schwab C, Tavernar L, et al. The Pathology of Severe COVID-19-Related Lung Damage. Dtsch Arztebl Int 2020;117:500–6.
17. Carsana L, Sonzogni A, Nasr A, et al. Pulmonary post-mortem findings in a series of COVID-19 cases from northern Italy: a two-centre descriptive study. Lancet Infect Dis 2020;20:1135–40.
18. Wu JH, Li X, Huang B, et al. [Pathological changes of fatal coronavirus disease 2019 (COVID-19) in the lungs: report of 10 cases by postmortem needle autopsy]. Zhonghua Bing Li Xue Za Zhi 2020;49:568–75.
19. Navarro Conde P, Alemany Monraval P, Medina Medina C, et al. Autopsy findings from the first known death from Severe Acute Respiratory Syndrome SARS-CoV-2 in Spain. Rev Esp Patol 2020;53:188–92.
20. Copin MC, Parmentier E, Duburcq T, et al. Time to consider histologic pattern of lung injury to treat critically ill patients with COVID-19 infection. Intensive Care Med 2020;46:1124–6.
21. von der Thusen J, van der Eerden M. Histopathology and genetic susceptibility in COVID-19 pneumonia. Eur J Clin Invest 2020;50:e13259.
22. Schwensen HF, Borreschmidt LK, Storgaard M, et al. Fatal pulmonary fibrosis: a post-COVID-19 autopsy case. J Clin Pathol. 2020:jclinpath-2020-206879.
23. Fox SE, Akmatbekov A, Harbert JL, et al. Pulmonary and cardiac pathology in African American patients with COVID-19: an autopsy series from New Orleans. Lancet Respir Med 2020;8:681–6.
24. Schaller T, Hirschbuhl K, Burkhardt K, et al. Postmortem Examination of Patients With COVID-19. JAMA 2020;323:2518–20.
25. Bharat A, Querrey M, Markov NS, et al. Lung transplantation for patients with severe COVID-19. Sci Transl Med 2020;12(574):eabe4282.
26. Lax SF, Skok K, Zechner P, et al. Pulmonary Arterial Thrombosis in COVID-19 With Fatal Outcome : Results From a Prospective, Single-Center, Clinicopathologic Case Series. Ann Intern Med 2020;173:350–61.
27. Rapkiewicz AV, Mai X, Carsons SE, et al. Megakaryocytes and platelet-fibrin thrombi characterize multi-organ thrombosis at autopsy in COVID-19: A case series. EClinicalMedicine 2020;24:100434.

28. Elsoukkary SS, Mostyka M, Dillard A, et al. Autopsy Findings in 32 Patients with COVID-19: A Single-Institution Experience. Pathobiology 2021;88:56–68.
29. Edler C, Schroder AS, Aepfelbacher M, et al. Dying with SARS-CoV-2 infection-an autopsy study of the first consecutive 80 cases in Hamburg, Germany. Int J Leg Med 2020;134:1275–84.
30. Wichmann D, Sperhake JP, Lutgehetmann M, et al. Autopsy Findings and Venous Thromboembolism in Patients With COVID-19: A Prospective Cohort Study. Ann Intern Med 2020;173:268–77.
31. Krueger T, van den Heuvel J, van Kampen-van den Boogaart V, et al. Pulmonary function three to five months after hospital discharge for COVID-19: a single centre cohort study. Sci Rep 2023;13:681.
32. Petito E, Franco L, Falcinelli E, et al. COVID-19 infection-associated platelet and neutrophil activation is blunted by previous anti-SARS-CoV-2 vaccination. Br J Haematol 2023;201:851–6.
33. Varga Z, Flammer AJ, Steiger P, et al. Endothelial cell infection and endotheliitis in COVID-19. Lancet 2020;395:1417–8.
34. Rovas A, Osiaevi I, Buscher K, et al. Microvascular dysfunction in COVID-19: the MYSTIC study. Angiogenesis 2021;24:145–57.
35. Goshua G, Pine AB, Meizlish ML, et al. Endotheliopathy in COVID-19-associated coagulopathy: evidence from a single-centre, cross-sectional study. Lancet Haematol 2020;7:e575–82.
36. Rendeiro AF, Ravichandran H, Bram Y, et al. The spatial landscape of lung pathology during COVID-19 progression. Nature 2021;593:564–9.
37. Heinrich F, Sperhake JP, Heinemann A, et al. Germany's first COVID-19 deceased: a 59-year-old man presenting with diffuse alveolar damage due to SARS-CoV-2 infection. Virchows Arch 2020;477: 335–9.
38. Melms JC, Biermann J, Huang H, et al. A molecular single-cell lung atlas of lethal COVID-19. Nature 2021;595:114–9.
39. Nienhold R, Ciani Y, Koelzer VH, et al. Two distinct immunopathological profiles in autopsy lungs of COVID-19. Nat Commun 2020;11:5086.
40. Tian S, Xiong Y, Liu H, et al. Pathological study of the 2019 novel coronavirus disease (COVID-19) through postmortem core biopsies. Mod Pathol 2020;33: 1007–14.
41. Barnes BJ, Adrover JM, Baxter-Stoltzfus A, et al. Targeting potential drivers of COVID-19: Neutrophil extracellular traps. J Exp Med 2020;217.
42. Mastellos DC, Pires da Silva BGP, Fonseca BAL, et al. Complement C3 vs C5 inhibition in severe COVID-19: Early clinical findings reveal differential biological efficacy. Clin Immunol 2020;220:108598.
43. Veras FP, Pontelli MC, Silva CM, et al. SARS-CoV-2-triggered neutrophil extracellular traps mediate COVID-19 pathology. J Exp Med 2020;217.
44. Radermecker C, Detrembleur N, Guiot J, et al. Neutrophil extracellular traps infiltrate the lung airway, interstitial, and vascular compartments in severe COVID-19. J Exp Med 2020;217.
45. Skendros P, Mitsios A, Chrysanthopoulou A, et al. Complement and tissue factor-enriched neutrophil extracellular traps are key drivers in COVID-19 immunothrombosis. J Clin Invest 2020;130:6151–7.
46. Petito E, Falcinelli E, Paliani U, et al. Association of Neutrophil Activation, More Than Platelet Activation, With Thrombotic Complications in Coronavirus Disease 2019. J Infect Dis 2021;223:933–44.
47. Mukhopadhyay S, Sinha S, Mohapatra SK. Analysis of transcriptomic data sets supports the role of IL-6 in NETosis and immunothrombosis in severe COVID-19. BMC Genom Data 2021;22:49.
48. Schurink B, Roos E, Radonic T, et al. Viral presence and immunopathology in patients with lethal COVID-19: a prospective autopsy cohort study. Lancet Microbe 2020;1:e290–9.
49. Dupont T, Caillat-Zucman S, Fremeaux-Bacchi V, et al. Identification of Distinct Immunophenotypes in Critically Ill Coronavirus Disease 2019 Patients. Chest 2021;159:1884–93.
50. Sposito B, Broggi A, Pandolfi L, et al. The interferon landscape along the respiratory tract impacts the severity of COVID-19. Cell 2021;184(19):4953–68.e16.
51. Unterman A, Sumida TS, Nouri N, et al. Single-cell multi-omics reveals dyssynchrony of the innate and adaptive immune system in progressive COVID-19. Nat Commun 2022;13:440.
52. McGonagle D, Sharif K, O'Regan A, et al. The Role of Cytokines including Interleukin-6 in COVID-19 induced Pneumonia and Macrophage Activation Syndrome-Like Disease. Autoimmun Rev 2020;19:102537.
53. Lee JS, Koh JY, Yi K, et al. Single-cell transcriptome of bronchoalveolar lavage fluid reveals sequential change of macrophages during SARS-CoV-2 infection in ferrets. Nat Commun 2021;12:4567.
54. Ren X, Wen W, Fan X, et al. COVID-19 immune features revealed by a large-scale single-cell transcriptome atlas. Cell 2021;184:5838.
55. Morrissey SM, Geller AE, Hu X, et al. A specific low-density neutrophil population correlates with hypercoagulation and disease severity in hospitalized COVID-19 patients. JCI Insight 2021;6.
56. Chua RL, Lukassen S, Trump S, et al. COVID-19 severity correlates with airway epithelium-immune cell interactions identified by single-cell analysis. Nat Biotechnol 2020;38:970–9.
57. Qin C, Zhou L, Hu Z, et al. Dysregulation of Immune Response in Patients With Coronavirus 2019 (COVID-19) in Wuhan, China. Clin Infect Dis 2020; 71:762–8.
58. Afzali B, Noris M, Lambrecht BN, et al. The state of complement in COVID-19. Nat Rev Immunol 2022; 22:77–84.

59. Holter JC, Pischke SE, de Boer E, et al. Systemic complement activation is associated with respiratory failure in COVID-19 hospitalized patients. Proc Natl Acad Sci U S A 2020;117:25018–25.

60. Georg P, Astaburuaga-Garcia R, Bonaguro L, et al. Complement activation induces excessive T cell cytotoxicity in severe COVID-19. Cell 2022;185: 493–512 e25.

61. Nalbandian A, Sehgal K, Gupta A, et al. Post-acute COVID-19 syndrome. Nat Med 2021;27:601–15.

62. Chopra V, Flanders SA, Vaughn V, et al. Variation in COVID-19 characteristics, treatment and outcomes in Michigan: an observational study in 32 hospitals. BMJ Open 2021;11:e044921.

63. Katzenstein TL, Christensen J, Lund TK, et al. Relation of Pulmonary Diffusing Capacity Decline to HRCT and VQ SPECT/CT Findings at Early Follow-Up after COVID-19: A Prospective Cohort Study (The SECURe Study). J Clin Med 2022;11.

64. Wu X, Liu X, Zhou Y, et al. 3-month, 6-month, 9-month, and 12-month respiratory outcomes in patients following COVID-19-related hospitalisation: a prospective study. Lancet Respir Med 2021;9:747–54.

65. Bharat A, Machuca TN, Querrey M, et al. Early outcomes after lung transplantation for severe COVID-19: a series of the first consecutive cases from four countries. Lancet Respir Med 2021;9: 487–97.

66. Kehara H, Mangukia C, Sunagawa G, et al. Lung Transplantation for COVID-19 Pulmonary Sequelae. Transplantation 2023;107:449–56.

67. Gschwend J, Sherman SPM, Ridder F, et al. Alveolar macrophages rely on GM-CSF from alveolar epithelial type 2 cells before and after birth. J Exp Med 2021;218.

68. Venet M, Ribeiro MS, Decembre E, et al. Severe COVID-19 patients have impaired plasmacytoid dendritic cell-mediated control of SARS-CoV-2. Nat Commun 2023;14:694.

69. Phetsouphanh C, Darley DR, Wilson DB, et al. Immunological dysfunction persists for 8 months following initial mild-to-moderate SARS-CoV-2 infection. Nat Immunol 2022;23:210–6.

70. Wang EY, Mao T, Klein J, et al. Diverse functional autoantibodies in patients with COVID-19. Nature 2021;595:283–8.

Interstitial Lung Abnormalities

Mary Beth Beasley, MD

KEYWORDS

- interstitial lung abnormalities • Interstitial lung disease • Usual interstitial pneumonia
- Idiopathic pulmonary fibrosis • Smoking-related interstitial fibrosis • Lung cancer

Key points

- Interstitial lung abnormalities (ILA) is a relatively recently defined radiographic term with 3 proposed subtypes: nonsubpleural, subpleural nonfibrotic, and subpleural fibrotic.
- Subpleural fibrotic ILA in particular are associated with an increased risk of progression to clinically significant interstitial lung disease (ILD).
- ILA have an association with a variety of increased morbidities apart from progression, particularly complications related to lung cancer treatment and outcome.
- Limited information about histologic correlates of ILA is available. Many ILA seem to be smoking-related fibrosis but histologic features of usual interstitial pneumonia (UIP) are also seen and seem to have a correlation with the subpleural fibrotic subtype, although further study is needed.
- Reporting and communication regarding ILA is important concerning developing management strategies given the increased risk of morbidities and complications in various areas compared with patients without ILA.

ABSTRACT

Interstitial lung abnormalities (ILA) is a radiographic term, which has recently undergone clarification of definition with creation of 3 subtypes. ILA is defined as incidental identification of computed tomography abnormalities in a patient who is not suspected of having an interstitial lung disease (ILD). A subset of ILA may progress to clinically significant ILD and is associated with morbidities not related to progression such as an increased incidence of sepsis-related acute respiratory distress syndrome (ARDS). ILA has been associated with an increased incidence of treatment-related complications in patients with lung cancer. Information on corresponding histology is limited; knowledge gaps exist concerning optimal patient management.

computed tomography (CT) abnormalities in a patient who is not suspected of having an interstitial lung disease (ILD). This term has been used to encompass a variety of findings and has been variously termed "interstitial lung changes at an early stage," "early ILD," "subclinical ILD," and "preclinical ILD."[1–4] In 2020, the Fleischner society issued a position paper in order to provide guidance for consistency in terminology and definition.[5] Once thought to be an incidental finding of limited consequence, ILA is emerging as an important factor about the potential development of clinically significant ILD as well as a risk factor for clinical complications and poor outcomes in several areas.[5–7]

The aim of this article is to review the current knowledge on the concept of ILA and the clinical significance of this finding, particularly concerning risks of progression and adverse clinical outcomes. Histologic correlates will be reviewed with an emphasis on current knowledge gaps and proposals for future directions concerning pathology.

OVERVIEW

Interstitial lung abnormalities (ILA) is a radiologic term based on the incidental identification of

Department of Pathology, Icahn School of Medicine at Mount Sinai, One Gustave Levy Place, Annenberg 15-76, New York, NY 10029, USA

E-mail address: Mary.beasley@mountsinai.org

Surgical Pathology 17 (2024) 215–225

https://doi.org/10.1016/j.path.2023.11.007

BACKGROUND

ILA is a relatively common finding, particularly in patients aged older than 60 years and has typically been reported in 4% to 9% of smokers and 2% to 7% of nonsmokers.[5,8] A 2023 meta-analysis reported a prevalence of ILA of 7% in lung cancer screening studies and 7% in studies of the general population, although the incidence in lung cancer screening cohorts has been reported as high as 14%.[9] The actual prevalence is thought to potentially be higher due to inconsistency of reporting and is predicted to increase as the use of lung cancer screening expands.[6,10]

ILA is strictly a radiologic definition and applies only to radiographic abnormalities occurring in a patient in whom ILD is not suspected. The definition of ILA itself does not imply the absence of symptoms or pulmonary function abnormalities. However, differentiation of ILA from clinical or subclinical ILD in patients with respiratory symptoms not initially thought to be due to ILD is determined by clinical evaluation.[5,6]

Most critically, a subset of patients with ILA will develop progressive disease or experience a greater incidence of complications unrelated to progression such as drug-induced pneumonitis, increased cancer-associated mortality, or development of respiratory distress syndrome. As such, appropriate identification of ILA may provide an opportunity to evaluate early treatment interventions and/or risk factor modification.[5–7,9]

DEFINITION OF INTERSTITIAL LUNG ABNORMALITIES

The Fleischner Society position paper defines ILA as incidental ground glass or reticular abnormalities, traction bronchiectasis, honeycombing and nonemphysematous cysts involving at least 5% of the cross-sectional area of any one lung zone and detected in an individual in whom ILD is not suspected (Table 1).

ILA is further divided into 3 subtypes: (1) nonsubpleural: ILA without predominant subpleural localization, (2) subpleural nonfibrotic: ILA with a predominant subpleural localization but without evidence of fibrosis (Fig. 1), and (3) subpleural fibrotic: ILA with predominant subpleural localization and with evidence of pulmonary fibrosis (fibrosis being characterized by the presence of architectural distortion with traction bronchiectasis or honeycombing, or both; Fig. 2).[5]

The last 2 subtypes, and particularly the subpleural fibrotic subtype, seem to have the most clinical significance based on current knowledge.[5–7] It

was acknowledged that the 5% cutoff was somewhat arbitrary but was retained to conform to earlier literature and to avoid inclusion of more minimal radiographic findings.[5]

Conversely, the incidental finding of "extensive disease," referring to the finding of disease involving 3 or more of the 6 zones of the bilateral lung, should be included in ILD rather than ILA.[6] Additionally, findings which are not considered ILA include the following: dependent lung atelectasis, focal paraspinal fibrosis in close contact with thoracic spine osteophytes, mild focal or unilateral opacities, interstitial edema, findings of aspiration, and smoking-related centrilobular nodularity in the absence of other findings. The last finding, while included in other earlier descriptions of ILA, was excluded from the Fleischner definition because it typically corresponds to respiratory bronchiolitis, a common finding, which is typically not progressive.[5–7] Apical caps and pleuroparenchymal fibroelastosis (PPFE)-like changes are also excluded from the definition of ILA. PPFE itself is a distinct radiographic pattern typically consisting of multiple subpleural areas of consolidation and traction bronchiectasis predominantly involving the upper lobes bilaterally, and it has not been systematically studied in asymptomatic patients.[6,7] Additionally, the term ILA is not applicable to an individual in whom an ILD might ordinarily be expected, such as an individual with a familial history of ILD or a history of connective tissue disease (CTD), for example, because they are not viewed as being incidental.[5] In cohorts of at-risk familial patients, the prevalence of radiographic abnormalities equivalent to ILA has been reported as 26%; however, because this is a population in which findings are expected, the use of the term "subclinical ILD" may be more appropriate although the terminology is evolving and the term "CTD-related ILA" has also been proposed for this subset of patients.[6,11]

RISK FACTORS FOR INTERSTITIAL LUNG ABNORMALITIES

The majority of studies have found that advanced age is strongly associated with ILA, as has tobacco smoke exposure.[5,6] The meta-analysis of Grant-Orser and colleagues also reported an association with male sex, older age, and lower forced vital capacity percent predicted.[9] Male sex has not shown an association in all studies, however. Metrics associated with exposure to traffic-related air pollution were reported in both the MESA Lung study and the Framingham Heart study.[12,13] Similar to some cases of idiopathic

Table 1
Definition of interstitial lung abnormalities

Definition of ILA	Incidental ground glass or reticular abnormalities, traction bronchiectasis, honeycombing, and nonemphysematous cysts involving at least 5% of the cross-sectional area of any one lung zone and detected in an individual in whom ILD is not suspected
Subtypes of ILA	• Nonsubpleural: ILA without predominant subpleural localization • Subpleural nonfibrotic: ILA with a predominant subpleural localization but without evidence of fibrosis • Subpleural fibrotic: ILA with predominant subpleural localization and with evidence of pulmonary fibrosis (fibrosis being characterized by the presence of architectural distortion with traction bronchiectasis or honeycombing, or both)
Radiographic findings that are not ILA	• Extensive disease involving 3 or more lung zones • Dependent lung atelectasis • Focal paraspinal fibrosis in contact with thoracic spine osteophytes • Mild focal or unilateral opacities, interstitial edema • Findings of aspiration • Smoking-related centrilobular opacities • Apical cap/PPFE-like changes

pulmonary fibrosis and familial ILD, ILA have been seen in association with the presence of MUC5B genetic polymorphisms.[14–16]

It should be noted that some degree of reticular abnormalities and fibrosis are not uncommon in older individuals and, in fact, have sometimes been regarded as part of the normal aging spectrum. However, observations of progression in older individuals and an increased risk of other morbidities independent of age support that ILA is still clinically relevant in older individuals.[6]

SIGNIFICANCE OF INTERSTITIAL LUNG ABNORMALITIES AND PROGRESSION TO INTERSTITIAL LUNG DISEASE

The main significance of ILA is the risk of progression to clinically significant ILD as well as increased risk of other complications.

Progression of ILA was reported to occur in up to 20% of cases during 2 years in the National Lung Cancer Screen trial[17] and in 73% during 5 years in the AGES-Reykjavik study[18] and is most commonly associated with subpleural fibrotic ILA, although progression has also been reported in patients with nonfibrotic ILA with basal and peripheral predominance. Subpleural reticular changes, lower lobe predominant changes and traction bronchiectasis have all be associated with progression. In a study by Putman, and colleagues, 100% of cases with honeycomb change

progressed during 5 years.[18] ILA with a nonsubpleural distribution are usually not progressive.[5,6,13,16,18] In addition to these radiographic elements, risk factors for the progression of ILA include inhalation exposures, medication use, radiation therapy, thoracic surgery, physiologic findings, and gas exchange abnormalities. It is recommended that individuals with one of more clinical or radiographic risk factors for progression be actively monitored with dedicated chest CT scans using thin section and pulmonary function testing.[6]

The impact of ILA on patient morbidity and mortality has been demonstrated in scenarios unrelated to disease progression and these findings are again more likely to be associated with basal and peripheral ILA as opposed to nonsubpleural ILA.[6] Several issues may arise in patients with lung cancer as discussed later but morbidities unrelated to progression are not limited to the lung cancer patient population. Patients with sepsis and ILA have been observed to have increased rates of ARDS and in-hospital mortality.[19] ILA have also been reported as an independent predictor of worse mortality in patients undergoing transcathether aortic valve replacement.[20]

IMPACT OF CORONAVIRUS DISEASE 2019 PANDEMIC

The coronavirus disease 2019 (COVID-19) pandemic resulted in millions of individuals being

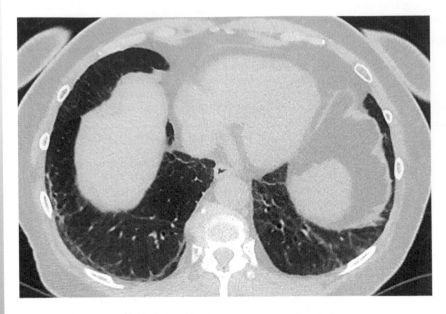

Fig. 1. Chest CT of subpleural nonfibrotic ILA. Increased subpleural reticular markings are present without evidence of honeycomb change or traction bronchiectasis. (*Image courtesy* of Adam Jacobi, MD, Mount Sinai Medical Center Department of Radiology.)

infected with various strains of severe acute respiratory syndrome coronavirus 2 and subsequently suffering from varying degrees of pulmonary injury. Residual radiographic abnormalities have been reported in a significant number of patients. Han and colleagues reported on 144 patients and observed ILA in 56 (39%) patients 2 years after infection but it was noted that the incidence of ILA decreased with 54% showing ILA at 6 months and 42% at 12 months.[21] Similarly, Noh, and colleagues recorded ILA in 150 patients with cancer who were hospitalized for COVID-19 and noted 70% had ILA at 3 months following discharge but only 26% had ILA at 6 months, and fibrotic ILA were more common at 6 months.[22] Hino and colleagues reported ILA in 32% of 132 patients following diagnosis of COVID-19, which seemed to be associated with the severity of COVID-19 pneumonia.[23] Whether these residual abnormalities are the equivalent to ILA concerning the risk of

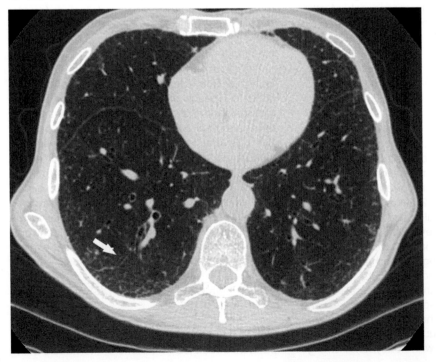

Fig. 2. Chest CT of subpleural fibrotic ILA. Increased subpleural markings are present but with the additional finding of traction bronchiectasis (*arrow*) and early suggestion of honeycomb change. (*Image courtesy* of Adam Jacobi, MD, Mount Sinai Medical Center Department of Radiology.)

progression is unclear. Given the extent of COVID-19 infection globally, residual lung abnormalities have the potential to complicate the interpretation of CT scans concerning ILA risk progression. Clarifying the similarities and differences between ILA and residual lung abnormalities from COVID-19 will require further study.[6]

INTERSTITIAL LUNG ABNORMALITIES AND LUNG CANCER

Issues associated with ILA and lung cancer include those involving risk of lung cancer, impact of ILA on prognosis in lung cancer, and increased incidence of complications due to lung cancer treatment. As with fibrotic ILD, ILA have been shown to have an association with the development of lung cancer, with some studies showing an increased incidence.[24,25] Patients with ILA and lung cancer have been shown to have a worse prognosis and an increased incidence of complication following cancer treatment, be it surgical or nonsurgical. Patients with ILA have been reported to experience increased lung cancer-associated mortality, including both early stage patients who have undergone resection and in advanced stage patients treated with chemotherapy. The reason for the former in particular is unclear; however, it is hypothesized that patient with ILA may be at increased risk for lung injury.[7,24] Iwasawa and colleagues[26] demonstrated that ILA was a predictor of poorer disease-free survival in patients with stage I and II lung cancer. ILA have been associated with a risk of postoperative pneumonia, ARDS, prolonged air leakage, and other postsurgical complications.[27] Systemic treatments, including chemotherapy, targeted therapies, immunotherapies, and antibody-drug conjugates, have all been associated with an increased risk of pneumonitis in patients with ILA. Preexiting ILA also seem to increase the risk of postradiation pneumonitis, although this issue needs further study as granularity regarding the definition and extent of ILA was not considered in all studies.[7] Nakashini and colleagues demonstrated that patients with ILA treated with either nivolumab or pembrolizumab experienced therapy-related ILD in 17% of cases, in contrast to the overall reported rate of approximately 5%.[28]

As such, ILA are emerging as an important comorbidity concerning lung cancer; however, although ILA should be considered in regard to treatment planning, there is no clear guidance on how to manage patients who have ILA and lung cancer at this time.

HISTOLOGIC CORRELATES

Literature describing pathologic correlates of ILA is emerging but remains limited in scope. The majority of publications are based on findings in pulmonary resection specimens, primarily done for lung cancer in current or former cigarette smokers. Such specimens have a high prevalence of background interstitial fibrosis, with Katzenstein and colleagues reporting clinically occult fibrosis occupying more than 25% of a resected lobe in 60% of cases. The majority of these cases showed smoking-related interstitial fibrosis (SRIF), although usual interstitial pneumonia (UIP), Langerhans cell histiocytosis, and asbestosis were also found.[29] Kawabata and colleagues also found a significant incidence of background smoking-related fibrosis termed "airspace enlargement with fibrosis" or respiratory-bronchiolitis, although some cases of UIP were also found.[30] Neither of these studies was specifically correlated with radiographic ILA, although the findings infer that subclinical fibrosis, and by extension ILA, in smokers potentially correlated primarily with smoking-related fibrosis.

Miller and colleagues evaluated histologic correlates of ILA in 424 lung nodule resections. In this study, 26 patients with known ILA showed fibrosis in 19, with UIP in 2. Interestingly, histologic fibrosis was found in 207 patients with no ILA or an indeterminate status radiographically. Overall, the findings were predominantly smoking-related.[31] Hung and colleagues evaluated 406 specimens from 397 patients and found fibrotic ILD in 10%, consisting of SRIF in 7%, UIP in 1% and nonspecific interstitial pneumonia or unclassified disease in the remaining 2%. ILA were found in 100% of the UIP cases but only 10% of the SRIF cases. This study found fibrotic changes in 51% of specimens with no ILA, although no cases of UIP lacked ILA.[32]

The study of Chae and colleagues is of particular note because histologic findings are correlated with radiographic subtype of ILA, and the study is based on a series of surgical lung biopsies as opposed to cancer resections. The authors evaluated 45 patients with ILA from 268 patients who underwent surgical lung biopsies between January 2004 and April 2019. The authors state that the patients underwent surgical lung biopsy because the patients were considered preclinical ILD subjects and underwent lung biopsy for more accurate diagnosis given the lack of management guidelines. The CT features were classified as subpleural nonfibrotic (n = 9) or subpleural fibrotic ILA (n = 36) with histologic findings characterized as "definite," "probable," or "indeterminate" for UIP or as an "alternate diagnosis" following ATS guidelines. In this series, 25 cases (69%) of subpleural fibrotic ILA showed definite or probable UIP and 1 case (11%) of subpleural nonfibrotic ILA showed definite or probable UIP. Eight of the subpleural fibrotic ILA were categorized as indeterminate for UIP and 3 as inconsistent with UIP/alternate diagnosis, whereas 4 cases each of subpleural nonfibrotic ILA were classified as indeterminate of inconsistent/alternate diagnosis. In this study, subpleural fibrotic ILA were associated with an increased risk of progression and death; however, the finding of a UIP pattern histologically did not correlate with progression. CT features of subpleural fibrotic ILA were also associated with an increased mortality.[33]

Although the above studies provide some insight into histologic correlates of ILA, significant knowledge gaps exist. Only the studies of Miller and colleagues, Hung and colleagues, and Chae and colleagues evaluated histologic findings in conjunction with knowledge of radiographic ILA, and only the article of Chae and colleagues specifically evaluates findings in the context of the subtype of ILA present. Given that the studies of both Miller and colleagues, and Hung and colleagues are conducted on lung resections performed primarily for lung cancer, there is the potential for significant skewing of findings toward smoking-related findings. Conversely, given it is not common practice for surgical lung biopsies to be conducted for ILA alone, and the authors state the patients were considered as preclinical ILD subjects, the study of Chae and colleagues is potentially skewed toward those with a greater chance of harboring true subclinical ILD. Additionally, the finding of progression correlating only with the radiologic finding of subpleural fibrotic ILA and not with a histologic UIP pattern is curious. This could be due to a variety of reasons including the retrospective nature of the study, the small number of cases overall, and of nonfibrotic subpleural ILA in particular, the minimal amount of detail on the patients in regard to potential clinical etiologies and lack of granularity on non-UIP histologies.

Ultimately, although it might be suspected that UIP histology would be encountered in subpleural fibrotic ILA, further study is needed in regard to histologic correlates in hopes of contributing to further insight into the patterns of fibrosis present and their implications in regard to progression. Additionally, the significance of converse scenario of fibrotic lung findings being present histologically but lacking ILA radiographically, as was noted in the studies of Miller and colleagues, and Hung and colleagues, warrants further evaluation.

WHAT DOES THIS MEAN FOR THE PATHOLOGIST?

Although uniformity of ILA identification and classification is encouraged for radiologists, a similar effort needs to occur concerning pathology. In spite of limitations about potential skew toward smoking-related changes, resection specimens for lung cancer provide the greatest opportunity for radiologic–pathologic correlation of ILA. This will require significant multidisciplinary effort and communication. Given the potential complications resulting from lung cancer treatment in patients with ILA, it is currently recommended that ILA be documented and considered in patient management. Ideally, information regarding ILA noted by the radiologist in the preoperative setting should also be conveyed to the pathologist, who could then take sections of the nonneoplastic lung corresponding to the areas of potential ILA in an attempt to provide histologic correlation/classification. Although this will likely require considerable effort, a shift in the approach to sectioning and reporting the nonneoplastic lung in resection specimens has the potential to make a great contribution. Typical grossing strategies ordinarily involve obtaining a sample of nonneoplastic lung; however, there is no current standard in regard to how many sections should be obtained or from where they should be obtained. Although correlation of gross evaluation and sectioning with CT findings would be optimal, careful attention to subpleural areas as opposed to random sections might provide greater opportunity for potential correlation with subpleural ILA, which are more likely to progress or be associated with other morbidities. This strategy, however, would not contribute to our understanding of nonsubpleural ILA pathology. Additionally, reporting background changes in lung parenchyma is not without challenges. Fibrosis may occur as a secondary change in the immediate vicinity of a tumor. As such, parenchyma should be evaluated at a reasonable distance from a tumor mass. Further, in the United States, reporting of findings in the nonneoplastic lung is not a required element in the College of American Pathologists (CAP) reporting checklist for carcinoma resections.[34] Understandably, the focus in such cases is on reporting critical elements related to the malignancy present but increased consistency and diligence in reporting nonneoplastic findings would not only allow for increased study and understanding of ILA but potentially alert clinicians to patients with a possible greater risk of complications.

Fig. 3. SRIF with associated emphysema. SRIF, characterized by fibrosis with a glassy hyalinized appearance, is a frequently reported finding in studies of histologic correlates of ILA. Hematoxylin-eosin stain (H&E) 40x

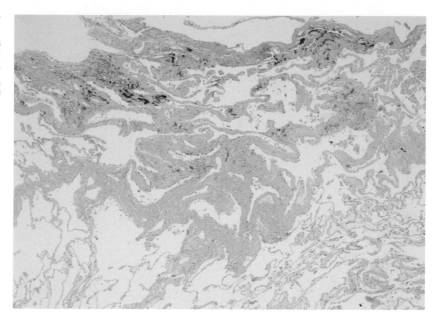

BACKGROUND LUNG FINDINGS CORRELATING WITH INTERSTITIAL LUNG ABNORMALITIES

Thus far, although a minor component of other histologies has been documented, reported histologic correlates of ILA have most frequently been smoking-related changes/SRIF or changes compatible with UIP.[31–33] SRIF is characterized by a glassy, hyalinized appearance and is frequently associated with areas of emphysema (**Fig. 3**). Respiratory bronchiolitis, consisting of accumulation of smoker's-type macrophages containing finely granular brown pigment within the alveolar spaces and bronchiolar lumens may also be present. Rarely, foci of Langerhans cell histiocytosis may also be encountered, characterized by peribronchiolar fibrosis, often exhibiting a "stellate" configuration. The areas of fibrosis contain a mixture of eosinophils, smoker's type macrophages, and Langerhans cells, which are typically polygonal cells with grooved nuclei, and will be positive for CD1a, S-100, and Langerin. Given the association with smoking, one of more of these findings may be present in the same specimen.

Features suggesting UIP warrant particular note given their apparent association with subpleural fibrotic ILA and the potential to represent occult subclinical ILD. Briefly, UIP is characterized by patchy fibrosis with a subpleural predominance, typically showing areas of severe and/or honeycomb fibrosis alternating with areas of spared parenchyma. The fibrosis exhibits temporal heterogeneity in the form of fibroblast foci (**Fig. 4**). Subpleural changes showing some but not all features of UIP may also be encountered (**Fig. 5**).

Both SRIF and UIP should be distinguished from subpleural apical caps, which are a common finding in lung cancer resections, particularly in the upper lobes. Apical caps are subpleural areas of fibroelastotic scar and are not considered ILA (**Fig. 6**).

KNOWLEDGE GAPS/FUTURE DIRECTIONS

It is important to note that the concept of ILA is relatively new and still evolving, and some studies predate the development of more uniform definition of ILA. As such, future updates are to be expected about reporting and potential management as further study is undertaken. Although subpleural fibrotic ILA seem to be associated with the greatest risk of progression and other complications, significant knowledge gaps exist in regard to our understanding of ILA including which patients will progress to clinically significant ILD, which patients develop significant complications unrelated to progression, what is the true significance of nonsubpleural and subpleural nonfibrotic ILA, what are the histologic correlates of ILA and how do they relate to risk, and what is the significance of histologic fibrosis in the absence of ILA, among others. As such, the development of a uniform approach and definition for diagnosis should provide an opportunity for clarity concerning issues regarding prevalence, progression, morbidity, and mortality. Greater understanding

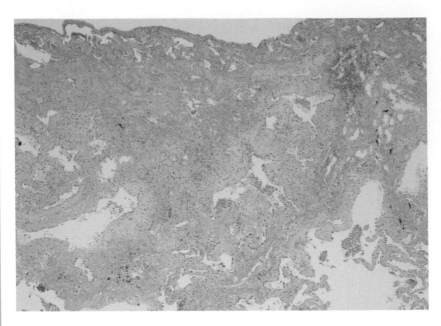

Fig. 4. Subpleural interstitial fibrosis with early honeycomb change and fibroblast foci, consistent with early UIP. Histologic features of UIP have also been reported as correlates of ILA, particularly the subpleural fibrotic type. H&E 40x

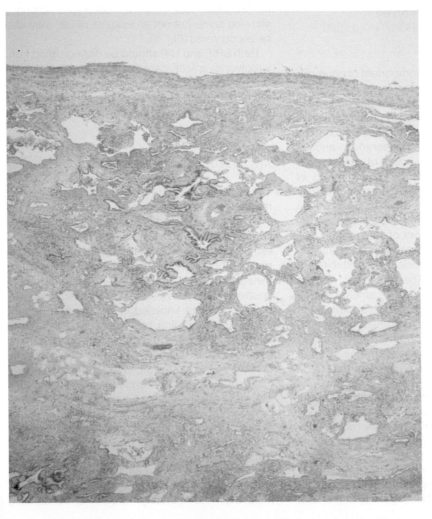

Fig. 5. More extensive subpleural fibrosis with early honeycomb change and fibroblast foci but with lymphoid aggregates and peribronchiolar metaplasia and small lymphoid aggregates, potentially suggesting UIP. H&E 2040x

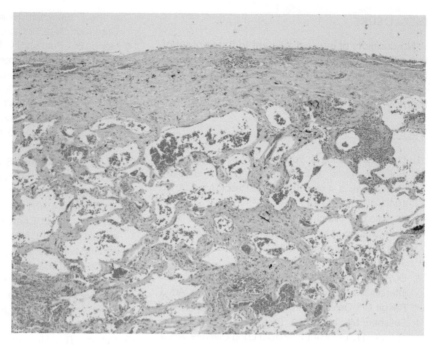

Fig. 6. Apical cap. Characterized by subpleural fibroelastotic scarring, apical caps are a frequent finding in lung cancer resections and are not considered part of the definition of ILA. H&E 40x.

of these issues will hopefully result in identification of risk factors and biomarkers for patients at risk of progression or other morbidities, as well as development of management strategies.

SUMMARY

The definition of ILA has been recently refined and subclassified into nonsubpleural, subpleural nonfibrotic, and subpleural fibrotic types. ILA have been associated with progression to clinically significant ILD and have also been associated with increased morbidities unrelated to disease progression, such as an increased incidence of ARDS in patients with sepsis. Patients with ILA who develop lung cancer have an increased risk of complications following thoracic surgery as well as an increased incidence of complications following all types of adjuvant therapies. A uniform approach to radiologic reporting should aid in further evaluating clinical risks and developing management strategies, with a 2-fold aim of identification and potential early intervention in patients likely to progress to ILD and the reduction of complications unrelated to progression. Greater information regarding histologic correlates is needed and can contribute to our understanding of ILA. Surgical resections offer the greatest opportunity for this evaluation but will require potential modification of grossing strategies and increased diligence in reporting findings in the nonneoplastic lung. Increased awareness of ILA and their significance combined with improved communication among radiology, pathology, and the clinical treatment team should help facilitate this effort.

CLINICS CARE POINTS

- ILA refers to incidental ground glass or reticular abnormalities, traction bronchiectasis, honeycombing, and nonemphysematous cysts involving at least 5% of the cross-sectional area of any one lung zone and detected in an individual in whom ILD is not suspected.

- Subpleural fibrotic ILA in particular are associated with a risk of progression to clinically significant ILD and are associated with other clinical morbidities unrelated to disease progression.

- Identification of ILA in a consistent uniform fashion will potentially lead to opportunities for earlier intervention in patients likely to develop ILD.

- The presence of ILA in patients with lung cancer is associated with an increased risk of complications concerning treatment, which requires potential development of management strategies.

DISCLOSURE

No conflicts of interest relevant to the content of the article; Unrelated conflicts: AbbVie (advisory board and consultant on MET testing in lung cancer); Astra-Zeneca (advisory board related to Her2 therapy in lung cancer).

REFERENCES

1. Tsushima K, Sone S, Yoshikawa S, et al. The radiological patterns of interstitial change at an early phase: over a 4-year follow-up. Respir Med 2010; 104(11):1712–21.
2. Washko GR, Hunninghake GM, Fernandez IE, et al. Lung volumes and emphysema in smokers with interstitial lung abnormalities. N Engl J Med 2011; 364(10):897–906.
3. Doyle TJ, Hunninghake GM, Rosas IO. Subclinical interstitial lung disease: why you should care. Am J Respir Crit Care Med 2012;185(11):1147–53.
4. Salisbury ML, Lynch DA. Toward Early Identification of Clinically Relevant Interstitial Lung Disease. Am J Respir Crit Care Med 2017;196(11):1368–9.
5. Hatabu H, Hunninghake GM, Richeldi L, et al. Interstitial lung abnormalities detected incidentally on CT: a Position Paper from the Fleischner Society. Lancet Respir Med 2020;8(7):726–37.
6. Hata A, Schiebler ML, Lynch DA, et al. Interstitial Lung Abnormalities: State of the Art. Radiology 2021;301(1):19–34.
7. Hata A, Hino T, Yanagawa M, et al. Interstitial Lung Abnormalities at CT: Subtypes, Clinical Significance, and Associations with Lung Cancer. Radiographics 2022;42(7):1925–39.
8. Washko GR, Lynch DA, Matsuoka S, et al. Identification of early interstitial lung disease in smokers from the COPDGene Study. Acad Radiol 2010;17(1):48–53.
9. Grant-Orser A, Min B, Elmrayed S, et al. Prevalence, Risk Factors, and Outcomes of Adult Interstitial Lung Abnormalities: A Systematic Review and Meta-Analysis. Am J Respir Crit Care Med 2023. https://doi.org/10.1164/rccm.202302-0271OC.
10. Oldham JM, Adegunsoye A, Khera S, et al. Underreporting of Interstitial Lung Abnormalities on Lung Cancer Screening Computed Tomography. Ann Am Thorac Soc 2018;15(6):764–6.
11. Salisbury ML, Hewlett JC, Ding G, et al. Development and Progression of Radiologic Abnormalities in Individuals at Risk for Familial Interstitial Lung Disease. Am J Respir Crit Care Med 2020;201(10):1230–9.
12. McGroder CF, Hansen S, Hinckley Stukovsky K, et al. Incidence of Interstitial Lung Abnormalities: The MESA Lung Study. Eur Respir J 2023. https://doi.org/10.1183/13993003.01950-2022.
13. Araki T, Putman RK, Hatabu H, et al. Development and Progression of Interstitial Lung Abnormalities in the Framingham Heart Study. Am J Respir Crit Care Med 2016;194(12):1514–22.
14. Hobbs BD, Putman RK, Araki T, et al. Overlap of Genetic Risk between Interstitial Lung Abnormalities and Idiopathic Pulmonary Fibrosis. Am J Respir Crit Care Med 2019;200(11):1402–13.
15. Kim JS, Manichaikul AW, Hoffman EA, et al. MUC5B, telomere length and longitudinal quantitative interstitial lung changes: the MESA Lung Study. Thorax 2023;78(6):566–73.
16. Moll M, Peljto AL, Kim JS, et al. A Polygenic Risk Score for Idiopathic Pulmonary Fibrosis and Interstitial Lung Abnormalities. Am J Respir Crit Care Med 2023. https://doi.org/10.1164/rccm.202212-2257OC.
17. Jin GY, Lynch D, Chawla A, et al. Interstitial lung abnormalities in a CT lung cancer screening population: prevalence and progression rate. Radiology 2013;268(2):563–71.
18. Putman RK, Gudmundsson G, Axelsson GT, et al. Imaging Patterns Are Associated with Interstitial Lung Abnormality Progression and Mortality. Am J Respir Crit Care Med 2019;200(2):175–83.
19. Putman RK, Hunninghake GM, Dieffenbach PB, et al. Interstitial Lung Abnormalities Are Associated with Acute Respiratory Distress Syndrome. Am J Respir Crit Care Med 2017;195(1):138–41.
20. Kadoch M, Kitich A, Alqalyoobi S, et al. Interstitial lung abnormality is prevalent and associated with worse outcome in patients undergoing transcatheter aortic valve replacement. Respir Med 2018;137: 55–60.
21. Han X, Chen L, Fan Y, et al. Longitudinal Assessment of Chest CT Findings and Pulmonary Function after COVID-19 Infection. Radiology 2023;307(2): e222888.
22. Noh S, Bertini C, Mira-Avendano I, et al. Interstitial lung abnormalities after hospitalization for COVID-19 in patients with cancer: A prospective cohort study. Cancer Med 2023. https://doi.org/10.1002/cam4.6396.
23. Hino T, Nishino M, Valtchinov VI, et al. Severe COVID-19 pneumonia leads to post-COVID-19 lung abnormalities on follow-up CT scans. Eur J Radiol Open 2023;10:100483. https://doi.org/10.1016/j.ejro.2023.100483.
24. Axelsson GT, Putman RK, Aspelund T, et al. The associations of interstitial lung abnormalities with cancer diagnoses and mortality. Eur Respir J 2020;56(6). https://doi.org/10.1183/13993003.02154-2019.
25. Whittaker Brown SA, Padilla M, Mhango G, et al. Interstitial Lung Abnormalities and Lung Cancer Risk in the National Lung Screening Trial. Chest 2019;156(6):1195–203.
26. Iwasawa T, Okudela K, Takemura T, et al. Computer-aided Quantification of Pulmonary Fibrosis in Patients with Lung Cancer: Relationship to Disease-free Survival. Radiology 2019;292(2):489–98.

27. Im Y, Park HY, Shin S, et al. Prevalence of and risk factors for pulmonary complications after curative resection in otherwise healthy elderly patients with early stage lung cancer. Respir Res 2019;20(1):136.

28. Nakanishi Y, Masuda T, Yamaguchi K, et al. Pre-existing interstitial lung abnormalities are risk factors for immune checkpoint inhibitor-induced interstitial lung disease in non-small cell lung cancer. Respir Investig 2019;57(5):451–9.

29. Katzenstein AL, Mukhopadhyay S, Zanardi C, et al. Clinically occult interstitial fibrosis in smokers: classification and significance of a surprisingly common finding in lobectomy specimens. Hum Pathol 2010;41(3):316–25.

30. Kawabata Y, Hoshi E, Murai K, et al. Smoking-related changes in the background lung of specimens resected for lung cancer: a semiquantitative study with correlation to postoperative course. Histopathology 2008;53(6):707–14.

31. Miller ER, Putman RK, Vivero M, et al. Histopathology of Interstitial Lung Abnormalities in the Context of Lung Nodule Resections. Am J Respir Crit Care Med 2018;197(7):955–8.

32. Hung YP, Hunninghake GM, Miller ER, et al. Incidental nonneoplastic parenchymal findings in patients undergoing lung resection for mass lesions. Hum Pathol 2019;86:93–101.

33. Chae KJ, Chung MJ, Jin GY, et al. Radiologic-pathologic correlation of interstitial lung abnormalities and predictors for progression and survival. Eur Radiol 2022;32(4):2713–23.

34. Schneider F, Butnor KB, Beasley MB, Dacic S. Protocol for the Examination of Resection Specimens From Patients With Primary Non-Small Cell Carcinoma, Small Cell Carcinoma, or Carcinoid Tumor of the Lung Version: 4.3.0.1 September 2022. College of American Pathologists.

Evolving Diagnostic Approach of Pulmonary Salivary Gland-type Tumors

Ridhi Sood, MD, DM[a], Deepali Jain, MD, FIAC, FRCPath[a],*

KEYWORDS

- Endobronchial tumor • Central airway tumor • Salivary gland-type tumor • Unusual lung histologies
- Rare pulmonary primaries

Key points

- Salivary gland-type tumors of the lung are rare.
- Histopathology is key to their diagnosis because they lack specific clinical and radiological features.
- Pulmonary salivary gland tumor subtypes bear resemblance to each other and other lung cancers.
- Special stains, immunohistochemistry, and key cytogenetic and molecular studies need to be used to accurately diagnose them.

ABSTRACT

Pulmonary salivary gland-type, although bear resemblance to their salivary gland counterparts, present a diagnostic challenge due to their rarity. Clinical features overlap with lung carcinoma; however, management strategies and outcomes are distinct. Onus falls on the pathologist to avoid misinterpretation of small biopsies especially in young, nonsmokers with slow growing or circumscribed endobronchial growths. A combination of cytokeratin, myoepithelial immunohistochemical markers, and identification of signature molecular alteration is invaluable in differentiation from lung cancers and subtyping the pulmonary salivary gland-type tumor.

BACKGROUND: NEED FOR REVIEW

Salivary gland-type tumors (SGTs) are diverse neoplasms that are uncommon outside the head and neck (H&N) region. Evidence suggests that SGTs originate from submucosal glands in the esophagus, skin, breast, cervix, trachea, and bronchi.[1,2] Pulmonary salivary gland-type tumors (PSGTs) are rare and account for less than 1% of lung tumors.[3,4]

Compared to other pulmonary neoplasms, PSGTs affect a younger demographic and often have central locations. Nonetheless, diagnosing PSGTs proves challenging due to shared clinical and radiological features with more common pulmonary carcinomas. Although the majority of PSGTs are also malignant, they have superior survival and drastically different management strategies compared with non–small cell lung carcinomas (NSCLCs). PSGTs are treated surgically, necessitating pathologic diagnosis, which is often the only method of diagnosis.

CLASSIFICATION OF PULMONARY SALIVARY GLAND-TYPE TUMORS

Fortunately, PSGTs shares the same histologic, immunohistochemical, and molecular features as their H&N counterparts, enabling similar classification. Comparison of the current World Health Organization (WHO) classifications (fifth edition) of salivary gland tumors of H&N[5] and thoracic tumors[6] depicted in **Fig. 1**. It is easy to visualize the wide variety of benign SGTs in the H&N compartment compared with those in the tracheobronchial tree. Only a fraction of SGT histologies

[a] Department of Pathology, All India Institute of Medical Sciences, New Delhi, 110029, India
* Corresponding author.
E-mail address: deepalijain76@aiims.edu

Surgical Pathology 17 (2024) 227–241
https://doi.org/10.1016/j.path.2023.11.001

occurs in the lung reflecting their low prevalence.[7,8] Mucoepidermoid carcinoma (MEC) and adenoid cystic carcinoma (AdCC) are the most common PSGTs, followed by epithelial-myoepithelial carcinoma (EMC), and hyalinizing clear cell carcinoma (HCCC). This contrasts with SGTs of H&N region where benign tumors (65%) outnumber the carcinomas (35%).[9] The most common benign tumor of the salivary gland, that is, pleomorphic adenoma (PA) is very uncommon at this site although they display similar *CTNNB1* (β-catenin):: Pleomorphic adenoma gene 1 (*PLAG1*) gene fusion and nuclear PLAG1 expression.[10] In the lung, PA can be confused with hamartoma, chondroma, myoepithelioma, and sclerosing pneumocytoma. Mucous cell adenoma, oncocytoma, and myoepithelioma are some of the other rare benign PSGTs.

DIAGNOSTIC CHALLENGES WITH LIMITED BIOPSY SAMPLES

Histopathological diagnosis is hindered by small size of lung biopsy. The central location of PSGTs enables endobronchial fine needle aspiration (EBNA), bronchial brush, washings, and bronchial lavages sampling[11,12] In addition to rapid on-site evaluation, biopsy imprint cytology can reduce "nondiagnostic" pathologic reports.

Pathologic characteristics of SGTs overlap architecturally and cytologically, confusing even experts in the field at times. This worsens when evaluating tissue samples from minor salivary gland.[13] The same can be extrapolated in pulmonary site due to (1) occurrence of native minor salivary gland tissue in the bronchopulmonary tissue; (2) overlapping histologic features between PSGTs and NSCLCs; and (3) small biopsy specimens which may not represent the lesion or be sufficient for molecular testing. In these cases, using terminologies such as "non–small cell carcinoma with features suggestive of salivary gland-type tumor" is recommended.[14] "Carcinoma NOS," however, cannot be applied because it pertains to NSCLCs lacking TTF1, p40, and neuroendocrine differentiation. Endobronchial resections counter these tissue issues, enabling early diagnosis. Studies analyzing molecular tumorigenesis of SGTs offer a range of "omics" and theranostic advancements. Availability of immunohistochemistry (IHC), fluorescence in-situ hybridization (FISH), and next–generation sequencing tests has redefined the diagnostic approach.

This review focuses on distinguishing morphologic features and ancillary tests of PSGTs, including IHC, cytogenetics, and molecular tests, which are crucial for prognostication and differentiating them from their mimics (**Box 1**). A pattern-based approach in diagnosing lung biopsies with SGT-like morphologic features is explored.

WHO Thoracic Tumors (5th Ed. 2021)
❖ Pleomorphic adenoma of the lung
❖ Adenoid cystic carcinoma of the lung
❖ Epithelial-myoepithelial carcinoma of the lung
❖ Mucoepidermoid carcinoma of the lung
❖ Hyalinizing clear cell carcinoma of the lung
❖ Myoepithelioma and myoepithelial carcinoma of the lung

WHO Head and neck Tumors (5th Ed. 2022)
Benign epithelial tumours
❖ Pleomorphic adenoma
❖ Basal cell adenoma
❖ Warthin tumour
❖ Oncocytoma
❖ Salivary gland myoepithelioma
❖ Canalicular adenoma
❖ Cystadenoma of the salivary glands
❖ Ductal papillomas
❖ Sialadenoma papilliferum
❖ Lymphadenoma
❖ Sebaceous adenoma
❖ Intercalated duct adenoma and hyperplasia
❖ Striated duct adenoma
❖ Sclerosing polycystic adenoma

WHO Head and neck Tumors (5th Ed. 2022)
Malignant epithelial tumours
❖ Mucoepidermoid carcinoma
❖ Adenoid cystic carcinoma
❖ Acinic cell carcinoma
❖ Secretory carcinoma
❖ Microsecretory adenocarcinoma
❖ Polymorphous adenocarcinoma
❖ Hyalinizing clear cell carcinoma
❖ Basal cell adenocarcinoma
❖ Intraductal carcinoma
❖ Salivary duct carcinoma
❖ Myoepithelial carcinoma
❖ Epithelial-myoepithelial carcinoma
❖ Mucinous adenocarcinoma
❖ Sclerosing microcystic adenocarcinoma
❖ Carcinoma ex pleomorphic adenoma
❖ Carcinosarcoma of the salivary glands
❖ Sebaceous adenocarcinoma
❖ Lymphoepithelial carcinoma
❖ Squamous cell carcinoma
❖ Sialoblastoma
❖ Salivary carcinoma NOS and emerging entities

Fig. 1. Classification of SGTs in lung and H&N. Data from the WHO classification of head and neck tumors[5] and thoracic tumors.[6] (*Adapted from* Speight PM, Barrett AW. Salivary gland tumors: diagnostic challenges and an update on the latest WHO classification. In: Fletcher CDM eds. Diagnostic istopathology. 5th ed. Elsevier Ltd; 2020. p. 147–58 and Resio BJ, Chiu AS, Hoag J, Dhanasopon AP, Blasberg JD, Boffa DJ. Primary Salivary Type Lung Cancers in the National Cancer Database. Ann Thorac Surg. 2018;105(6):1633-9.)

> **Box 1**
> **Diagnostic highlights of primary pulmonary salivary gland-type carcinomas**
>
> Mucoepidermoid carcinoma
>
> - Occurs centrally, can originate in peripheral lung when high grade
> - Triad of cells is pathognomic; however, the squamoid cells of MEC lack keratinization
> - Mucin stains and immunostains p63, CK7, and TTF1 are diagnostically helpful
> - Break Apart FISH for *MAML2* oncogene is highly specific for diagnosis although its absence does not exclude the diagnosis
> - Molecular alterations: HER2 and EGFR can be seen in overlapping with adenocarcinoma of lung
>
> Adenoid cystic carcinoma
>
> - Classic location is tracheal (>>bronchi), with submucosal growth
> - Charcterstically bilayered with cells arranged in cribriform pattern and BM-like material production
> - Molecular alteration: *MYB-NFIB* fusion; testing via FISH or IHC (lacks specificity)
>
> Myoepithelial neoplasm
>
> - Monolayered, lack ducts and tubules
> - Diverse cytologic (clear, spindled, epithelioid, or plasmacytoid) and architectural (lobules, cords, trabeculae, sheets, and so forth) appearance
> - Stromal dominance: hyalinized, myxoid, or chondroid
> - Molecular alterations (rearrangement, amplification, or mutation) in *EWSR1* gene
>
> Epithelial myoepithelial carcinoma
>
> - Bilayered
> - Forms ducts or tubules
> - *HRAS* mutations
>
> Hyalinizing clear cell carcinoma
>
> - Single cell type
> - Solid nests with prominent and diffuse cytoplasmic clearing
> - Stromal dominance: fibrotic or hyalinized
> - Molecular alterations in *EWSR1-ATF1* fusion
>
> *Abbreviations:* MEC, mucoepidermoid carcinoma, CK: cytokeratin; TTF1, thyroid transcription factor 1; FISH, fluorescence in situ hybridization; MAML2, Mastermind-like protein 2; HER2, human epidermal growth factor receptor 2; EGFR, epidermal growth factor receptor; MYB: MYB proto-oncogene; NFIB, nuclear factor I/B; IHC, immunohistochemistry; HRAS, Harvey Rat sarcoma virus; EWSR1, Ewing Sarcoma breakpoint region 1; ATF1, activating transcription factor 1.

UNIQUE CLINICOPATHOLOGICAL FEATURES OF INDIVIDUAL PULMONARY SALIVARY GLAND-TYPE TUMORS

MUCOEPIDERMOID CARCINOMA

Clinicoradiological features

MECs are one of the most common SGTs accounting for 56% to 78% of all PSGTs.[15–17] Although rare in adults, they account for 10% to 20% of pediatric malignant lung tumors. These tumors can originate centrally, from the airways (trachea and main and segmental bronchi), or peripherally within lung parenchyma.[18] Grossly, these tumors can be sessile, polypoid, or pedunculated with a circumscribed border. When centrally located, these tumors show an "air crescent sign" on computerized tomography, whereas the peripheral MECs lack characteristic radiological findings.

Histopathology and cytomorphology

MECs are characterized by a combination of mucus-secreting, squamous and intermediate cells. There is limited evidence supporting the

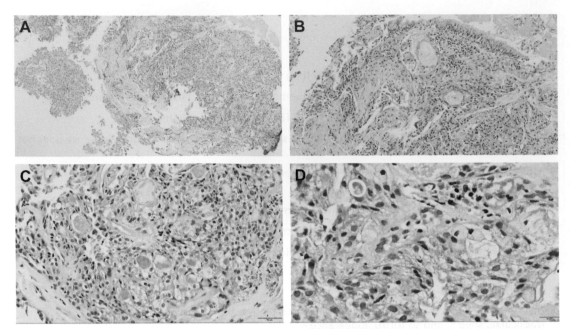

Fig. 2. Case of low-grade MEC showing (*A*) microcysts (hematoxylin-eosin [H&E], 100×) and (*B*) subepithelial pattern of infiltration (H&E, 200×). (*C*) Heterogenous population of mucous, clear, and intermediate cells (H&E, 400×) (*D*) lack cytologic atypia and mitosis (H&E, 400×).

2-tiered grading system (based on cytologic atypia) for pulmonary MECs given the rarity of high-grade lung MECs. Nonetheless, it is recommended by the WHO for thoracic tumors.[19] Low-grade MECs predominantly show cysts lined by bland columnar mucinous cells with infrequent mitoses (**Fig. 2**). Conversely, high-grade MECs contain a higher proportion of solid nests of pleomorphic squamoid and intermediate cells with scarce mucin-secreting cells (**Fig. 3**). Most (~75%) high-grade tumors are peripherally located[20] and prone to parenchymal infiltration, recurrence, and nodal metastasis. A 3-tiered grading system used by Deb and colleagues demonstrated that high-grade MECs had a significantly worse prognosis than low-grade or intermediate-grade MECs.[21] Differentials and mimics of pulmonary MECs are spread across the histologic spectrum highlighted in **Fig. 4**.

Only a few case reports have described aspiration findings of pulmonary MECs,[22] although their central locations make preoperative cytologic sampling more likely. Doxtader and colleagues (2019) diagnosed 3 MECs diagnosed during 10 years using EBNA.[12] The smears showed mucinous background with flat sheets of uniform (intermediate) cells devoid of cilia, exhibiting mild nuclear atypia, and scant cytoplasm. Scattered within these cellular groups are mucocytes (highlighted on mucin stains) and squamoid cells have a central nucleus with

moderate amount of light pink-purple cytoplasm (**Fig. 5**). Clearing and oncocytic changes can be encountered although keratinization should be consistently absent.[23,24]

Ancillary studies

Immunohistochemistry: MECs express both high and low molecular weight cytokeratin (CK) according to their cellular constituents; that is, intermediate and squamoid cells are positive for CK5/6, CK7, and CK19 while intermediate and mucous cells express CK7.[25] Epithelial mucins (MUC) are expressed in all grades, with MUC5AC being the most consistent. Squamous differentiation markers, including p63 (more sensitive) and p40 (more specific), are expressed in the intermediate and squamoid tumor cells. The latter are also positive in adenosquamous carcinoma (AdSC) and squamous cell carcinoma (SCC).[26] Thyroid transcription factor 1 (TTF1) and napsin A are 2 immunostains invaluable in ruling out primary lung adenocarcinoma as MECs are consistently negative. MECs are SOX10 negative, which helps distinguish them from other PSGTs. Several authors have investigated the utility of Ki-67 index for discriminating high-grade and low-grade MECs, although there is no recommend cutoff.[27,28]

Cytogenetics and molecular analysis: translocation (q21; p13) producing cyclic adenosine 3′,

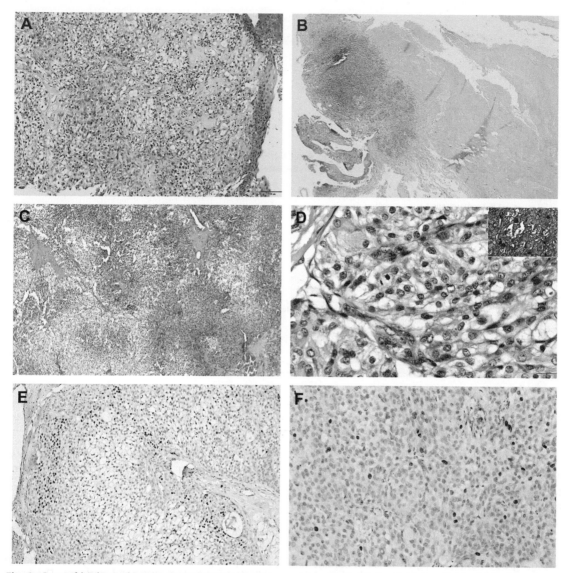

Fig. 3. Case of high-grade MEC showing (*A*) extensive squamous metaplasia of surface lining and subepithelial infiltration by a tumor arranged as solid nests (H&E, 200×) along with (*B*) large areas of necrosis (H&E, 40×). (*C*) Cytologically, predominance of squamoid and intermediate cells is seen (H&E, 200×) along with (*D*) few scattered mucous cells (inset shows Alcian blue stain highlighting mucocytes; H&E, 400×). (*E*) p63 expression in squamoid cells (DAB, 200×) and (*F*) high Ki67 proliferation index (DAB, 400×).

5'-monophosphate (cAMP) response element-binding protein (CREB)-regulated transcription coactivator 1 (CRTC1) and Mastermind-like transcriptional coactivator 2 (MAML2) fusion protein is found in 33% to 86% of pulmonary MECs.[29–31] This fusion protein activates cyclic adenosine 3', 5'-monophosphate (cAMP) signaling and disrupts notch signaling.[32] Initial research in salivary gland MEC indicated improved overall survival with MAML2 rearrangement but later studies refuted this finding.[33,34] Similar studies have not been carried out in pulmonary MEC. Real-time reverse transcriptase-polymerase chain reaction (RT-PCR) and FISH readily detect *CRTC1::MAML2* fusion transcript (see **Fig. 5**). Human epidermal growth factor receptor 2 (HER2) protein overexpression and gene amplification testing is routinely practiced as prognostic and predictive biomarker in salivary MECs. However, studies on pulmonary MECs do not replicate the same.[29] Wang and colleagues sequenced 25 pulmonary MECs and highlighted low somatic mutation rate (<5 mutations/mega-base pair) and narrower mutational diversity than salivary MECs.[16]

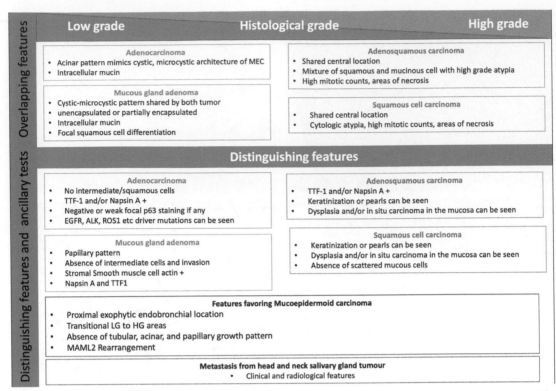

Fig. 4. Diagnostic features of histologic mimickers MEC of the lung. ALK, Anaplastic lymphom Kinase; EGFR, Epidermal growth factor receptor; HG, High grade; LG, Low grade; MAML2, mastermind like transcriptional co-activator2; MEC, Mucoepidermoid carcinoma; ROS1, ROS proto-oncogene 1.

Differential diagnosis

TTF-1 and napsin A IHC expression differentiates MECs from adenocarcinomas and AdSC. However, only histology can distinguish squamous cell carcinoma (SCC), majority of which originate centrally like MECs. Morphologic criteria favoring high-grade MEC over SCC include (1) low-grade to high-grade transition, (2) absence of carcinoma in-situ, and (3) lack of individual cell keratinization and squamous pearl formation. **Figure 4** shows characteristic feature of MEC and its differentials. MAML2 rearrangement supports MEC diagnosis; however, absence does not exclude MECs.

ADENOID CYSTIC CARCINOMA

Clinicoradiological features

AdCCs comprise 15% to 50% of all PSGTs,[15,17] although in few studies, their prevalence exceeded that of pulmonary MECs.[20,35] Majority (>90%) develop in the trachea with rare tumors occurring in segmental bronchi. In fact, peripheral involvement indicates metastasis over primary disease.[36] Lobar collapse and atelectasis accompany large-sized tumors. Radiologically, nodular, or heterogeneously thickened walls are seen which are in keeping with its characteristic submucosal growth

(**Fig. 6**). Visualizing submucosal spread grossly is difficult, lowering R0 resection rates and hence increasing recurrence.[37]

Histopathology and cytomorphology

Analogous to their salivary counterparts, they are bilayered with inner "basaloid" luminal and abluminal "myo-epithelial" cellular phenotype arranged in cribriform, tubular, and solid patterns. Predominance of the latter portends worse prognosis. Presence of basement membrane (BM)-like basophilic matrix (**Fig. 7**) composed of collagen IV, laminin, and heparan sulfate is pathognomonic. Individual cells are small, with hyperchromatic, angulated nuclei, scarce mitosis, and scant cytoplasm. These "basaloid" cells form tight 3D spheres with bright magenta BM-like material highlighted on Romanowsky Giemsa stain and pale blue green on Papanicolaou stain.

Ancillary studies

Immunohistochemistry: Luminal cells express CK7, and CD117 while myoepithelial markers viz. p63, p40, CK5/6, smooth muscle actin (SMA), smooth muscle myosin heavy chain (SMMHC), calponin, S-100, or glial fibrillary acidic protein stain the abluminal cells. Pan CK and SOX10 are

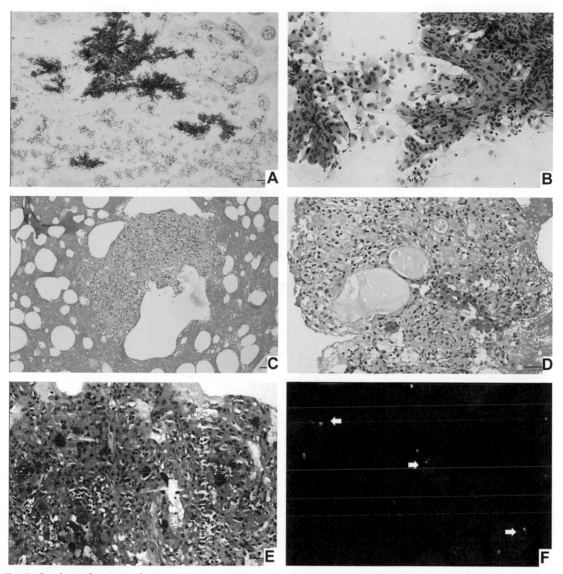

Fig. 5. Cytologic features of MEC. (*A*) Fragments and singly disposed epithelial cells (Papanicolaou stain, 100×). (*B*) Varying degrees of squamous and mucinous differentiation (Papanicolaou stain, 200×). (*C, D*) Cell block showing similar findings (H&E). (*E*) Deep blue acid mucin highlighted on Alcian blue stain, 200×. (*F*) Positive break-apart FISH for MAML2; with one intact gene and one rearranged (*white arrows*).

positive in both cell types. Mitotically active and undifferentiated AdCCs can lack myoepithelial markers and hence pose diagnostic traps. Ki-67 proliferation index is lower in AdCC than basaloid SCCs and can be applied when differential is between these tumors.[11] Myeloblastosis (MYB) protein antibody, a product of *MYB*-Nuclear factor 1B (*NFIB*) translocation,[38] is sensitive but not specific and can be positive in EMC as well. It serves as a reliable diagnostic and prognostic biomarker especially in undifferentiated AdCCs.

Cytogenetics and molecular analysis: t(6;9) (q22–23;p23–24) and less frequently t(8;9) leads to the formation of *MYB::NFIB* fusion product.

These translocations are seen in 30% to 100% of salivary and tracheobronchial AdCCs. Roden and colleagues observed MYB rearrangement to be 100% specific in distinguishing pulmonary AdCCs from NSCLCs and small-cell carcinomas.[39] It is worthwhile to note that only a subset of MYB IHC positive tumors harbor *MYB* translocations. Molecular therapies targeting *MYB*-activated pathways are being explored.

Differential diagnosis

In the absence of characteristic tubular or cribriform architecture, distinction from NSCLCs and other PSGTs is difficult especially because p63

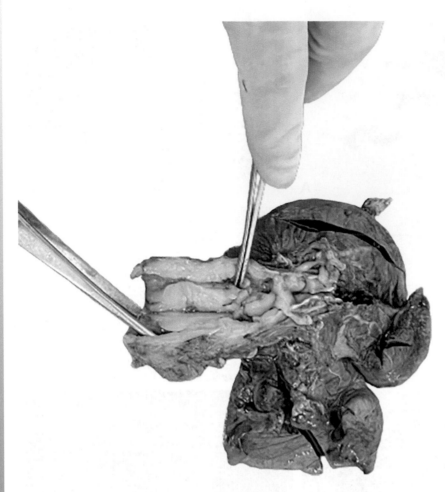

and CD117 can be expressed in many of the high-grade lung carcinoma. For instance, CD117 is positive in small cell carcinoma and SCC, whereas p63 can stain SCC and adenocarcinomas.[40] The *MYB* rearrangement is specific for AdCC and may be useful in cases of diagnostic ambiguity.

MYOEPITHELIOMA AND MYOEPITHELIAL CARCINOMA OF THE LUNG

Clinicoradiological features

Pulmonary myoepithelial neoplasms (PMNs) were first described by Higashiyama and colleagues in 1998 and account for 0.1% to 0.2% of all lung cancers. Although less than 50 cases have been reported in literature, their incidence is higher in Asians. Their central location entails radiological differentials of carcinoid, papilloma, AdSC and SCC.[41] Nonetheless, these tumors can also occur in the peripheral compartment. Parenchymal pulmonary myoepithelial neoplasm (PMN) had infiltrative borders and a larger size compared with centrally located tumors.[42]

Histopathology and cytomorphology

PMNs comprise of a pure myoepithelial proliferation lacking ducts and tubular structures and show extreme cytologic and architectural diversity. Arrangement in lobules, nodules, cords, trabeculae, or reticular patterns can be seen (Fig. 8). The characteristic increasing zonal cellularity center to periphery aids in distinction from AdCC. Cytologic spectrum includes round-oval, clear, epithelioid, spindled, or plasmacytoid morphology. Matrix production by myoepithelial tumor cells gives rise to hyalinized, myxoid or chondroid stroma. Histologic features favoring myoepithelial carcinoma over myoepithelioma are larger tumor size, infiltrative growth, lack of encapsulation, cytologic atypia, necrosis, increased mitotic activity, necrosis, and distant metastasis.

Ancillary testing

Immunohistochemistry: PMN express all myoepithelial markers. Caution should be exercised in the interpretation of TTF-1 in entrapped pneumocytes

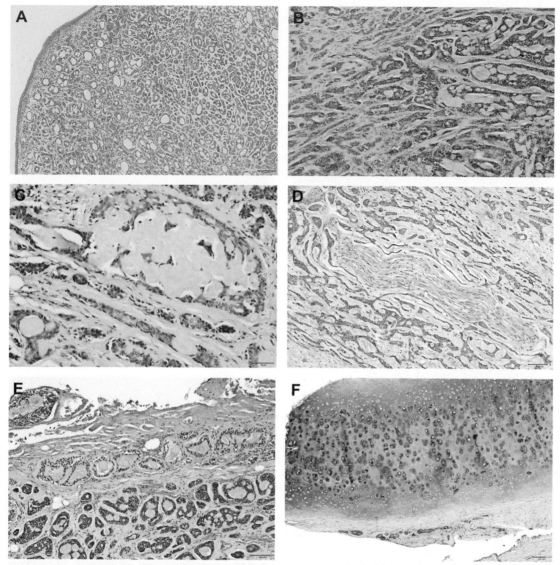

Fig. 7. Case of adenoid cystic carcinoma showing (*A, B*) intramucosal epithelial proliferation arranged in a cribriform pattern containing myxoid hyaline material (H&E, [40× (*A*) and 100× (*B*)]). (*C*) Myxoid hyaline material (H&E, 200×). (*D*) Perineural invasion is a typical finding in adenoid cystic carcinoma of the lung (H&E, 100×). (*E, F*) Involvement of soft tissue and tracheal ring margins (H&E, [200× (*E*) and 100× (*F*)]).

because adenocarcinoma cells especially in small and crushed samples.

Cytogenetics and molecular analysis: The pulmonary myoepithelial tumors show Ewing Sarcoma breakpoint region 1 (EWSR1) and fused in sarcoma (FUS) rearrangement similar to their soft tissue and salivary gland counterparts.[43,44]

Differential diagnosis

The differential diagnosis includes other myoepithelial rich tumors such as EMC. EMCs have an additional epithelial cell layer better visualized on IHC. Myoepithelial tumors exhibiting clearing,

sclerosis, or desmoplasia can resemble HCCC. In this instance, myoepithelial immunostains (negative in HCCC and positive in myoepithelial neoplasms) are valuable. Distinction of metastatic myoepithelial carcinoma from other primary sites, however, can only be achieved clinically.

EPITHELIAL MYOEPITHELIAL CARCINOMA

Clinicoradiological features

As the name suggests, EMC exhibits dual differentiation. Until 2018, fewer than 60 EMCs of the lung were reported.[41] Incidence is estimated to be 3.8% to 8% among PSGTs. Although malignant,

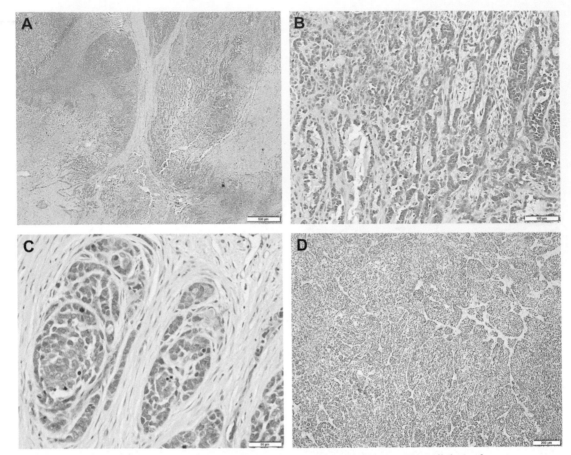

Fig. 8. Pulmonary myoepithelial carcinoma: (*A*) Lobules and islands with increasing cellularity from center to periphery (H&E, 100×), (*B*) plasmacytoid cells arranged in cords separated by loose myxoid stroma (H&E, 200×), (*C*) mild degree of atypia and occasional mitotic figure (H&E, 400×), and (*D*) Diffuse SOX10 expression.

EMCs behave indolently with ~10% developing recurrences and metastases.[45]

Histopathology and cytomorphology

EMCs are biphasic, histologic diverse tumors with inner tightly grouped "luminal" epithelial-type cells, and outer "abluminal" layer of myoepithelial-type cells.[42] The latter can dominate and form solid nests. All morphologic variations of myoepithelial cells, that is, cytoplasmic clearing (commonest), basaloid, sebaceous, oncocytic, and keratinized squamous, can be seen (**Fig. 9**). Architectural deviations in form of papillae,[46] small ducts, and solid nests can be seen.

Ancillary tests

Immunohistochemistry: CD117 can be positive in the myoepithelial component of EMC although TTF-1 and HMB-45 are uniformly negative in both cell types.[8,47]

Cytogenetics and molecular analysis: Harvey Rat sarcoma virus (HRAS) mutation are seen in more than 80% salivary gland EMC[48] and can be used to distinguish pulmonary EMC from NSCLC. Yet, due to EMC's rarity at this location, the frequency, specificity, and relationship of histologic differences to HRAS mutations remain limited. PIK3CA, KRAS, and BRAFV600 E are other point mutations in these tumors.

Differential diagnosis

EMC require distinction from benign and malignant pulmonary clear cell tumors such as myoepithelioma, myoepithelial carcinoma, HCCC, MEC, and rare PAs. PMN and HCCC can be distinguished by virtue of single cell composition and other biphasic PSGTs such as AdCC can be differentiated by the presence of basaloid cells rather than clear cells. Presence of squamoid cells and MAML2 rearrangement rules out MEC. When dealing with metastasis from H&N primaries, acinic cell carcinoma and oncocytic tumors can enter the differentials. Erroneous diagnosis of metastatic clear cell and papillary carcinomas originating

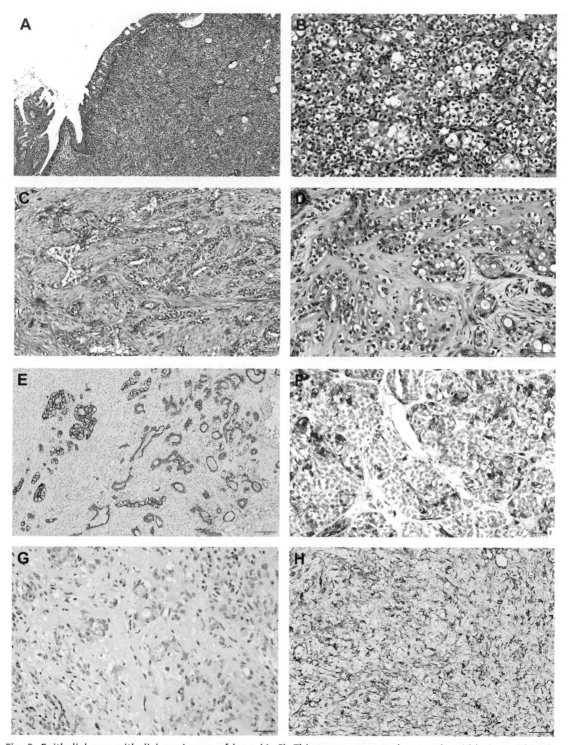

Fig. 9. Epithelial-myoepithelial carcinoma of lung (*A, B*). This tumor presented as a polypoid lesion within the bronchial lumen (note surface respiratory epithelium with focal squamous metaplasia; H&E, [100× (*A*) and 200× (*B*)]). (*C*) Nests of clear and basaloid cells (H&E, 200×). (*D*) The tubules are lined by dual-layered cells surrounded by hyalinized stroma (H&E, 400×). Immunostains expressed in luminal cells using (*E*) cytokeratin 7 and myoepithelial cells by (*F*) SMA, (*G*) p63, and (*H*) SMMHC (DAB, magnifications [200× (*E*), 400× (*F, G*), and 200× (*H*)]).

from renal, ovarian, and uterine primaries as well as benign or malignant perivascular epithelioid cell tumor (PEComa) and melanoma could be rendered without IHC. Similarly, glycogen-rich SCC and mucin-rich adenocarcinomas also pose diagnostic challenges.

HYALINIZING CLEAR CELL CARCINOMA

Clinicoradiological features

Fewer than 15 pulmonary HCCC have been reported in recent literature.[49,50] Recent changes in WHO's blue book of thoracic tumors and H&N tumors have changed the nomenclature from "clear cell carcinoma" to "HCCC."[51] Epidemiologically, these tumors have a female predominance. Clinically, their behavior is indolent and rarely do they recur or metastasize. A series of 5 HCCCs diagnosed collectively at our institute and Mayo clinic revealed 1 case with nodal metastases.[52]

Histopathology and cytomorphology

These tumors infiltrate as solid sheets, nests, trabeculae, and cords of polygonal cells with abundant pale eosinophilic to clear cytoplasm (Fig. 10). Mucinous and squamous differentiation may be observed generating overlap with MEC and SCC. SCC, however, shows a higher degree of cytologic pleomorphism, frequent mitosis, and necrosis while nuclear atypia is moderate at best in HCCC. Hyalinization or desmoplasia of the stromal partitions separating the clear cells is another salient diagnostic feature.

Ancillary tests

Immunohistochemistry: Tumor cells express p40, p63, CK5/6, and CK7 overlapping with PSGTs and SCC often necessitating FISH analysis.

Cytogenetics and molecular analysis: EWSR1 rearrangement is observed in 80% to 90% HCCCs, and despite its promiscuity, is absent in other histologic mimics at this site.[53] Specific transcript analysis (with partner genes activating transcription factor 1 [ATF1] or cAMP responsive element modulator [CREM]) using RT-PCR or sequencing is confirmatory as other primary pulmonary tumors harboring same fusions do not share histologic or immunophenotypic features with HCCCs.[54]

Differential diagnosis

Given the rarity of lung HCCC, it is essential to exclude metastasis. Histologic, immunophenotypic, cytogenetic, and molecular characteristics of HCCC are akin to their H&N equivalent. A central endobronchial location and the absence of a history of alternative primary favor a pulmonary origin. The differential diagnosis of HCCC includes other clear cell tumors of the lung such as the following:

(1) PSGTs such as myoepithelioma, myoepithelial carcinoma, and EMC express S100, calponin, and SMA, which are negative in HCCC. Exclusion of high-grade MEC may require FISH analysis.
(2) Adenocarcinoma can be excluded using TTF-1 IHC while distinction from SCC is morphologic as elaborated before.
(3) Other immunostains such as HMB45, S100 and SOX10 can be applied which will stain the tumor cells of PEComa.
(4) Metastatic clear cell carcinomas including renal cell carcinoma, ovarian and uterine clear cell carcinoma share CK positivity with PSGT, however, lack p40 and p63 expression. PAX8 with or without AMACR and HNF-beta are other helpful immunostains which are negative in PSGT.[55]

PATTERN BASED APPROACH TO DIAGNOSE SALIVARY GLAND-TYPE TUMORS ON LUNG BIOPSY

PSGTs can be approached by architecture (tubular, solid, cystic-microcystic, and cribriform), cell composition (single or dual cell type), or stromal

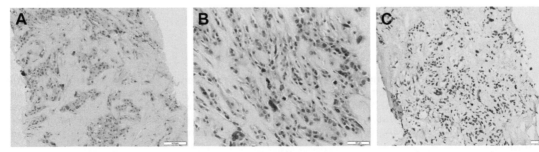

Fig. 10. Pulmonary hyalinizing clear cell carcinoma: Small nests of small-sized cuboidal cells with pale eosinophilic cytoplasm surrounded by hyalinized stroma (H&E, [200× (A), 400× (B)]). (C) Diffuse p40 positive (DAB, 200×).

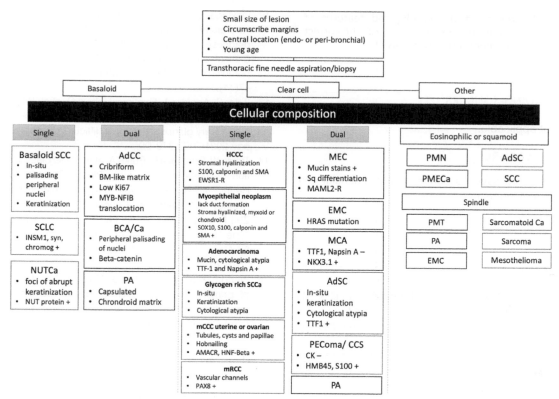

Fig. 11. Differentials diagnosis and ancillary testing based on cytologic features of pulmonary salivary glands tumors. AdCC, adenoid cystic carcinoma; AdSC, adenosquamous carcinoma; BCA/Ca, basal cell adenoma/carcinoma; Ca, carcinoma; CCS, clear cell sarcoma; EMC, epithelial myoepithelial carcinoma; HCCC, hyalinizing clear cell carcinoma; MCA, mucous cell adenoma; mCCC: metastatic clear cell carcinoma, MEC, mucoepidermoid carcinoma; mRCC, metastatic renal cell carcinoma; PA, pleomorphic adenoma; PEComa, perivascular epithelioid cell neoplasms; PMN, Pulmonary myoepithelial neoplasm; SCC, squamous cell carcinoma; SCLC, small cell lung cancer.

component (BM-like, hyalinized, chrondroid, or chondromyxoid). Because of small biopsy size, often the cytologic features viz. clear, basaloid, eosinophilic, or squamoid guide the diagnostic workup. Flowchart in **Fig. 11** can be applied to fine needle aspiration biopsy (FNAB)/biopsy specimens. Pathologists should consider the following before diagnosing PSGTs in limited biopsies.

1. Ruling out metastasis from extrapulmonary SGTs requires clinical inputs.
2. TTF1-positive pneumocytes can proliferate extensively in infiltrative PGSTs. Care must be taken to recognize and discriminate entrapped pneumocytes from tumor cells.
3. Presence of p40 expression in abluminal/scattered pattern raises suspicion of SGTs.
4. Using the terminology "adenocarcinoma, NOS" for suspected PSGTs is not advisable. Rather, for inconclusive biopsies, adding a note flagging features suspicious of SGTs followed by multidisciplinary meetings to decide management plan.

SUMMARY

PSGTs are often misdiagnosed as NSCLC or metastasis on small biopsies. A high index of suspicion in nonsmokers with a slow-growing, circumscribed tumor of the tracheobronchial tree is essential to avoid misdiagnosis. Following microscopic recognition of PSGT pattern with an appropriate panel of key IHC, cytogenetic and molecular tests is essential for accurate tumor typing and prognostication.

CLINICS CARE POINTS

- PSGT are uncommon, and often misdiagnosed as NSCLC clinically, radiologically and on histopathology.

- Application of diagnostic ancillary tests on recognising histological clues and patterns is invaluable for distinction.

- Awareness of the highlighted features of these tumours can direct towards the correct management, and prognosis.

FUNDING SOURCES

Not applicable.

DISCLOSURE

Authors have no commercial or financial conflicts of interest.

REFERENCES

1. Bennett AK, Mills SE, Wick MR. Salivary-type Neoplasms of the Breast and Lung. Semin Diagn Pathol 2003;20(4):279–304.
2. Yordanov A, Karamanliev M, Tantchev L, et al. Mucoepidermoid Carcinoma of the Uterine Cervix—Single-Center Study Over a 10-Year Period. Medicina (B Aires) 2020;56(1):37–9.
3. Molina JR, Aubry MC, Lewis JE, et al. Primary salivary gland-type lung cancer. Cancer 2007;110(10): 2253–9.
4. Heitmiller RF, Mathisen DJ, Ferry JA, et al. Mucoepidermoid lung tumors. Ann Thorac Surg 1989;47(3): 394–9.
5. Speight PM, Barrett AW. Salivary gland tumours: diagnostic challenges and an update on the latest WHO classification. In: Fletcher CDM, editor. Diagnostic Histopathology. 5th edition. Elsevier Ltd; 2020. p. 147–58.
6. WHO Classification of Tumours Editorial Board. Thoracic tumours (Internet). Lyon (France): International Agency for Research on Cancer; 2021 (cited 2023 july 17). (WHO classification of tumours series, 5th ed.; vol. 5). Available from: https://tumourclassification.iarc.who.int/chapters/35.
7. Resio BJ, Chiu AS, Hoag J, et al. Primary Salivary Type Lung Cancers in the National Cancer Database. Ann Thorac Surg 2018;105(6):1633–9.
8. Falk N, Weissferdt A, Kalhor N, et al. Primary Pulmonary Salivary Gland-type Tumors. Adv Anat Pathol 2016;23(1):13–23.
9. Alsanie I, Rajab S, Cottom H, et al. Distribution and Frequency of Salivary Gland Tumours: An International Multicenter Study. Head Neck Pathol 2022; 16(4):1043–54.
10. Asahina M, Hayashi T, Takamochi K, et al. Identification of CTNNB1-PLAG1 gene rearrangement in a patient with pulmonary pleomorphic adenoma. Virchows Arch 2020;477(5):739–42.
11. Wang M, Gilani S, Xu H, et al. Salivary Gland-type Tumors of the Lung. Arch Pathol Lab Med 2021; 145(11):1379–86.
12. Doxtader EE, Shah AA, Zhang Y, et al. Primary salivary gland-type tumors of the tracheobronchial tree diagnosed by transbronchial fine needle aspiration: Clinical and cytomorphologic features with histopathologic correlation. Diagn Cytopathol 2019; 47(11):1168–76.
13. Ihrler S, Agaimy A, Guntinas-Lichius O, et al. Why is the histomorphological diagnosis of tumours of minor salivary glands much more difficult? Histopathology 2021;79(5):779–90.
14. Travis W, Brambilla E, Burke A, et al. WHO classification of tumours of the lung, Pleura, Thymus and Heart. 4th edition. Lyon, France: International Agency for Research on Cancer; 2015. p. 2015.
15. Zhu F, Liu Z, Hou Y, et al. Primary Salivary Gland–Type Lung Cancer: Clinicopathological Analysis of 88 Cases from China. J Thorac Oncol 2013;8(12): 1578–84.
16. Wang F, Xi SY, Hao WW, et al. Mutational landscape of primary pulmonary salivary gland-type tumors through targeted next-generation sequencing. Lung Cancer 2021;160:1–7.
17. Garg P, Sharma G, Rai S, et al. Primary salivary gland-type tumors of the lung: A systematic review and pooled analysis. Lung India 2019;36(2):118.
18. Liu X, Adams AL. Mucoepidermoid Carcinoma of the Bronchus: A Review. Arch Pathol Lab Med 2007;131(9):1400–4.
19. Husain AN, Nicholson AG, Farver C. Mucoepidermoid carcinoma of the lung. In: Dacic S, Thompson LD, editors. WHO classification of tumours Editorial board thoracic tumours. 5th edition. Lyon (France): International Agency for Research on Cancer; 2021.
20. Zhang Y, Liu X, Gu Y, et al. Clinical, laboratory, pathological, and radiological characteristics and prognosis of patients with pulmonary salivary gland-type tumors. J Cancer Res Clin Oncol 2023;149(7): 4025–39.
21. Deb PQ, Suster D. Outcome of primary pulmonary salivary gland-type carcinoma. Am J Clin Pathol 2021;156:S150.
22. Puzyrenko A, Shponka V, Sheinin Y, et al. Primary pulmonary mucoepidermoid carcinoma: Cytohistologic correlation and review of the literature. Ann Diagn Pathol 2021;51:151698.
23. Ló Pez-Terrada D, Bloom MGK, Cagle PT, et al. Oncocytic Mucoepidermoid Carcinoma of the Trachea. Arch Pathol Lab Med 1999;123(7):635–7.
24. Zhu Y, Li Y, Guo L, et al. Clinicopathological practice in the differential diagnosis of mucoepidermoid carcinoma from neoplasms with mucinous component. Chronic Dis Transl Med 2023;9(1):29–38.
25. Azevedo RS, de Almeida OP, Kowalski LP, et al. Comparative Cytokeratin Expression in the Different Cell Types of Salivary Gland Mucoepidermoid Carcinoma. Head Neck Pathol 2008;2(4):257–64.

26. Kim NI, Lee JS. Greater specificity of p40 compared with p63 in distinguishing squamous cell carcinoma from adenocarcinoma in effusion cellblocks. Cyto-Journal 2020;17:13.

27. Hou J, Wang H, Zhang G, et al. Mucoepidermoid Carcinoma of the Lung: Report of 29 Cases. Zhongguo Fei Ai Za Zhi 2017;20(3):168–74.

28. Huo Z, Wu H, Li J, et al. Primary Pulmonary Mucoepidermoid Carcinoma: Histopathological and Molecular genetic Studies of 26 Cases. PLoS One 2015; 10(11):e0143169.

29. Hu S, Gong J, Zhu X, et al. Pulmonary Salivary Gland Tumor, Mucoepidermoid Carcinoma: A Literature Review. J Oncol 2022;2022:1–10.

30. Salem A, Bell D, Sepesi B, et al. Clinicopathologic and genetic features of primary bronchopulmonary mucoepidermoid carcinoma: the MD Anderson Cancer Center experience and comprehensive review of the literature. Virchows Arch 2017;470(6):619–26.

31. Roden AC, García JJ, Wehrs RN, et al. Histopathologic, immunophenotypic and cytogenetic features of pulmonary mucoepidermoid carcinoma. Mod Pathol 2014;27(11):1479–88.

32. Wu L, Liu J, Gao P, et al. Transforming activity of MECT1-MAML2 fusion oncoprotein is mediated by constitutive CREB activation. EMBO J 2005;24(13): 2391–402.

33. Seethala RR, Chiosea SI. MAML2 Status in Mucoepidermoid Carcinoma Can No Longer Be Considered a Prognostic Marker. Am J Surg Pathol 2016;40(8): 1151–3.

34. Cipriani NA, Lusardi JJ, McElherne J, et al. Mucoepidermoid Carcinoma: A Comparison of Histologic Grading Systems and Relationship to MAML2 Rearrangement and Prognosis. Am J Surg Pathol 2019; 43(7):885–97.

35. Kim BG, Lee K, Um SW, et al. Clinical outcomes and the role of bronchoscopic intervention in patients with primary pulmonary salivary gland-type tumors. Lung Cancer 2020;146:58–65.

36. Kitada M, Ozawa K, Sato K, et al. Adenoid cystic carcinoma of the peripheral lung: a case report. World J Surg Oncol 2010;8(1):74.

37. Kumar V, Soni P, Garg M, et al. A Comparative Study of Primary Adenoid Cystic and Mucoepidermoid Carcinoma of Lung. Front Oncol 2018;8:153.

38. Vallonthaiel AG, Jain D, Singh V, et al. c-Myb Overexpression in Cytology Smears of Tracheobronchial and Pulmonary Adenoid Cystic Carcinomas. Acta Cytol 2017;61(1):77–83.

39. Roden AC, Greipp PT, Knutson DL, et al. Histopathologic and Cytogenetic Features of Pulmonary Adenoid Cystic Carcinoma. J Thorac Oncol 2015;10(11):1570–5.

40. Yatabe Y, Dacic S, Borczuk AC, et al. Best Practices Recommendations for Diagnostic Immunohistochemistry in Lung Cancer. J Thorac Oncol 2019; 14(3):377–407.

41. Song DH, Choi IH, Ha SY, et al. Epithelial-myoepthelial carcinoma of the tracheobronchial tree: The prognostic role of myoepithelial cells. Lung Cancer 2014;83(3):416–9.

42. Leduc C, Zhang L, Öz B, et al. Thoracic Myoepithelial Tumors. Am J Surg Pathol 2016;40(2):212–23.

43. Skálová A, Agaimy A, Vanecek T, et al. Molecular Profiling of Clear Cell Myoepithelial Carcinoma of Salivary Glands With EWSR1 Rearrangement Identifies Frequent PLAG1 Gene Fusions But No EWSR1 Fusion Transcripts. Am J Surg Pathol 2021; 45(1):1–13.

44. ElNaggar Adel K, Chan John KC, Grandis Jennifer R, et al. WHO classification of Head and Neck tumors. Lyon: IARC Press; 2017. p. 107.

45. Nakashima Y, Morita R, Ui A, Iihara K, Yazawa T. Epithelial-myoepithelial carcinoma of the lung: a case report. Surg Case Rep 2018;4(1):74.

46. Guleria P, Madan K, Kumar S, et al. Pulmonary epithelial myoepithelial carcinoma with papillary architecture: an uncommon morphology of a rare tumour. Pathology 2019;51(4):443–5.

47. Pelosi G, Fraggetta F, Maffini F, et al. Pulmonary Epithelial-Myoepithelial Tumor of Unproven Malignant Potential: Report of a Case and Review of the Literature. Mod Pathol 2001;14(5):521–6.

48. Urano M, Nakaguro M, Yamamoto Y, et al. Diagnostic Significance of HRAS Mutations in Epithelial-Myoepithelial Carcinomas Exhibiting a Broad Histopathologic Spectrum. Am J Surg Pathol 2019; 43(7):984–94.

49. Grosjean V, Fournel P, Picot T, et al. Hyalinizing clear cell carcinoma of the lung with EWSR1::CREM fusion. Histopathology 2023;83(2):333–5.

50. Takamatsu M, Sato Y, Muto M, et al. Hyalinizing clear cell carcinoma of the bronchial glands: presentation of three cases and pathological comparisons with salivary gland counterparts and bronchial mucoepidermoid carcinomas. Mod Pathol 2018;31(6):923–33.

51. Nicholson AG, Tsao MS, Beasley MB, et al. The 2021 WHO Classification of Lung Tumors: Impact of Advances Since 2015. J Thorac Oncol 2022;17(3): 362–87.

52. Thakur S, Nambirajan A, Larsen BT, et al. Primary Pulmonary Hyalinizing Clear Cell Carcinoma: Case Series With Review of Literature. Int J Surg Pathol 2022;1–8.

53. García JJ, Jin L, Jackson SB, et al. Primary pulmonary hyalinizing clear cell carcinoma of bronchial submucosal gland origin. Hum Pathol 2015;46(3): 471–5.

54. Zhang Y, Han W, Zhou J, et al. Primary lung hyalinizing clear cell carcinoma: a diagnostic challenge in biopsy. Diagn Pathol 2022;17(1):35.

55. Falk N, Weissferdt A, Kalhor N, et al. Primary Pulmonary Salivary Gland-type Tumors: A Review and Update. Adv Anat Pathol 2016;23(1):13–23.

Sarcoma of the Lung and Mediastinum

Ken-ichi Yoshida, MD, PhD[a], Akihiko Yoshida, MD, PhD[b,c],*

KEYWORDS

• Lung • Mediastinum • Sarcoma • Diagnosis

Key points

• Primary sarcoma of the lung and mediastinum is rare.

• The diagnosis requires careful exclusion of sarcomatoid carcinoma, sarcomatoid mesothelioma, and metastases from extra-thoracic sites.

• Immunohistochemical workups are usually necessary for diagnosis.

• Molecular investigations may be required in select cases.

ABSTRACT

Primary sarcoma of the lung and mediastinum is rare. The diagnosis requires careful exclusion of sarcomatoid carcinoma, sarcomatoid mesothelioma, and metastases from extra-thoracic sites. This review summarizes the key morphologic, immunohistochemical, and molecular characteristics of sarcomas that are encountered in the lung and mediastinum. The tumor types discussed are synovial sarcoma, well-differentiated/dedifferentiated liposarcoma, myxoid pleomorphic liposarcoma, intimal sarcoma of the pulmonary artery, inflammatory myofibroblastic tumor, epithelioid hemangioendothelioma, primary pulmonary myxoid sarcoma, malignant peripheral nerve sheath tumor, Ewing sarcoma, and *CIC*-rearranged sarcoma. Relevant differential diagnoses are also addressed.

sarcomatoid mesothelioma, especially when the phenotype is undifferentiated and not compatible with specific sarcoma types in elderly patients. Clinical information (eg, smoking history, asbestos exposure) and imaging should be reviewed and discussed with clinicians. Cohesive tumor clusters, glandular/papillary architecture, and keratinization should be sought. Keratin expression can be the only clue to suspect carcinoma/mesothelioma, and broad-spectrum keratins (eg, AE1/AE3, MNF116) should be liberally used, although true sarcoma can be extensively positive for keratin.[1] Thyroid transcription factor 1 (TTF1), p40, and claudin-4 are important positive markers of epithelial differentiation, whereas WT1 and HEG1 are useful mesothelial markers; however, the sensitivity of these markers is limited in sarcomatoid variants.[2,3] Metastatic sarcomas from extra-thoracic sites must also be ruled out. The presence of multiple nodules in the lung is suggestive of metastasis, although solitary metastasis is not uncommon. Rigorous history taking may be necessary because metastasis can occur many years after the resection of a primary sarcoma. This review summarizes the key histologic and molecular findings of the primary sarcoma

INTRODUCTION

Primary sarcoma of the lung and mediastinum is rare. The diagnosis requires careful exclusion of more common sarcomatoid carcinoma and

---

[a] Department of Diagnostic Pathology and Cytology, Osaka International Cancer Institute, Osaka, Japan;
[b] Department of Diagnostic Pathology, National Cancer Center Hospital, 5-1-1, Tsukiji, Chuo-ku, Tokyo 104-0045, Japan; [c] Rare Cancer Center, National Cancer Center, Tokyo, Japan
* Corresponding author.
E-mail address: akyoshid@ncc.go.jp

Surgical Pathology 17 (2024) 243–255
https://doi.org/10.1016/j.path.2023.11.008
1875-9181/24/© 2023 Elsevier Inc. All rights reserved.

types that are encountered in the lung and mediastinum.

SYNOVIAL SARCOMA

OVERVIEW

Synovial sarcoma (SS) is one of the most common types of primary sarcoma that arise in the thorax. Thoracic SSs occur in all ages, with a peak in the 4th to 5th decades of life. Thoracic SS shows a poorer prognosis than its soft tissue counterpart,[4–6] probably because of its late discovery and challenging diagnosis and resection. Pain and dyspnea are the most common symptoms.

MICROSCOPIC FINDINGS

SSs can be either monophasic or biphasic. Monophasic SS shows cellular fascicles of monomorphic spindle cells (Fig. 1A), whereas biphasic SS is composed of varying proportions of spindle and glandular epithelial components (Fig. 1B). The glands often contain eosinophilic secretions.

Monophasic SS involving the lung may entrap native pneumocytes, which should be distinguished from the biphasic pattern. The poorly differentiated pattern, which superimposes either on the monophasic or biphasic type, is characterized by high nuclear atypia, increased mitosis, necrosis, and/or round cell histology (Fig. 1C). Immunohistochemically, SS is at least focally positive for keratin, epithelial membrane antigen (EMA), TLE1, and CD99, although none of them is entirely specific. Most cases are negative for CD34. CD56 and synaptophysin can be positive. The epithelial component in biphasic SS is positive for claudin-4.[7] The poorly differentiated pattern can be negative for keratin. SS often demonstrates reduced SMARCB1 (INI1) expression.[8] The recently developed SS18::SSX fusion-specific antibody is highly sensitive and specific (Fig. 1D).[9]

MOLECULAR FINDINGS

SS harbors a specific chromosomal translocation, t(X;18)(p11;q11), resulting in *SS18::SSX1/2/4*

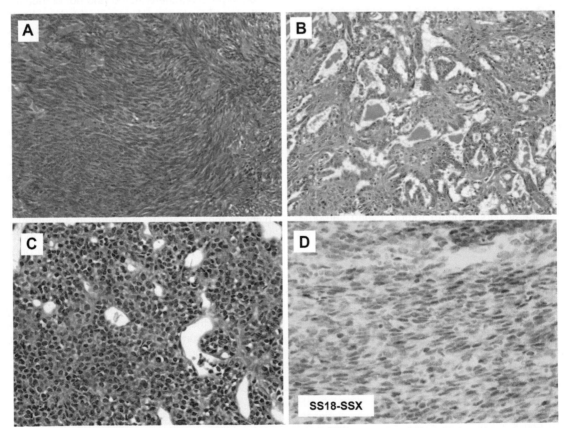

Fig. 1. Synovial sarcoma. (*A*) The monophasic variant shows fascicles of uniform long spindle cells. (*B*) The biphasic variant additionally demonstrates glands containing eosinophilic secretions. (*C*) The poorly differentiated pattern features small round cells. (*D*) Immunohistochemical reactivity using SS18::SSX fusion-specific antibody is useful for diagnosis.

fusions. Rare *SSX1* fusions to non-*SS18* partners have been reported.[10]

DIFFERENTIAL DIAGNOSIS

Malignant peripheral nerve sheath tumor (MPNST) often shows more pleomorphic cytology than SS, and the majority of the cases demonstrate the immunohistochemical loss of trimethylation at lysine 27 of histone 3 (H3K27me3). *Solitary fibrous tumor*, which usually affects the visceral pleura and will be discussed elsewhere in this volume, may rarely occur within the lung parenchyma or the mediastinum. The tumor often shows CD34 expression and is consistently positive for STAT6, reflective of *NAB2::STAT6* fusion. *Type A thymoma* is diffusely positive for p40. The differential diagnosis of biphasic SS includes *adenocarcinoma*, *pleomorphic carcinoma,* and *biphasic malignant mesothelioma*. Highly monotonous cytology and eosinophilic glandular secretion should prompt the consideration of SS. Poorly differentiated SS should be differentiated from other small round cell tumors (eg, *small cell carcinoma*, *Ewing sarcoma*). The detection of the specific fusion gene *SS18::SSX* or its protein product is the most reliable ancillary method.

LIPOSARCOMA

OVERVIEW

All liposarcoma subtypes have been reported in the thorax. Among them, well-differentiated/dedifferentiated liposarcoma (WD-/DD-LPS) is the most common, and myxoid pleomorphic liposarcoma characteristically affects the mediastinum.[11] These subtypes are described in detail. In general, mediastinal liposarcomas are large but may remain asymptomatic for long periods. Shortness of breath, cough, and pain are common symptoms.

WELL-DIFFERENTIATED/DEDIFFERENTIATED LIPOSARCOMA

WD-LPS is a locally aggressive tumor that has no metastatic potential unless it undergoes dedifferentiation. WD-LPS involving the thymus is sometimes referred to as "thymoliposarcoma" (**Fig.** 2A). Lipoma-like, sclerosing, and inflammatory patterns may coexist in a single tumor. The lipoma-like pattern is composed of mature adipocytes of varying sizes with irregular fibrous bands that harbor atypical stromal cells with hyperchromasia and pleomorphism. The sclerosing pattern comprises abundant fibrous stroma that may obscure the adipose tissue component. The inflammatory pattern features prominent lymphoplasmacytic, histiocytic, and/or neutrophilic infiltrates (**Fig.** 2B). DD-LPS arises from WD-LPS as a usually non-lipogenic, often high-grade sarcoma. The border with well-differentiated components can be abrupt or gradual. Dedifferentiated components frequently resemble undifferentiated pleomorphic sarcoma (**Fig.** 2C) or myxofibrosarcoma. Heterologous differentiation (eg, bone, cartilage, smooth muscle, skeletal muscle) may be present. Lipoblastic differentiation resembling pleomorphic liposarcoma may occur.[12] Immunohistochemistry for MDM2 and CDK4 is often positive in DD-LPS (**Fig.** 2D, E). However, the staining sensitivity for WD-LPS is variable. High-level *MDM2* amplification is a consistent finding of these types of liposarcoma and helps in difficult cases.

MYXOID PLEOMORPHIC LIPOSARCOMA

Myxoid pleomorphic liposarcoma is a newly recognized, extremely rare, and aggressive subtype that commonly affects children and adolescents with a predilection for the mediastinum.[11,13] Histologically, the tumor exhibits mixed histologic features of myxoid liposarcoma and pleomorphic liposarcoma. Most commonly, pleomorphic large lipoblastic cells are distributed among uniform smaller cells in the background of myxoid stroma and arborizing capillaries (**Fig.** 3). *TP53* and *RB1* are commonly altered,[15,16] resulting in p53 overexpression and Rb loss, respectively. *MDM2* amplification and *DDIT3* rearrangement are lacking, leading to negative MDM2 and DDIT3 staining, respectively. Genome-wide loss of heterozygosity is characteristic.[17]

DIFFERENTIAL DIAGNOSIS

WD-LPS should be distinguished from benign adipocytic neoplasms. *Lipoma* and *thymolipoma* lack atypical stromal cells. *Atypical spindle cell/pleomorphic lipomatous tumors*, which are rare in the mediastinum, typically show the loss of Rb expression.[18] *Fat-forming solitary fibrous tumor* is positive for STAT6. CD34 is commonly expressed in WD-LPS and is not helpful for differential diagnosis. The sclerosing and inflammatory patterns should be distinguished from non-neoplastic fibrosis, including *sclerosing mediastinitis* and *lymphoid neoplasm* by paying attention to scattered large atypical stromal cells. DD-LPS is mimicked by *undifferentiated pleomorphic sarcoma*, *myxofibrosarcoma*, *leiomyosarcoma*, and *MPNST*. The combined overexpression of MDM2 and CDK4 characterizes WD-LPS and DD-LPS. Isolated MDM2 positivity is a relatively nonspecific finding.[19] *MDM2* amplification may need to be confirmed in challenging cases. Myxoid

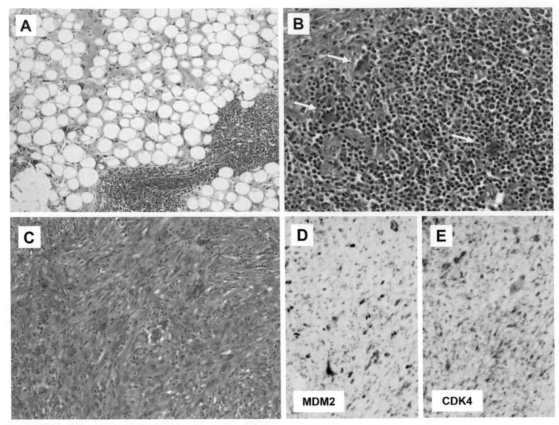

Fig. 2. Well-differentiated/dedifferentiated liposarcoma. (A) Lipoma-like well-differentiated liposarcoma involving the thymus ("thymoliposarcoma"). (B) The inflammatory pattern of well-differentiated liposarcoma contains massive inflammation and a few scattered atypical cells (arrows). (C) Dedifferentiated liposarcoma is often high-grade pleomorphic sarcoma. MDM2 (D) and CDK4 (E) immunohistochemical co-expression is characteristic.

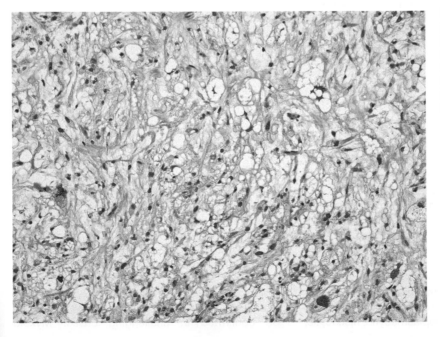

Fig. 3. Myxoid pleomorphic liposarcoma. The tumor demonstrates spindle cells within a myxoid and hypervascular stroma and harbors scattered large pleomorphic lipoblasts.

pleomorphic liposarcoma should be distinguished from myxoid liposarcoma, which is the most common liposarcoma type in children. Myxoid liposarcoma typically lacks pleomorphic cells and demonstrates *DDIT3* rearrangement and DDIT3 expression.[20]

INTIMAL SARCOMA

OVERVIEW

Intimal sarcoma (IS) is an aggressive sarcoma arising from the great vessels. Thoracic IS often involves the pulmonary artery and its branches. Recent evidence suggests that cardiac undifferentiated sarcomas, which often affect the left atrium, share similar genetic and epigenetic profiles with IS and are increasingly considered to represent cardiac "intimal" sarcoma.[21,22] IS occurs in patients with a mean age of 40 to 50 years and has a slight female predilection. The most common presenting symptom is dyspnea, followed by chest or back pain. The tumor may occlude the vascular lumen and result in pulmonary embolism, infarction, or pulmonary hypertension.

MICROSCOPIC FINDINGS

IS presents as an intraluminal mass attached to the vessel wall (**Fig. 4**A). The tumor often spreads along the vascular intima, and in most examples, the entire lumen is affected with or without focal extravascular components. The tumor consists of pleomorphic spindle cell proliferation with varying degrees of cytologic atypia and pleomorphism (**Fig. 4**B). Myxoid changes are common.[23] Although most of them are high-grade tumors, low-grade histology may be present. Heterologous differentiation (eg, bone, cartilage, skeletal muscle) is uncommon. Immunohistochemical profiles are inconsistent. However, the tumors overexpress MDM2 in greater than 70% of cases (**Fig. 4**C), which is reflective of the underlying *MDM2* amplification.[12,13]

MOLECULAR FINDINGS

MDM2, *CDK4*, *PDGFRA*, and *KIT* amplifications are highly recurrent.[24–26] *CDKN2A/B* loss can also be observed.

DIFFERENTIAL DIAGNOSIS

IS must be differentiated from the hematogenous spread of *metastatic sarcoma* from the somatic soft tissues, and clinical history is instrumental to differentiating between them. Correlation with imaging and operative findings is essential to confirm the intravascular/intracardiac location of the tumor. Immunohistochemical overexpression of MDM2 and CDK4 may support IS in an appropriate clinical context. However, it is not entirely sensitive, nor is it specific in relation to other *MDM2*-amplified sarcomas (eg, DD-LPS).

INFLAMMATORY MYOFIBROBLASTIC TUMOR

OVERVIEW

Inflammatory myofibroblastic tumor (IMT) is a rarely metastasizing intermediate neoplasm. IMT commonly involves the lung, whereas mediastinal examples are rare. Children and young adults are predominantly affected. Pulmonary tumors can cause chest pain and dyspnea, which may be associated with fever, weight loss, and malaise.

MICROSCOPIC FINDINGS

IMT consists of a fascicular proliferation of uniform spindle cells with amphophilic fibrillary cytoplasm. Nuclear atypia is often minimal and mitosis is uncommon. The stroma is variably myxoid or collagenous, rich in chronic inflammatory infiltrates (**Fig. 5**A). An aggressive variant, epithelioid inflammatory myofibroblastic sarcoma (EIMS), is characterized by the presence of epithelioid cells with large nucleoli and a prominent neutrophilic infiltrate (**Fig. 5**B),[27] although this is predilected to the abdominal cavity and rare in the thorax. Immunohistochemically, tumor cells are variably positive for smooth muscle actin and desmin. Keratin can be expressed, sometimes diffusely, in one-third of cases. *ALK*-rearranged IMT is positive for ALK (**Fig. 5**C), and the staining pattern depends on the *ALK* partners.[28] Sensitive ALK antibody clones (eg, 5A4, D5F3) are recommended for accurate detection.[28] *ROS1*-rearranged IMT shows ROS1 expression.[29]

MOLECULAR FINDINGS

ALK rearrangement occurs in ∼60% of IMT, more commonly in children and young adults. Numerous *ALK* partner genes have been identified. *RANBP2::ALK* or *RRBP1::ALK* fusions characterize EIMS, associated with a nuclear membranous/perinuclear cytoplasmic ALK expression,[27,30] respectively. *ROS1*, *NTRK3*, *RET*, or *PDGFRB* rearrangements are present in a subset.[28,31,32] Collectively, kinase fusions have been identified in ∼85% of IMT.[32] Alternative transcription initiation is another mechanism of *ALK* activation.[33] The kinase activation provides therapeutic opportunities with small-molecule inhibition in selected patients.

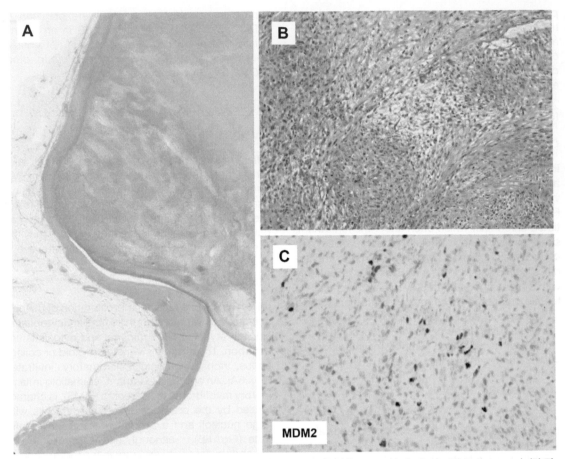

Fig. 4. Intimal sarcoma of the pulmonary artery. (A) The tumor arises from and is limited within the vessel. (B) The tumor shows pleomorphic spindle cell proliferation with focal myxoid features. (C) MDM2 immunostaining is positive.

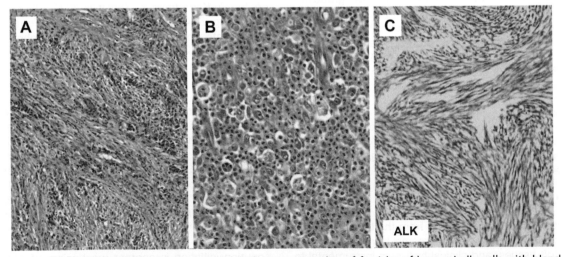

Fig. 5. Inflammatory myofibroblastic tumor. (A) The tumor consists of fascicles of long spindle cells with bland nuclei in the background of lymphoplasmacytic infiltration. (B) Epithelioid inflammatory myofibroblastic sarcoma showing scattered epithelioid cells within prominent neutrophilic infiltration. (C) Most tumors are positive for ALK, which is reflective of *ALK* rearrangement.

DIFFERENTIAL DIAGNOSIS

Organizing pneumonia is characterized by pale-staining fibroblastic nodules filling the peripheral airway (Masson bodies). *IgG4-related disease* typically harbors storiform fibrosis and obliterative phlebitis and it may occur alongside other manifestations (eg, autoimmune pancreatitis).[34,35] High serum IgG4 is a characteristic feature. The number of IgG4-positive plasma cells in tissues is increased; however, this alone is not sufficient for the diagnosis of IgG4-related disease. *Leiomyosarcoma* shows more eosinophilic cytoplasm, blunt-ended nuclei, greater nuclear atypia, and pleomorphism. The specific smooth muscle marker, h-caldesmon, is positive in most cases of leiomyosarcoma. However, a recently characterized *inflammatory leiomyosarcoma of the lung* is negative for h-caldesmon.[36] *Desmoid fibromatosis* shows less inflammation and aberrant nuclear β-catenin expression. A recently proposed *clear cell stromal tumor of the lung* may harbor prominent inflammation; however, it is characterized by at least focal cytoplasmic clearing and *YAP1::TFE3* fusion.[37] *Sarcomatoid carcinoma* with inflammation should be distinguished by coexisting classic carcinoma components.[38] Differential diagnosis should be facilitated by ALK or ROS1 immunohistochemistry. However, *ALK*-rearranged sarcomatoid carcinoma of the lung mimicking ALK-positive IMT is a rare pitfall.[39]

EPITHELIOID HEMANGIOENDOTHELIOMA

OVERVIEW

Epithelioid hemangioendothelioma (EHE) is a malignant vascular neoplasm. EHE commonly affects the lung, liver, bone, and soft tissue; however, any site can be involved. EHE in the lung was initially described as an "intravascular bronchiolo-alveolar tumor,"[40] and it often develops multiple bilateral nodules. EHE has a peak incidence in the 4th to 5th decade of life, and it has a female predilection. Thoracic EHE may cause pain, cough, dyspnea, or hemoptysis, but it can be asymptomatic.

MICROSCOPIC FINDINGS

Pulmonary EHE often consists of coalescent micropolypoid nodules that fill the alveolar spaces (**Fig. 6**A). They have variably chondromyxoid or hyaline stroma, with hypocellular centers and more cellular peripheries. Embedded within the matrix are cords or nests of epithelioid cells (**Fig. 6**B), with a glassy eosinophilic cytoplasm and occasional intracytoplasmic vacuoles ("blister cells"). Calcification/ossification may be present.

Angiocentric growth leading to vascular occlusion could be observed as well. A true vasoformative pattern is lacking in *WWTR1::CAMTA1*-positive EHEs, whereas *YAP1::TFE3*-positive tumors exhibit solid sheets of epithelioid cells with voluminous cytoplasms and well-formed vascular spaces. EHE usually shows few mitoses and mild nuclear atypia; however, in a minority of cases, there is increased cytologic atypia, high mitotic activity, and/or tumor cell necrosis (**Fig. 6**C), and these findings are associated with aggressive behaviors.[41] Immunohistochemically, EHEs are positive for endothelial markers, including ERG, CD31, CD34, FLI1, and D2-40. *CAMTA1*- and *TFE3*-rearranged EHE variants show diffuse nuclear expression of CAMTA1[42,43] (**Fig. 6**D) and TFE3,[44,45] respectively.

MOLECULAR FINDINGS

WWTR1::CAMTA1 fusion is the genetic hallmark of ~90% of EHE.[46,47] Less than 10% of cases harbor *YAP1::TFE3* fusions,[44,45] and a rare subset (often in the heart) harbors *WWTR1* fusions to non-*CAMTA1* genes.[41,48]

DIFFERENTIAL DIAGNOSIS

Unlike *pulmonary hamartoma* and *chondroma*, EHE does not show true hyaline cartilage. *Carcinoma, carcinoid,* and *mesothelioma* should be distinguished from EHE with hypercellular atypical histology using vascular endothelial markers (eg, ERG, CD31). Keratin may be positive in EHE. Synaptophysin can be expressed in aggressive EHEs, which can mimic large-cell neuroendocrine carcinoma.[41] The expression of claudin-4, TTF1, or p40 is not observed in EHE; however, HEG1, a marker for mesothelioma, can be expressed in EHE.[49] *Sclerosing pneumocytoma* consistently shows TTF1-positive round cells. CAMTA1 and TFE3 immunohistochemistry help exclude *angiosarcoma*, *pseudomyogenic hemangioendothelioma*, and *epithelioid hemangioma*, all of which may show epithelioid histology. *Metastatic epithelioid sarcoma*, which is often positive for CD34 and ERG, shows the loss of SMARCB1 expression.

PRIMARY PULMONARY MYXOID SARCOMA

OVERVIEW

Primary pulmonary myxoid sarcoma (PPMS) is an extremely rare, low-grade sarcoma occurring in the lungs of middle-aged adults with a slight female predilection.[50] Common symptoms include cough and hemoptysis; however, imaging studies may incidentally detect the tumors. Most PPMSs

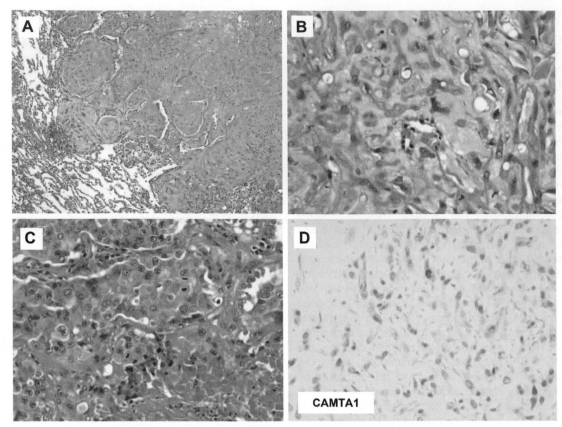

Fig. 6. Epithelioid hemangioendothelioma with *WWTR1::CAMTA1* fusion. (*A*) Pulmonary tumors often demonstrate micropolypoid growth filling the alveolar spaces. (*B*) The tumor shows the corded or isolated growth of epithelioid cells within myxohyaline stroma. (*C*) Atypical histologic features include high nuclear atypia, frequent mitosis, and necrosis. (*D*) The tumor is immunohistochemically positive for CAMTA1.

are indolent and cured by surgery, with rare examples developing recurrence or metastasis. The tumor has histologic and genetic overlap with the myxoid variant of angiomatoid fibrous histiocytoma, which fuels nosologic controversy.[51,52] Angiomatoid fibrous histiocytoma of conventional type can also occur in the lung.[53]

MICROSCOPIC FINDINGS

PPMS exhibits a characteristic multinodular growth composed of spindle, stellate, or polygonal cells in a reticular or cord-like pattern within an abundant myxoid stroma (Fig. 7). Most tumors involve the central airway, often showing endobronchial growth. Peripheral fibrosis or a fibrous pseudocapsule may be noted. Lymphoplasmacytic infiltration of varying degrees is a common finding. Mild to moderate cytologic atypia or focal necrosis can be present, and mitoses are few. Immunohistochemically, tumor cells are often

focally positive for EMA but negative for S100 protein and desmin.

MOLECULAR FINDINGS

Most PPMSs harbor *EWSR1::CREB1* fusion.[50,54] The alternative *EWSR1::ATF1* fusion has rarely been reported.[52,55]

DIFFERENTIAL DIAGNOSIS

Metastatic *extraskeletal myxoid chondrosarcoma* shows more eosinophilic cytoplasm, focal reactivity to S100 protein and/or neuroendocrine markers (eg, INSM1, synaptophysin), and *NR4A3* fusion. *Myoepithelial tumor* tends to show more heterogeneous myxohyaline stroma, and it often tests positive for keratin, S100 protein, and muscle markers, with a subset harboring *EWSR1* rearrangement.[56] *Pulmonary tumors with notochordal differentiation* show mucoid stroma and the corded growth of

Fig. 7. Primary pulmonary myxoid sarcoma. The tumor shows the reticular growth of uniform spindle cells within an abundant myxoid stroma.

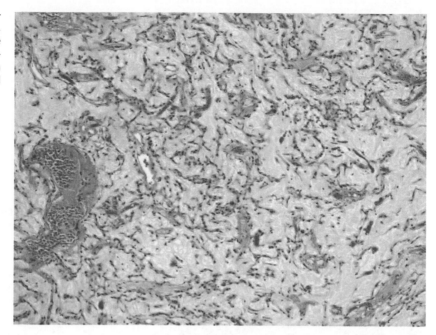

bland epithelioid cells that are positive for keratin, S100 protein, and brachyury.[57,58]

OTHER SARCOMAS

MALIGNANT PERIPHERAL NERVE SHEATH TUMOR

MPNST can occur from a peripheral nerve in the mediastinum (eg, phrenic nerve, vagus nerve) or a preexisting neurofibroma. The tumor may be neurofibromatosis type 1-associated, sporadic, or radiation-induced. The tumor consists of swirling fascicles of mildly pleomorphic spindle cells in alternating cellularity (**Fig. 8**A). Conventional MPNST can be focally positive for S100 or SOX10; however, both are negative in many cases. The complete loss of H3K27me3 is observed in ~60% of MPNST cases (**Fig. 8**B), which reflects the underlying mutations in *EED* or *SUZ12*,[59,60] although H3K27me3 loss is not entirely specific for MPNST.[61] As a differential diagnosis, *cellular schwannoma* and *neurofibroma* with atypical features diffusely express S100 and SOX10 and retain H3K27me3 expression. *Leiomyosarcoma* is reactive for smooth muscle markers (eg, smooth muscle actin, desmin, h-caldesmon).

EWING SARCOMA

Ewing sarcoma is characterized by diffuse sheets of uniform small round cells (**Fig. 9**A). The tumor cells often demonstrate diffuse strong membranous reactivity to CD99 (**Fig. 9**B). NKX2.2 and PAX7 are more specific markers, and the combination of these three markers usually provides distinction from other small round cell mimics.[62] Neuroendocrine marker expression (eg, synaptophysin, INSM1) is variable. The genetic hallmark is *EWSR1/FUS::ETS* fusion. As a differential diagnosis, *small cell carcinoma* shows less uniform cytology, darker chromatin, and molding, whereas TTF1 is often positive and Rb loss is frequent. Keratin expression in ~30% of cases of Ewing sarcoma and focal NKX2.2 positivity in a subset of small cell carcinoma are pitfalls.[62] *Neuroblastoma* is often positive for PHOX2B.[63,64] *NUT carcinoma*, which often harbors *BRD4/3::NUTM1* fusion, is characterized by the diffuse speckled reactivity of NUT protein.[65]

CIC-REARRANGED SARCOMA

CIC-rearranged sarcoma most often harbors *CIC::DUX4* fusion and is characterized by diffuse sheets of relatively uniform but mildly pleomorphic round-to-epithelioid cells (**Fig. 10**). Focal myxoid changes are common. The tumors are immunohistochemically positive for ETV4 and WT1 and negative for NKX2.2.[62] Differentials include *carcinoma*, *mesothelioma*, *Ewing sarcoma*, *germ cell tumor*, and *lymphoma*. *Thoracic SMARCA4-deficient undifferentiated tumor*, now mostly considered as an undifferentiated/dedifferentiated form of non-small cell lung carcinoma, is defined by SMARCA4 loss, often along with SMARCA2 loss and variable reactivity to SALL4, SOX2, and CD34.[66,67]

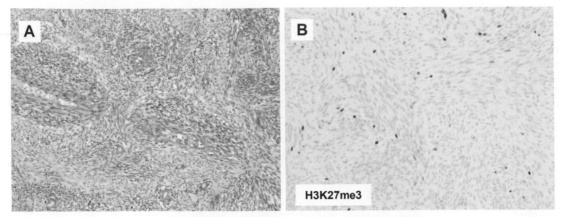

Fig. 8. Malignant peripheral nerve sheath tumor. (*A*) The tumor consists of swirling fascicles of spindle cells with frequent perivascular hypercellularity. (*B*) The loss of trimethylation at lysine 27 of histone 3 is observed in the majority of cases.

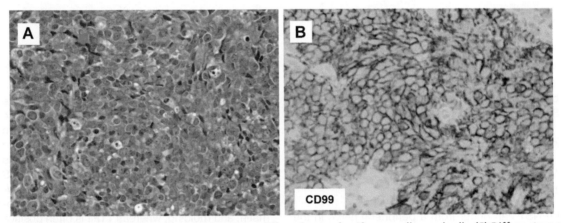

Fig. 9. Ewing sarcoma. (*A*) The tumor demonstrates diffuse sheets of uniform small round cells. (*B*) Diffuse strong membranous reactivity of CD99 is characteristic.

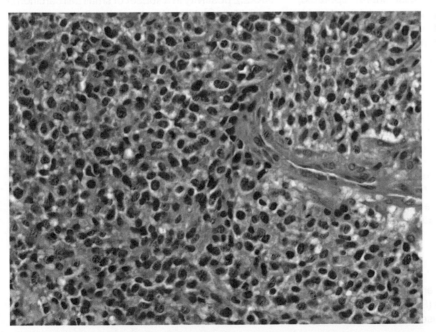

Fig. 10. CIC-rearranged sarcoma. The tumor forms diffuse sheets of relatively uniform but mildly pleomorphic round cells.

CLINICS CARE POINTS

- Primary sarcoma is rare in the lung and mediastinum.

- Sarcomatoid carcinoma, sarcomatoid mesothelioma, and metastatic sarcoma from extra-thoracic sites are much more common and should be carefully excluded before primary sarcoma is considered.

- Immunohistochemical workups are usually necessary for diagnosis.

- Molecular investigations may be required in select cases.

DISCLOSURE

This work was supported in part by JSPS, Japan KAKENHI, Japan (Grant Numbers JP21K06919). The authors have nothing to disclose pertaining to this work.

REFERENCES

1. Iwata J, Fletcher CD. Immunohistochemical detection of cytokeratin and epithelial membrane antigen in leiomyosarcoma: a systematic study of 100 cases. Pathol Int 2000;50:7–14.

2. Churg A, Naso JR. Hypothesis: HEG1 and claudin-4 staining will allow a diagnosis of epithelioid and biphasic mesothelioma versus non-small-cell lung carcinoma with only two stains in most cases. Histopathology 2023;82:385–92.

3. Hiroshima K, Wu D, Koh E, et al. Membranous HEG1 expression is a useful marker in the differential diagnosis of epithelioid and biphasic malignant mesothelioma versus carcinomas. Pathol Int 2021;71:604–13.

4. Bégueret H, Galateau-Salle F, Guillou L, et al. Primary intrathoracic synovial sarcoma: A clinicopathologic study of 40 t(X;18)-positive cases from the French Sarcoma Group and the Mesopath Group. Am J Surg Pathol 2005;29:339–46.

5. Hartel PH, Fanburg-Smith JC, Frazier AA, et al. Primary pulmonary and mediastinal synovial sarcoma: A clinicopathologic study of 60 cases and comparison with five prior series. Mod Pathol 2007;20:760–9.

6. Lan T, Chen H, Xiong B, et al. Primary pleuropulmonary and mediastinal synovial sarcoma: A clinicopathologic and molecular study of 26 genetically confirmed cases in the largest institution of southwest China. Diagn Pathol 2016;11:1–14.

7. Ordonez NG. Value of claudin-4 immunostaining in the diagnosis of mesothelioma. Am J Clin Pathol 2013;139:611–9.

8. Ito J, Asano N, Kawai A, et al. The diagnostic utility of reduced immunohistochemical expression of SMARCB1 in synovial sarcomas: a validation study. Hum Pathol 2016;47:32–7.

9. Baranov E, McBride MJ, Bellizzi AM, et al. A Novel SS18-SSX Fusion-specific Antibody for the Diagnosis of Synovial Sarcoma. Am J Surg Pathol 2020; 44:922–33.

10. Yoshida A, Arai Y, Satomi K, et al. Identification of novel SSX1 fusions in synovial sarcoma. Mod Pathol 2022;35:228–39.

11. Boland JM, Colby TV, Folpe AL. Liposarcomas of the mediastinum and thorax: A clinicopathologic and molecular cytogenetic study of 24 cases, emphasizing unusual and diverse histologic features. Am J Surg Pathol 2012;36:1395–403.

12. Mariño-Enríquez A, Fletcher CDM, Cin PD, et al. Dedifferentiated liposarcoma with "homologous" lipoblastic (pleomorphic liposarcoma-like) differentiation: clinicopathologic and molecular analysis of a series suggesting revised diagnostic criteria. Am J Surg Pathol 2010; 34:1122–31.

13. Alaggio R, Coffin CM, Weiss SW, et al. Liposarcomas in young patients: a study of 82 cases occurring in patients younger than 22 years of age. Am J Surg Pathol 2009;33:645–58.

15. Creytens D, Folpe AL, Koelsche C, et al. Myxoid pleomorphic liposarcoma—a clinicopathologic, immunohistochemical, molecular genetic and epigenetic study of 12 cases, suggesting a possible relationship with conventional pleomorphic liposarcoma. Mod Pathol 2021;34:2043–9.

16. Hofvander J, Jo VY, Ghanei I, et al. Comprehensive genetic analysis of a paediatric pleomorphic myxoid liposarcoma reveals near-haploidization and loss of the RB1 gene. Histopathology 2016;69:141–7.

17. Dermawan JK, Hwang S, Wexler L, et al. Myxoid pleomorphic liposarcoma is distinguished from other liposarcomas by widespread loss of heterozygosity and significantly worse overall survival: a genomic and clinicopathologic study. Mod Pathol 2022;35:1644–55.

18. Marino-Enriquez A, Nascimento AF, Ligon AH, et al. Atypical spindle cell lipomatous tumor: clinicopathologic characterization of 232 cases demonstrating a morphologic spectrum. Am J Surg Pathol 2017;41: 234–44.

19. Binh MB, Sastre-Garau X, Guillou L, et al. MDM2 and CDK4 immunostainings are useful adjuncts in diagnosing well-differentiated and dedifferentiated liposarcoma subtypes: a comparative analysis of 559 soft tissue neoplasms with genetic data. Am J Surg Pathol 2005;29:1340–7.

20. Scapa JV, Cloutier JM, Raghavan SS, et al. DDIT3 Immunohistochemistry Is a Useful Tool for the Diagnosis of Myxoid Liposarcoma. Am J Surg Pathol 2021;45:230–9.

21. Koelsche C, Benhamida JK, Kommoss FKF, et al. Intimal sarcomas and undifferentiated cardiac sarcomas carry mutually exclusive MDM2, MDM4, and CDK6 amplifications and share a common DNA methylation signature. Mod Pathol 2021;34: 2122–9.

22. Neuville A, Collin F, Bruneval P, et al. Intimal sarcoma is the most frequent primary cardiac sarcoma: clinicopathologic and molecular retrospective analysis of 100 primary cardiac sarcomas. Am J Surg Pathol 2014;38:461–9.

23. Yamada Y, Kinoshita I, Miyazaki Y, et al. Myxoid type and non-myxoid type of intimal sarcoma in large vessels and heart: review of histological and genetic profiles of 20 cases. Virchows Arch 2022;480:919–25.

24. Bode-Lesniewska B, Zhao J, Speel EJM, et al. Gains of 12q13-14 and overexpression of mdm2 are frequent findings in intimal sarcomas of the pulmonary artery. Virchows Arch 2001;438:57–65.

25. Dewaele B, Floris G, Finalet-Ferreiro J, et al. Coactivated platelet-derived growth factor receptor {alpha} and epidermal growth factor receptor are potential therapeutic targets in intimal sarcoma. Cancer Res 2010;70:7304–14.

26. Koyama T, Shimizu T, Kojima Y, et al. Clinical activity and exploratory resistance mechanism of milademetan, an MDM2 inhibitor, in intimal sarcoma with MDM2 amplification: an open-label phase 1b/2 study. Cancer Discov 2023;3:1814–25.

27. Mariño-Enríquez A, Wang WL, Roy A, et al. Epithelioid inflammatory myofibroblastic sarcoma: An aggressive intra-abdominal variant of inflammatory myofibroblastic tumor with nuclear membrane or perinuclear ALK. Am J Surg Pathol 2011;35:135–44.

28. Yamamoto H, Yoshida A, Taguchi K, et al. ALK, ROS1 and NTRK3 gene rearrangements in inflammatory myofibroblastic tumours. Histopathology 2016;69:72–83.

29. Hornick JL, Sholl LM, Dal Cin P, et al. Expression of ROS1 predicts ROS1 gene rearrangement in inflammatory myofibroblastic tumors. Mod Pathol 2015;28: 732–9.

30. Lee JC, Li CF, Huang HY, et al. ALK oncoproteins in atypical inflammatory myofibroblastic tumours: novel RRBP1-ALK fusions in epithelioid inflammatory myofibroblastic sarcoma. J Pathol 2017;241:316–23.

31. Antonescu CR, Suurmeijer AJH, Zhang L, et al. Molecular characterization of inflammatory myofibroblastic tumors with frequent ALK and ROS1 gene fusions and rare novel RET rearrangement. Am J Surg Pathol 2015;39:957–67.

32. Lovly CM, Gupta A, Lipson D, et al. Inflammatory myofibroblastic tumors harbor multiple potentially actionable Kinase fusions. Cancer Discov 2014;4: 889–95.

33. Chang JC, Zhang L, Drilon AE, et al. Expanding the molecular characterization of thoracic inflammatory myofibroblastic tumors beyond ALK gene rearrangements. J Thorac Oncol 2019;14:825–34.

34. Zen Y, Kitagawa S, Minato H, et al. IgG4-positive plasma cells in inflammatory pseudotumor (plasma cell granuloma) of the lung. Hum Pathol 2005;36: 710–7.

35. Matsui S, Hebisawa A, Sakai F, et al. Immunoglobulin G4-related lung disease: clinicoradiological and pathological features. Respirology 2013;18:480–7.

36. Kao YC, Kuo CT, Kuo PY, et al. Pulmonary "inflammatory leiomyosarcomas" are indolent tumors with diploid genomes and no convincing rhabdomyoblastic differentiation. Am J Surg Pathol 2022;46: 424–33.

37. Agaimy A, Stoehr R, Michal M, et al. Recurrent YAP1-TFE3 gene fusions in clear cell stromal tumor of the lung. Am J Surg Pathol 2021;45:1541–9.

38. Wick MR, Ritter JH, Nappi O. Inflammatory sarcomatoid carcinoma of the lung: report of three cases and clinicopathologic comparison with inflammatory pseudotumors in adult patients. Hum Pathol 1995; 26:1014–21.

39. Mason EF, Fletcher CD, Sholl LM. 'Inflammatory myofibroblastic tumour'-like dedifferentiation of anaplastic lymphoma kinase-rearranged lung adenocarcinoma. Histopathology 2016;69:510–5.

40. Dail DH, Liebow AA, Gmelich JT, et al. Intravascular, bronchiolar, and alveolar tumor of the lung (IVBAT) an analysis of twenty cases of a peculiar sclerosing endothelial tumor. Cancer 1983;51:452–64.

41. Shibayama T, Makise N, Motoi T, et al. Clinicopathologic characterization of epithelioid hemangioendothelioma in a series of 62 cases: a proposal of risk stratification and identification of a synaptophysin-positive aggressive subset. Am J Surg Pathol 2021;45:616–26.

42. Shiba E, Harada H, Yabuki K, et al. CAMTA1 is a useful immunohistochemical marker for diagnosing epithelioid haemangioendothelioma. Histopathology 2015;67:827–35.

43. Doyle LA, Fletcher CDM, Hornick JL. Nuclear expression of CAMTA1 distinguishes epithelioid hemangioendothelioma from histologic mimics. Am J Surg Pathol 2016;40:94–102.

44. Antonescu CR, Le Loarer F, Mosquera JM, et al. Novel YAP1-TFE3 fusion defines a distinct subset of epithelioid hemangioendothelioma. Genes Chromosomes Cancer 2013;52:775–84.

45. Dermawan JK, Azzato EM, Billings SD, et al. YAP1-TFE3-fused hemangioendothelioma: a multi-institutional clinicopathologic study of 24 genetically-confirmed cases. Mod Pathol 2021;34:2211–21.

46. Errani C, Zhang L, Sung YS, et al. A novel WWTR1-CAMTA1 gene fusion is a consistent abnormality in epithelioid hemangioendothelioma of different anatomic sites. Genes Chromosomes Cancer 2011; 50:644–53.

47. Tanas MR, Sboner A, Oliveira AM, et al. Identification of a disease-defining gene fusion in epithelioid hemangioendothelioma. Sci Transl Med 2011;3.

48. Suurmeijer AJH, Dickson BC, Swanson D, et al. Variant WWTR1 gene fusions in epithelioid hemangioendothelioma-A genetic subset associated with cardiac involvement. Genes Chromosomes Cancer 2020;59:389–95.

49. Tsuji S, Washimi K, Kageyama T, et al. HEG1 is a novel mucin-like membrane protein that serves as a diagnostic and therapeutic target for malignant mesothelioma. Sci Rep 2017;7:45768.

50. Thway K, Nicholson AG, Lawson K, et al. Primary pulmonary myxoid sarcoma with EWSR1-CREB1 fusion: a new tumor entity. Am J Surg Pathol 2011;35:1722–32.

51. Smith SC, Palanisamy N, Betz BL, et al. At the intersection of primary pulmonary myxoid sarcoma and pulmonary angiomatoid fibrous histiocytoma: Observations from three new cases. Histopathology 2014; 65:144–6.

52. Gui H, Sussman RT, Jian B, et al. Primary pulmonary myxoid sarcoma and myxoid angiomatoid fibrous histiocytoma: A unifying continuum with shared and distinct features. Am J Surg Pathol 2020;44:1535–40.

53. Thway K, Nicholson AG, Wallace WA, et al. Endobronchial pulmonary angiomatoid fibrous histiocytoma: two cases with EWSR1-CREB1 and EWSR1-ATF1 fusions. Am J Surg Pathol 2012;36:883–8.

54. Jeon YK, Moon KC, Park SH, et al. Primary pulmonary myxoid sarcomas with EWSR1-CREB1 translocation might originate from primitive peribronchial mesenchymal cells undergoing (myo)fibroblastic differentiation. Virchows Arch 2014;465:453–61.

55. Nishimura T, Ii T, Inamori O, et al. Primary pulmonary myxoid sarcoma with EWSR1::ATF1 fusion: a case report. Int J Surg Pathol 2022;31:88–91.

56. Leduc C, Zhang L, Oz B, et al. Thoracic myoepithelial tumors: a pathologic and molecular study of 8 cases with review of the literature. Am J Surg Pathol 2016;40:212–23.

57. Kikuchi Y, Yamaguchi T, Kishi H, et al. Pulmonary tumor with notochordal differentiation: report of 2 cases suggestive of benign notochordal cell tumor of extraosseous origin. Am J Surg Pathol 2011;35: 1158–64.

58. Kikuchi Y, Nakatani Y, Yamaguchi T. Where is the primary site of the extra-axial chordoma masquerading as lung cancer? Clin Lung Cancer 2021;22:e655–7.

59. Asano N, Yoshida A, Ichikawa H, et al. Immunohistochemistry for trimethylated H3K27 in the diagnosis of malignant peripheral nerve sheath tumours. Histopathology 2017;70:385–93.

60. Prieto-Granada CN, Wiesner T, Messina JL, et al. Loss of H3K27me3 expression is a highly sensitive marker for sporadic and radiation-induced MPNST. Am J Surg Pathol 2016;40:479–89.

61. Makise N, Sekimizu M, Konishi E, et al. H3K27me3 deficiency defines a subset of dedifferentiated chondrosarcomas with characteristic clinicopathological features. Mod Pathol 2019;32:435–45.

62. Yoshida A. Ewing and Ewing-like sarcomas: A morphological guide through genetically-defined entities. Pathol Int 2023;73:12–26.

63. Nonaka D, Wang BY, Edmondson D, et al. A study of gata3 and phox2b expression in tumors of the autonomic nervous system. Am J Surg Pathol 2013;37: 1236–41.

64. Hung YP, Lee JP, Bellizzi AM, et al. PHOX2B reliably distinguishes neuroblastoma among small round blue cell tumours. Histopathology 2017;71:786–94.

65. Haack H, Johnson LA, Fry CJ, et al. Diagnosis of NUT midline carcinoma using a NUT-specific monoclonal antibody. Am J Surg Pathol 2009;33:984–91.

66. Yoshida A, Kobayashi E, Kubo T, et al. Clinicopathological and molecular characterization of SMARCA4-deficient thoracic sarcomas with comparison to potentially related entities. Mod Pathol 2017;30:797–809.

67. Rekhtman N, Montecalvo J, Chang JC, et al. SMARCA4-deficient thoracic sarcomatoid tumors represent primarily smoking-related undifferentiated carcinomas rather than primary thoracic sarcomas. J Thorac Oncol 2020;15:231–47.

Nonmesothelial Spindle Cell Tumors of Pleura and Pericardium

Huihua Li, MD, PhD[a], Aliya N. Husain, MD[b],
David Moffat, MD[c], Sonja Klebe, MD, PhD[c],*

KEYWORDS

• Sarcomatoid mesothelioma • Spindle cell tumor • Pleura • Pericardium • Sarcoma • Metastasis

---

Key points

- Description of most common nonmesothelial spindle cell tumors involving pleura and pericardium
- Practice points for distinguishing mesothelioma from nonmesothelial spindle cell tumors of pleura and pericardium
- Clinical significance of nonmesothelial spindle cell tumors of pleura and pericardium

---

ABSTRACT

Spindle cell lesions of the pleura and pericardium are rare. Distinction from sarcomatoid mesothelioma, which has a range of morphologic patterns, can be difficult, but accurate diagnosis matters. This article provides practical guidance for the diagnosis of pleural spindle cell neoplasms, focusing on primary lesions.

OVERVIEW

Despite its anatomic and histologic simplicity relative to its close neighbor, the lung, many primary tumors and tumor-like lesions occur in the pleura. Most are rare, and this article focuses on the spindle-cell lesions that cause diagnostic difficulty because of their overlapping morphologic features and immunohistochemical profiles. The differences in prognosis; advances in treatment options, with targeted therapies being available for some of the selected conditions; and medicolegal implications mean that accurate diagnosis is critical. This article focuses on those conditions that may mimic sarcomatoid mesothelioma, especially primary pleural tumors and some of the metastatic malignancies that affect the pleura. **Table 1** summarizes clinical and histopathological features of sarcomatoid mesothelioma and nonmesothelial spindle cell tumors of pleura.

The importance of clinical information cannot be overstated; metastases to the pleura are more common than primary tumors, and this includes metastases from sarcomas. Clinical suspicion for mesothelioma may be high if there is known asbestos exposure, but the history of exposure by itself does not play a significant role for diagnosis. Both mesothelioma and lung cancer can be induced by asbestos; mesotheliomas may occur in patients with no (known) history of exposure to asbestos, and tumors unrelated to asbestos exposure may occur in asbestos-exposed individuals. The diagnosis of a cytokeratin-negative sarcomatoid mesothelioma may be a probabilistic diagnosis if all other diagnostic avenues have been exhausted and the alternatives excluded.

GROSS FEATURES, INCLUDING RADIOLOGICAL FEATURES

At the time of diagnosis, pathologists typically rely on radiological features as a surrogate for macroscopic appearance. Importantly, imaging findings

[a] Department of Pathology, Duke University Medical Center, Durham, NC 27710, USA; [b] Department of Pathology, University of Chicago, Chicago, IL 60637, USA; [c] Department of Anatomical Pathology, SA Pathology and Flinders University, Flinders Medical Centre, Bedford Park, South Australia 5042, Australia
* Corresponding author.
E-mail address: Sonja.Klebe@sa.gov.au

Surgical Pathology 17 (2024) 257–270
https://doi.org/10.1016/j.path.2024.01.001

Table 1
Summary of clinical and histopathologic features for spindle cell tumors of pleura and pericardium

	Clinical Features	Histologic Features	Immunohistochemistry Practical Points	Molecular Alterations
Sarcomatoid mesothelioma	Adults; diffuse nodularity; solitary nodules; rare	Variable morphology; paucicellular cases dominated by storiform fibrosis (desmoplastic variant)	CK + ve; variably + ve for D2-40, Calretinin, and WT1; GATA3 commonly + ve; SMA ± ve; TLE1 ± ve; FLI1+ve; Loss of MTAP > BAP1	Mutations in TP53, NF2, and CDKN2A; TMB typically low
Sarcomatoid carcinoma	Adults; may mimic mesothelioma radiologically and clinically		CK + ve; Claudin-4 ± ve; Calretinin can be +ve	TMB typically high
SFT benign/malignant	Adults	variable cellularity; patternless growth; staghorn vessels; collagenous stroma	CD34 and STAT6 +ve; maybe CD99 +ve; CK -ve; GATA3 +ve[a]	NAB2-STAT6 fusion; TERT promoter mutations may affect prognosis
EHE	Adults; large mass; bloody effusions	Variably pleomorphic; occasional myxoid stroma; sometimes with heterologous elements	CD31 is the most specific vascular marker; use at least 2 vascular markers; MDM2 and CDK4 +ve in most cases	Amplification of 12q13-15 including MDM2
Angiosarcoma	Adults; large mass; bloody effusions; rapidly progressive; Hx of radiation	Spindle to epithelioid cells; pleomorphism	CD31 is the most specific vascular marker; use at least 2 vascular markers; beware of FLI1 (+ve in 95% of mesotheliomas); maybe CK + ve	TMB may be low
IMT	Typically in young adults	Loose fascicles of spindle cells; mixed inflammatory infiltrate; edematous to myxoid stroma	+ve for ALK, ROS1, or pan-TRK; CK −/+ve; SMA −/+ve	ALK fusion most common; seldom fusion of ROS1, RET, PDGFRB or NTRK3
Desmoid fibromatosis	Adults; female predilection; clinical history if FAP	Elongated fascicles of uniform spindle cells; thin-walled vessels with perivascular edema	Nuclear β-catenin staining in 80% of cases; SMA + ve; CK -ve	CTNNB1 somatic mutation; rarely APC germline mutation

Synovial sarcoma	Young adult; deep soft tissues of extremities, pleura, or other sites	Monophasic: fascicles of spindle cells; biphasic: admixture of spindle and epithelioid components; poorly differentiated: mimic other small round blue cell tumors	+ve for *SS18-SSX* fusion-specific IHC; TLE1, CD99, EMA, GATA3, Calretinin maybe + ve	*SS18* fusion to one of the *SSX* genes
Dedifferentiated liposarcoma	Adults	Nonlipogenic sarcoma ± well differentiated liposarcoma	STAT6 may be +ve	*MDM2* amplification
CIC-rearranged sarcoma	Typically in young adults		Maybe Calretinin + ve	CIC-translocation
PPMS/PAFH	Young to middle aged; may involve pleura/appear to arise from pleura	Lobulated architecture; myxoid stroma (DDx mesothelioma); spindle or polygonal tumor cells in cord-like or reticulated pattern with mild-to-moderate atypia	CK-ve; vascular markers -ve; desmin + ve; EMA + ve	*EWSR1-CREB1EWSR1-ATF1*
Pleomorphic sarcoma (previously called MFH)	Any age	Prominent pleomorphism throughout the tumor	Positive stains not typically contributory; CK -ve	TMB low
SMARCA4 deficient undifferentiated tumor	Adults; smoking history		Claudin 4 -ve	*SMARCA4* deficient

Abbreviations: CK, cytokeratin; DDx, Differential diagnosis; EHE, epithelioid hemangioendothelioma; FAP, familial adenomatous polyposis; Hx, History; IMT, inflammatory myofibroblastic tumor; MFH, malignant fibrous histiocytoma; -ve, Negative; +ve, Positive; PAFH, pulmonary angiomatoid fibrous histiocytoma; PPMS, primary pulmonary myxoid sarcoma; SFT, solitary fibrous tumor; TMB, Tumor mutation burden.
[a] Small case numbers.

may be nonspecific (**Fig.** 1A); rather it is disease evolution that provides critical clues to diagnosis.[1] Malignant pleural thickening is typically nodular (>1 cm), often with circumferential involvement, and may involve the mediastinal pleura. However, pseudomesotheliomatous carcinoma is well recognized (**Fig.** 1B). Localized mesotheliomas are rare but do occur. Some of the other conditions discussed here are typically well-circumscribed solitary lesions (**Fig.** 1C, D).[2] Fluorine-18 fluorodeoxyglucose positron emission tomography-computed tomography (18F-FDG PET-CT) cannot reliably differentiate benign from malignant pleural thickening, or differentiate primary from secondary malignancy. Pleural plaques may be calcified or noncalcified and can present as focal areas of pleural thickening. The presence or absence of distant or lymph node metastases at the time of diagnosis is not a useful discriminator; metastasis in mesothelioma is often clinically underrecognized but is in fact common, with extrapleural dissemination found in 87.7% and

lymph node involvement in 53.3% of 318 autopsy cases, with tumor dissemination in extra thoracic sites in 55.4%, including liver (31.9%), spleen (10.8%), thyroid (6.9%), and the brain (3.0%).[3] Imaging and macroscopic appearances may be helpful but must be interpreted in conjunction with pathology assessment.

MICROSCOPIC FEATURES

Sarcomatoid mesothelioma shows a wide range of appearances, ranging from highly pleomorphic (**Fig.** 2A, B) to bland, hypercellular to paucicellular (**Fig.** 2D). Most sarcomatoid mesotheliomas show expression of cytokeratins, but expression of calretinin is variable (30% to 79%), with positive labeling for CK5/6 seen in only 29%, and podoplanin (D2-40) in 51% to 57% of sarcomatoid mesotheliomas.[4–6] Labeling for WT1 can be helpful, but there is heterogeneity of results with this antibody, which may be related to different clones and protocols used. Molecular investigations have

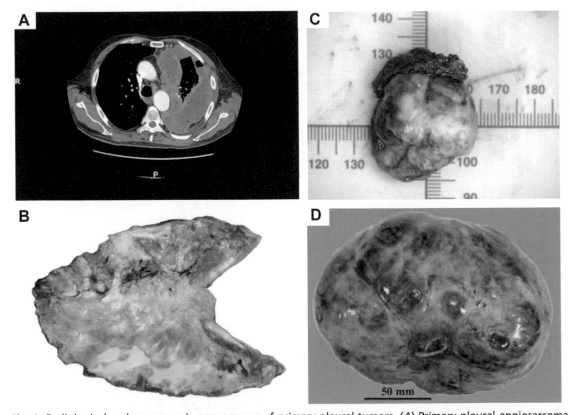

Fig. 1. Radiological and macroscopic appearances of primary pleural tumors. (*A*) Primary pleural angiosarcoma presenting with circumferential pleural thickening, mimicking mesothelioma. (*B*) Pseudomesotheliomatous carcinoma infiltrating chest wall and in between ribs, with calcified pleural plaques indicative of above-background asbestos exposure also being present. (*C*) Pleural localized mesothelioma is rare but may present as resectable solitary mass. (*D*) Solitary fibrous tumor presenting as well-circumscribed lesion. Note the typical pedicle containing a vascular leash at the bottom of the lesion.

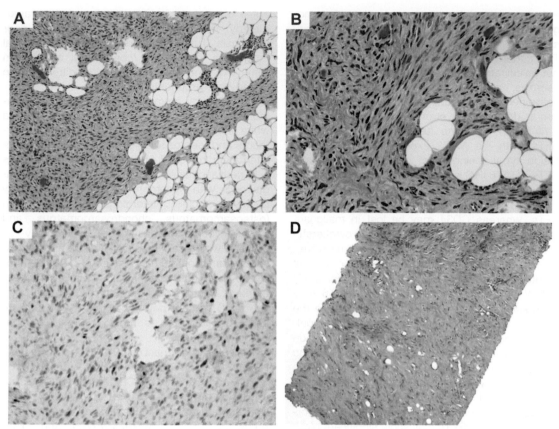

Fig. 2. Pleural sarcomatoid mesothelioma showing a wide range of morphologic appearances. (*A, B*) Pleomorphic, hypercellular sarcomatoid mesothelioma infiltrating into the adipose tissue (low and high magnifications). (*C*) Neoplastic mesothelial cells are extensively positive for GATA3. (*D*) Desmoplastic mesothelioma composed of bland spindle cells with haphazard growth pattern and separated by dense collagenous stroma.

advanced since a diagnostic algorithm was suggested by the International Mesothelioma Panel,[7] and additional markers have been explored, most notably GATA3, BAP1, and *CDKN2A/ MTAP*. GATA3 was initially used for identifying breast and urothelial carcinomas, but recent studies suggest its use for sarcomatoid mesothelioma diagnosis, with labeling reported in 58% to 100% of cases.[8–10] Labeling for GATA3 is not entirely specific for sarcomatoid mesothelioma, as these studies also reported labeling in 15% to 47% of sarcomatoid carcinomas[10,11] and some solitary fibrous tumors. Diffuse labeling for GATA3 (Fig. 2C) in the appropriate clinical context can support a diagnosis of mesothelioma, but the reverse does not apply; lack of labeling for GATA3 does not exclude a diagnosis of mesothelioma.

Sarcomatoid mesothelioma commonly shows *CDKN2A* homozygous deletion, and MTAP immunohistochemistry (IHC) is increasingly used as a surrogate for this somatic variant. However, *CDKN2A* deletion is not specific for mesothelioma and may be seen in other types of tumors,

including sarcomas[12] and inflammatory myofibroblastic tumors.[13] Deletion of *CDKN2A* in isolation is not diagnostic of sarcomatoid mesothelioma. The same applies for BAP1; loss of labeling indicates malignancy at the molecular level, and may be useful as part of a panel, but it is not specific for mesothelioma.

PRIMARY PLEURAL TUMORS

SOLITARY FIBROUS TUMOR

Solitary fibrous tumors (SFTs) are rare localized spindle-cell fibroblastoid neoplasms. Intrathoracic SFTs are typically pedunculated and arise from the visceral pleura (~80%) (see Fig. 1D). Their size ranges from a few millimeters to more than 400 mm in diameter and several kilograms in weight.[14] They arise at any age, but incidence peaks between the fourth and sixth decades of life, SFTs are rare under the age of 10. SFTs may be symptomatic because of hypoglycemia related to production of insulin-like growth factor (Doege-

Potter syndrome), have symptoms related to tumor growth, or be discovered incidentally. Morphology may vary in different areas of the same tumor. The patternless pattern of Stout is best known, but calcification, ossification, cystic degeneration, necrosis, and hemorrhage are common, and entrapped mesothelium may lead to misinterpretation as desmoplastic stroma in mesothelioma.

NAB2-STAT6 gene fusions are diagnostic of SFTs, with the NAB2 exon 4-STAT6 exon 2/3 fusion types being most common for thoracic SFTs. STAT6 IHC is a sensitive and specific surrogate for all STAT6 gene fusions. Positive labeling for STAT6 is present in benign and malignant SFTs, whereas CD34 may be lost in malignant SFTs. The fibroblastoid cells lack cytokeratin (CK) expression (present in sarcomatoid mesotheliomas, including localized ones). Other positive markers include vimentin and less consistently BCL-2 and CD99.[15,16] Importantly, STAT6 may be present in other mesenchymal lesions in the thorax, including desmoid fibromatosis and pulmonary artery intimal sarcoma, and correlation with imaging is essential.[17,18] STAT6 fusion testing may be required to resolve difficult cases. SFTs may also show labeling for CD117.[19] Schwannomas may mimic SFTs morphologically but can be excluded by lack of labeling for S-100. Importantly, malignant SFTs may show significant pleomorphism, and SFTs are not exclusive to the thorax/pleural metastasis from extrathoracic SFTs (Fig. 3).

The reported rates of malignancy in SFT range from 10.3% to 57%.[20,21] A meta-analysis of studies using criteria proposed by England and colleagues showed an unexpectedly high rate of malignancy of 29.0%.[22] Factors most consistently linked to adverse prognosis include a mitotic count greater than 4 per 10 high power fields, tumor size greater than 10 cm, necrosis, hypercellularity, cellular atypia, dedifferentiation, sessile tumor, invasion of adjacent structures, and areas of overtly sarcomatous tissue. TERT promoter mutations and presence of pleural effusions may also be significant for prognosis. There are no evidence-based treatment guidelines, but the data suggest long-term surveillance after surgical resection of SFT, even after complete resection. Models for risk stratification are still under investigation.[23]

MALIGNANT PERIPHERAL NERVE SHEATH TUMOR

Malignant peripheral nerve sheath tumor (MPNST) is derived from Schwann cells and often arises from a pre-existing benign nerve sheath tumor or in a patient with neurofibromatosis type 1 (NF1),

but it may occur in sporadically or after radiotherapy. These are aggressive tumors with poor prognosis. Tumor size greater than 5 cm, local recurrence, high-grade morphology, association with NF1, and rhabdomyoblastic differentiation are adverse prognostic factors.[24]

In the pleura, metastatic MPNST is more common than a primary.[25] Tumors show typically a white and fleshy cut surface, with areas of hemorrhage and necrosis. Microscopically, there are alternating hypocellular and hypercellular areas with perivascular accentuation composed of spindle cells with hyperchromatic, wavy, or focally buckled nuclei. Heterologous differentiation (osteosarcomatous, chondrosarcomatous, and rhabdomyosarcomatous components) may be present, which can cause confusion, as it is also seen in sarcomatoid mesothelioma.[26] The heterologous elements label for their appropriate markers. Immunohistochemistry is typically positive for S100 and patchily for SOX10. Complete loss of H3K27me3 is more common in high-grade MPNSTs.

The epithelioid variant of MPNST is not associated with NF1; it shows diffuse staining for S100 and SOX10 and loss of SMARCB1 expression, resulting in INI1 loss. In contrast, conventional MPNSTs show frequent and concurrent inactivating mutations in 3 pathways: NF1, CDKN2A/CDKN2B, and PRC2 core components (EED or SUZ12).

EPITHELIOID HEMANGIOENDOTHELIOMA

Epithelioid haemangioendothelioma (EHE) is included here, because despite its name, it may show spindle cells areas (which may be the only sampled component in a small biopsy). It is a distinctive malignant angioformative neoplasm, with the neoplastic cells often arranged as solid sheets or in a linear fashion, embedded in a hyaline or myxohyaline stroma.[27] The most common presentation is with pleural thickening and effusion, mimicking mesothelioma, secondary malignancy, and benign pleural fibrosis. It is more common in males, and histories of radiation or asbestos exposure are reported.[28] Abortive vascular differentiation may be found, and the neoplastic cells may possess empty-appearing intracytoplasmic vacuoles, nuclear inclusions, or myxoid stroma. Typically, tumors show WWTR1-CAMTA1 or YAP1-TFE3 fusion.

ANGIOSARCOMA

Pleural angiosarcoma is extremely rare, with fewer than 60 reported cases,[29] and may be metastatic or primary (see Fig. 1A; Fig. 4), but it is the most

Fig. 3. Metastatic solitary fibrous tumor (SFT) presenting in pleura. The patient had a history of SFT in the thigh 5 years prior to presentation with a pleural mass. (*A*) H&E appearance showing significant pleomorphism. (*B*) Positive labeling for STAT6 in metastatic SFT in pleura.

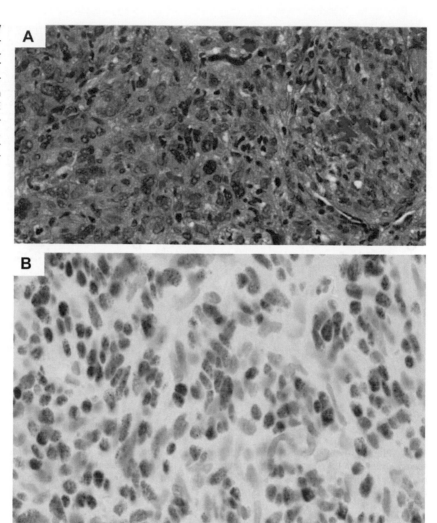

common primary cardiac sarcoma. Associated effusions are hemorrhagic, and the tumor shows a fleshy and hemorrhagic cut surface. The vasoformative nature of the tumor may be demonstrated morphologically or by immunohistochemistry. Tumor cells may appear biphasic. At least 1 positive immunohistochemical marker of vascular differentiation (CD31, ERG, CD34, Factor VIII, or FLI-1) is required to for the diagnosis of angiosarcoma, but the authors suggest use of at least 2 vascular markers. CD31 is the most sensitive and specific immunohistochemical marker, and the authors advise caution with the use of FLI-1, which is positive in 95% of mesotheliomas.[30] Mesothelioma may also occasionally show vasoformation and express vascular markers, but areas typical of mesothelioma are usually found elsewhere.[31] Epithelial markers including CAM5.2, CK7, CK8, and CK18 may be expressed; expression is typically focal and more common in epithelioid variants.

These markers may also be positive in hemangioendothelioma and are typically positive in mesothelioma. Radiation/lymphoedema-associated angiosarcomas are typically MYC-positive. Survival is poor, similar to mesothelioma, and both respond to immunotherapy, so clinical progression or therapy response is less useful as an aid for distinction.[28,32]

INFLAMMATORY MYOFIBROBLASTIC TUMOR

Inflammatory myofibroblastic tumor (IMT) shows intermediate malignant potential and a tendency for local recurrence with rare reports of distant metastases. Cytokeratin reactivity is not uncommon in IMTs.[33] Although ALK mutation is the hallmark of IMT, rare pleural (and more commonly peritoneal) mesotheliomas show ALK rearrangement.[34] IMTs may harbor *CDKN2A* deletions,[13] as do some other sarcomas.[12] Morphology, lack of

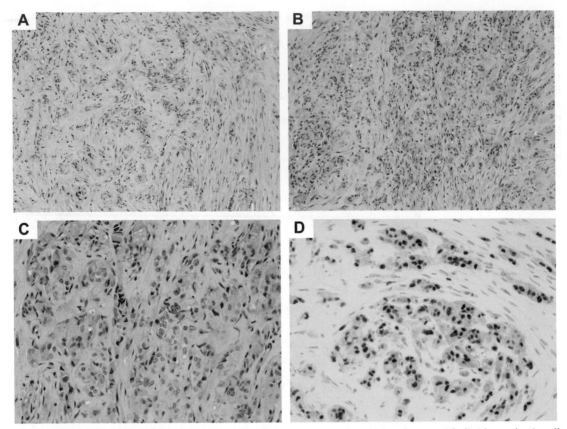

Fig. 4. Pleural involvement of metastatic epithelioid angiosarcoma. (*A, B*) The plump epithelioid neoplastic cells form vague vascular channels, some of which contain erythrocytes (low and intermediate magnifications). (*C*) The neoplastic cells have abundant eosinophilic cytoplasm and prominent nucleoli (high magnification). (*D*) ERG nuclear staining is positive in malignant cells.

infiltration, and clinical behavior can help in diagnosis of IMT, and the prominent inflammatory infiltrate in conjunction with ALK expression would be unusual for mesothelioma. IMTs are characterized by a relatively bland proliferation of myofibroblastic spindle cells in a loose mixed or hyaline stroma, with an associated mixed inflammatory infiltrate. Mitoses may be present, including atypical ones, and the appearances may be reminiscent of nodular fasciitis type (**Fig. 5**).

DESMOID FIBROMATOSIS

Desmoid tumors of the chest wall are well recognized in the literature and may impinge on the pleura, but primary desmoid tumors of the pleura are extremely rare. They may occur at any age,[35] and be large or small, and the cut surface is bosselated firm and white. The lesions typically extend into fat or skeletal muscle, and the most useful IHC marker is β-catenin; however, they also label for vimentin, smooth muscle and muscle-specific actin, and desmin, whereas CD34 and S-100 are

negative[36] (**Fig. 6**, patient with desmoid and subsequent sarcomatoid mesothelioma 9 years later).

SYNOVIAL SARCOMA

Synovial sarcoma (SS) is characterized by a distinctive t(X;18) chromosomal translocation with the fusion genes, *SYT-SSX1* or *SYT-SSX2*.[37] Typical pleural SS occurs at a younger age (mean approximately 44 years) than pleural mesothelioma. Pleural SS is sometimes surrounded by a fibrous pseudocapsule and often shows cystic degeneration, but multinodularity and diffuse growth occur. At a practical level, the authors consider that a clear and confident diagnosis of pleural SS requires demonstration of the t(X;18) translocation, which is not found in mesothelioma,[38] and for fluorescence in situ hybridization (FISH)-negative cases other molecular methods should be considered that may be more sensitive.[39,40] The value of IHC for distinction from mesothelioma is somewhat limited, since both mesothelioma and SS may label for cytokeratins, calretinin, and TLE1.[41,42] SS

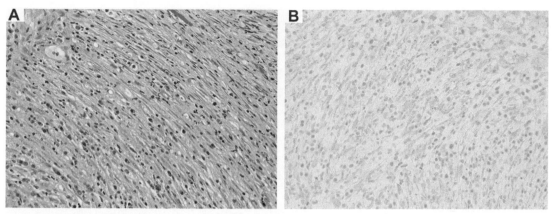

Fig. 5. Intrathoracic inflammatory myofibroblastic tumor (IMT). (*A*) Spindle-shaped neoplastic cells admixed with lymphoplasmacytic inflammatory cells. (*B*) The neoplastic cells have weak ALK cytoplasmic staining. Molecular studies demonstrated *EML4-ALK* fusion.

comprises 2 histologic subtypes: monophasic or biphasic. Monophasic SS is entirely composed of monotonous ovoid to spindle cells (**Fig. 7**)[43] whereas the biphasic subtype is composed of both spindle and epithelial components.

EXTRAGASTROINTESTINAL STROMAL TUMOR OF THE PLEURA

Extragastrointestinal stromal tumors (EGISTs) of the pleura are exceedingly rare[44] and thought to arise from the interstitial cell of Cajal (ICC) or

ICC-like cells. Correct diagnosis is important, as (depending on the mutation present) tumors may respond to imatinib.[45] Patients are young to middle-aged, and the lesions are well-circumscribed, with a tan-pink, fleshy, focal hemorrhagic and necrotic cut surface.[46] Tumors exhibit varied morphology including spindle-cell shaped (70%), epithelioid, and mixed type, and dedifferentiated EGISTs may appear anaplastic. The most helpful IHC markers are cKIT (CD117), but cKIT may also be positive in some mesotheliomas[19] and DOG1. SDHB loss can be

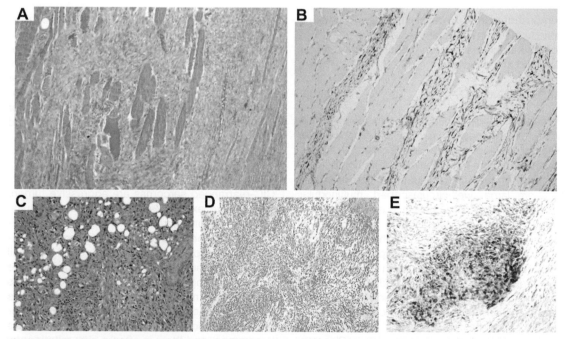

Fig. 6. Images from the same patient who presented with a desmoid fibromatosis (*A*) in the chest wall. This tumor showed β-catenin labeling (*B*). Nine years later, the patient had another chest wall lesion, which was sarcomatoid mesothelioma, (*C*) showing labeling for pancytokeratin (*D*) and calretinin (*E*).

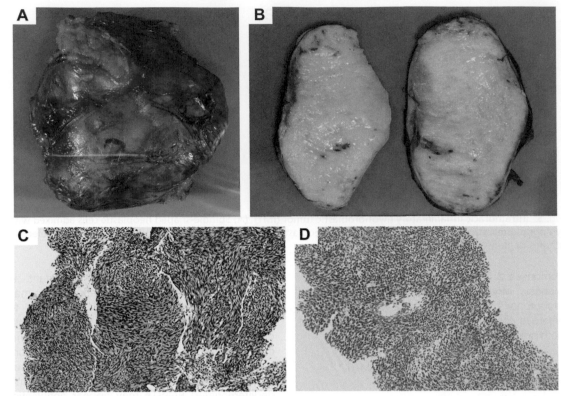

Fig. 7. A large anterior mediastinal synovial sarcoma. (*A, B*) This pedunculated large anterior mediastinal mass (12.5 cm) showing tan-white fleshy cut surface with focal necrosis. Biopsy demonstrated monotonous spindle cell proliferation (*C*) with TLE1 immunostaining diffusely positive (*D*). Molecular studies showed *SS18-SSX1* fusion, which confirmed the diagnosis of synovial sarcoma.

demonstrated in *SDH*-deficient GISTs. The lesions may be recurrent and can metastasize, and prognostic parameters include mitotic activity, tumor size, and anatomic site.[47]

LIPOSARCOMA

Primary pleural liposarcoma, including well-differentiated liposarcoma, myxoid liposarcoma, pleomorphic liposarcoma, and dedifferentiated liposarcoma, is rare but is the most common primary sarcoma of the mediastinum.[48] Macroscopically they are large, well-circumscribed, multinodular masses, and their heterogeneity is evident on imaging studies. In well-differentiated liposarcoma, a fibrillary sclerotic background or chronic inflammatory background may be seen. Lipoblasts are not required for diagnosis. Distinction from pleural lipoma requires IHC for MDM2. Dedifferentiated liposarcoma shows an abrupt transition to high-grade sarcoma, whereas myxoid liposarcoma contains a mixture of spindle cells, lipoblasts, myxoid stroma, and thin-walled chicken wire vasculature. Pleomorphic liposarcoma is a high-grade sarcoma with multivacuolated pleomorphic lipoblasts. MDM2

and/or CDK4 nuclear expression is present in well-differentiated and dedifferentiated liposarcomas, and *MDM2* and/or *CDK4* gene amplification may be shown by molecular studies, whereas *DDIT3* gene rearrangement (*FUS-DDIT3* or *EWSR1-DDIT3* gene fusion) is seen in in myxoid liposarcoma. All mediastinal liposarcomas have poor prognosis, characterized by local recurrences and metastatic disease.[48,49]

CIC-REARRANGED SARCOMA

CIC-rearranged sarcomas are aggressive tumors that involve extraskeletal sites in young adults, usually extremities or the trunk, although a rare primary pleural origin is reported.[50] Ewing sarcoma-like tumors typically have a small round blue cell appearance, but the CIC-rearranged tumors have a more heterogeneous cytology with focal areas of spindle cell morphology. Other variable features include myxoid stroma, lobulated growth, nucleolar prominence, and clear cytoplasm. Necrosis is common, and there is often a high mitotic rate. Immunohistochemically, they tend to exhibit patchy positivity for CD99. WT1, FLI-1 and ETV4

Table 2
Immunohistochemical studies for distinguishing pleural mesothelioma from most common non-mesothelial spindle cell tumors

Spindle Cell Tumors	Keratin	Calretinin/D2-40/WT1	GATA3	S100/SOX10	STAT6	ALK	β-catenin	TLE-1	CD117/DOG1	MDM2	CD31/ERG	Claudin-4	HMB45/MelanA
Sarcomatoid mesothelioma	+/−	+/−	+ (more diffuse)	−	−	−	−/(+)	+/−	−/(+)	−	−	−/+	−
SFT	−	−	−/+	+	+	−	−	−	−/(+)	−	−	−	−
MPNST	−/(+)	−	−	+ (focal)	−	−	−	−	−	−	−	−	−
EHE	−/(+)	−	−	−	−	−	−	−	−	−	+	−	−
Angiosarcoma	−/(+)	−	−	−	−	−	−	−	−	−	+	−	−
IMT	−/(+)	−	−	−	−	+	−	−	−	−	−	−	−
Desmoid	−	−	−	−	−/(+)	−	+	−	−	−	−	−	−
Synovial sarcoma	−/(+)	−	−	−	−	−	−	+	−	−	−	−	−
EGIST of the pleura	−	−	−	−	−	−	−	−	+	−	−	−	−
Liposarcoma	−	−	−	−	−	−	−	−	−	+	−	−	−
Sarcomatoid carcinoma	+	−/Calretinin+	+/−	−	−	−	−	−	−	−	−	+	−
Metastatic RCC	+	−	−	−	−	−	−	−	−	−	−	+/−	−
Metastatic melanoma	−	−	−	+	−	−	−	−	−	−	−	−	+

Abbreviations: EGIST: extragastrointestinal stromal tumor; EHE: epithelioid hemangioendothelioma; IMT: inflammatory myofibroblastic tumor; MPNST: malignant peripheral nerve sheath tumor; RCC: renal cell carcinoma; SFT: solitary fibrous tumor.

are often positive. Calretinin, NUT, and TLE1 positivity is also described, a potential diagnostic pitfall. Ninety-five percent of cases have a *DUX4* gene fusion partner, while other fusion partners include *FOXO4*, *LEUTX*, *NUTM1*, and *NUTM2A*.

PRIMARY PULMONARY MYXOID SARCOMA/ANGIOMATOID FIBROUS HISTIOCYTOMA

Primary pulmonary myxoid sarcoma (PPMS) and pulmonary angiomatoid fibrous histiocytoma (PAFH) have overlapping clinicopathological, morphologic, and molecular features.[51] They are multinodular tumors that have a variably myxoid stroma and lymphoid cuff, and they may involve the pleura. PAFH is usually positive immunohistochemically for EMA and Desmin, although these markers are more variable in PPMS. Both entities are negative for cytokeratins. Most harbor an *EWSR1-CREB1* fusion, while an *EWSR1-ATF1* fusion is found in others (particularly PAFH). PPMS is regarded as a low-grade malignant tumor that rarely metastasizes while PAFH follows a benign course.

METASTASES

Metastases are far more common in the pleura than primary tumors, but a detailed discussion is beyond the scope of this article. Suffice it to say that metastatic malignant melanoma and sarcomatoid renal cell carcinoma may be especially challenging on small biopsies, not least because they may show loss of BAP1 and MTAP. Most commonly used immunohistochemical markers for renal cell carcinoma such as PAX8, CAIX,[52] and CD10 can also be positive in sarcomatoid mesothelioma. Clinical history is essential for all cases of metastatic pleural malignancy.

SUMMARY

Spindle cell lesions of the pleura and pericardium comprise a spectrum of benign and malignant tumors and a range of reactive conditions (not discussed in this article). Their diagnosis is challenging but critical because of important prognostic, therapeutic, and medicolegal implications for the patient. This article described how pathologists can be aided by ancillary techniques (with summary of immunohistochemical studies for most common pleural spindle cell tumors in **Table 2**), particularly in relation to increasing knowledge of molecular events in these fascinating lesions.

CLINICS CARE POINTS

- History of asbestos exposure is not diagnostic of mesothelioma.
- GATA3 may be useful for diagnosis of sarcomatoid mesothelioma but may also label sarcomatoid carcinoma and SFTs.
- *CDKN2A*/MTAP and BAP1 may be helpful as part of a panel, but loss of either is not specific for mesothelioma.
- TLE1 may label mesothelioma and cannot replace molecular studies for t(x:18), which are required for definitive diagnosis of synovial sarcoma.
- Angiosarcomas may label for cytokeratins, and mesothelioma may label for vascular markers. Molecular studies may be helpful.
- Cytokeratin-negative mesothelioma exists but is a diagnosis of exclusion.

DISCLOSURE

S. Klebe prepares medicolegal reports on diagnosis and causation of asbestos-related disease to the courts and tribunals of Australia.

REFERENCES

1. Desimpel J, Vanhoenacker FM, Carp L, et al. Tumor and tumorlike conditions of the pleura and juxtapleural region: review of imaging findings. Insights Imaging 2021;12(1):97.
2. Kobashi Y, Matsushima T, Irei T. Clinicopathological analysis of lung cancer resembling malignant pleural mesothelioma. Respirology 2005;10(5):660–5.
3. Finn RS, Brims FJH, Gandhi A, et al. Postmortem findings of malignant pleural mesothelioma: a two-center study of 318 patients. Chest 2012;142(5):1267–73.
4. Oramas DM, Zaleski M, Moran CA. Sarcomatoid mesothelioma: a clinicopathological and immunohistochemical study of 64 cases. Int J Surg Pathol 2021;29(8):820–5.
5. Husain AN, Colby TV, Ordonez NG, et al. Guidelines for pathologic diagnosis of malignant mesothelioma 2017 update of the consensus statement from the International Mesothelioma Interest Group. Arch Pathol Lab Med 2018;142(1):89–108.
6. Klebe S, Brownlee NA, Mahar A, et al. Sarcomatoid mesothelioma: a clinical-pathologic correlation of 326 cases. Mod Pathol 2010;23(3):470–9.

7. Marchevsky AM, LeStang N, Hiroshima K, et al. The differential diagnosis between pleural sarcomatoid mesothelioma and spindle cell/pleomorphic (sarcomatoid) carcinomas of the lung: evidence-based guidelines from the International Mesothelioma Panel and the MESOPATH National Reference Center. Hum Pathol 2017;67:160–8.

8. Miettinen M, McCue PA, Sarlomo-Rikala M, et al. GATA3: a multispecific but potentially useful marker in surgical pathology: a systematic analysis of 2500 epithelial and nonepithelial tumors. Am J Surg Pathol 2014;38(1):13–22.

9. Prabhakaran S, Hocking A, Kim C, et al. The potential utility of GATA binding protein 3 for diagnosis of malignant pleural mesotheliomas. Hum Pathol 2020;105:1–8.

10. Berg KB, Churg A. GATA3 Immunohistochemistry for distinguishing sarcomatoid and desmoplastic mesothelioma from sarcomatoid carcinoma of the lung. Am J Surg Pathol 2017;41(9):1221–5.

11. Terra S, Roden AC, Aubry MC, et al. Utility of immunohistochemistry for MUC4 and GATA3 to aid in the distinction of pleural sarcomatoid mesothelioma from pulmonary sarcomatoid carcinoma. Arch Pathol Lab Med 2021;145(2):208–13.

12. Lucchesi C, Khalifa E, Laizet Y, et al. Targetable alterations in adult patients with soft-tissue sarcomas: insights for personalized therapy. JAMA Oncol 2018; 4(10):1398–404.

13. Bennett JA, Croce S, Pesci A, et al. Inflammatory myofibroblastic tumor of the uterus: an immunohistochemical study of 23 cases. Am J Surg Pathol 2020; 44(11):1441–9.

14. Chang YL, Lee YC, Wu CT. Thoracic solitary fibrous tumor: clinical and pathological diversity. Lung Cancer 1999;23(1):53–60.

15. Doyle LA, Vivero M, Fletcher CD, et al. Nuclear expression of STAT6 distinguishes solitary fibrous tumor from histologic mimics. Mod Pathol 2014;27(3): 390–5.

16. Tsubochi H, Endo T, Sogabe M, et al. Solitary fibrous tumor of the thymus with variegated epithelial components. Int J Clin Exp Pathol 2014;7(11):7477–84.

17. Demicco EG, Harms PW, Patel RM, et al. Extensive survey of STAT6 expression in a large series of mesenchymal tumors. Am J Clin Pathol 2015; 143(5):672–82.

18. Hassan A SP, Connor J, Kingston N, et al. Pulmonary artery intimal sarcoma presenting as lung mass. Human Pathology Reports 2023;31:300694.

19. Butnor KJ, Burchette JL, Sporn TA, et al. The spectrum of Kit (CD117) immunoreactivity in lung and pleural tumors: a study of 96 cases using a single-source antibody with a review of the literature. Arch Pathol Lab Med 2004;128(5):538–43.

20. Bylicki O, Rouviere D, Cassier P, et al. Assessing the multimodal management of advanced solitary fibrous tumors of the pleura in a routine practice setting. J Thorac Oncol 2015;10(2):309–15.

21. Guo W, Xiao HL, Jiang YG, et al. Retrospective analysis for thirty-nine patients with solitary fibrous tumor of pleura and review of the literature. World J Surg Oncol 2011;9:134.

22. Mercer RM, Wigston C, Banka R, et al. Management of solitary fibrous tumours of the pleura: a systematic review and meta-analysis. ERJ Open Res 2020;6(3).

23. Ricciardi S, Giovanniello D, Carbone L, et al. Malignant solitary fibrous tumours of the pleura are not all the same: analysis of long-term outcomes and evaluation of risk stratification models in a large single-centre series. J Clin Med 2023;12(3).

24. Le Guellec S, Decouvelaere AV, Filleron T, et al. Malignant peripheral nerve sheath tumor is a challenging diagnosis: a systematic pathology review, immunohistochemistry, and molecular analysis in 160 patients from the French Sarcoma Group Database. Am J Surg Pathol 2016;40(7):896–908.

25. Amrith BP, Pasricha S, Jajodia A, et al. A rare case of malignant peripheral nerve sheath tumor of pleura and review of literature. Indian J Pathol Microbiol 2021;64(1):158–60.

26. Klebe S, Mahar A, Henderson DW, et al. Malignant mesothelioma with heterologous elements: clinicopathological correlation of 27 cases and literature review. Mod Pathol 2008;21(9):1084–94.

27. Hammar SP, Henderson DW, Klebe S, et al. In: Neoplasms of the pleuraDail and hammar's pulmonary pathology. 3rd edition. New York: Springer; 2008.

28. Zhang PJ, Livolsi VA, Brooks JJ. Malignant epithelioid vascular tumors of the pleura: report of a series and literature review. Hum Pathol 2000;31(1):29–34.

29. Sedhai YR, Basnyat S, Golamari R, et al. Primary pleural angiosarcoma: case report and literature review. SAGE Open Med Case Rep 2020;8, 2050313X20904595.

30. Hui S, Guo-Qi Z, Xiao-Zhong G, et al. IMP3 as a prognostic biomarker in patients with malignant peritoneal mesothelioma. Hum Pathol 2018;81:138–47.

31. Pulford E, Hocking A, Griggs K, et al. Vasculogenic mimicry in malignant mesothelioma: an experimental and immunohistochemical analysis. Pathology 2016; 48(7):650–9.

32. Wang X, Wei J, Zeng Z, et al. Primary pleural epithelioid angiosarcoma treated successfully with anti-PD-1 therapy: a rare case report. Medicine (Baltim) 2021;100(35):e27132.

33. Harik LR, Merino C, Coindre JM, et al. Pseudosarcomatous myofibroblastic proliferations of the bladder: a clinicopathologic study of 42 cases. Am J Surg Pathol 2006;30(7):787–94.

34. Hung YP, Dong F, Watkins JC, et al. Identification of ALK rearrangements in malignant peritoneal mesothelioma. JAMA Oncol 2018;4(2):235–8.

35. Wilson RW, Gallateau-Salle F, Moran CA. Desmoid tumors of the pleura: a clinicopathologic mimic of localized fibrous tumor. Mod Pathol 1999;12(1): 9–14.

36. Andino L, Cagle PT, Murer B, et al. Pleuropulmonary desmoid tumors: immunohistochemical comparison with solitary fibrous tumors and assessment of beta-catenin and cyclin D1 expression. Arch Pathol Lab Med 2006;130(10):1503–9.

37. Henderson DW, Reid G, Kao SC, et al. Challenges and controversies in the diagnosis of malignant mesothelioma: part 2. Malignant mesothelioma subtypes, pleural synovial sarcoma, molecular and prognostic aspects of mesothelioma, BAP1, aquaporin-1 and microRNA. J Clin Pathol 2013; 66(10):854–61.

38. Weinbreck N, Vignaud JM, Begueret H, et al. SYT-SSX fusion is absent in sarcomatoid mesothelioma allowing its distinction from synovial sarcoma of the pleura. Mod Pathol 2007;20(6):617–21.

39. Begueret H, Galateau-Salle F, Guillou L, et al. Primary intrathoracic synovial sarcoma: a clinicopathologic study of 40 t(X;18)-positive cases from the French Sarcoma Group and the Mesopath Group. Am J Surg Pathol 2005;29(3):339–46.

40. Stimmler LM, Sykes P, Snell L, et al. Molecular tools for diagnosis of synovial sarcomas: correlation of RT-PCR and FISH on paraffin embedded material. Pathology 2010;42(Suppl 1):S84.

41. Matsuyama A, Hisaoka M, Iwasaki M, et al. TLE1 expression in malignant mesothelioma. Virchows Arch 2010;457(5):577–83.

42. Klebe S, Prabhakaran S, Hocking A, et al. Pleural malignant mesothelioma versus pleuropulmonary synovial sarcoma: a clinicopathological study of 22 cases with molecular analysis and survival data. Pathology 2018;50(6):629–34.

43. Hozain AE, Corvin C, Li H, et al. Mediastinal synovial sarcoma 14 years after talc pleurodesis for spontaneous pneumothorax. Annals of Thoracic Surgery Short Reports 2023;1(3):515–8.

44. Yi JH, Sim J, Park BB, et al. The primary extragastrointestinal stromal tumor of pleura: a case report and a literature review. Jpn J Clin Oncol 2013;43(12):1269–72.

45. Joensuu H, Wardelmann E, Sihto H, et al. Effect of KIT and PDGFRA mutations on survival in patients with gastrointestinal stromal tumors treated with adjuvant imatinib: an exploratory analysis of a randomized clinical trial. JAMA Oncol 2017;3(5):602–9.

46. Long KB, Butrynski JE, Blank SD, et al. Primary extragastrointestinal stromal tumor of the pleura: report of a unique case with genetic confirmation. Am J Surg Pathol 2010;34(6):907–12.

47. Miettinen M, Lasota J. Gastrointestinal stromal tumors: pathology and prognosis at different sites. Semin Diagn Pathol 2006;23(2):70–83.

48. Boland JM, Colby TV, Folpe AL. Liposarcomas of the mediastinum and thorax: a clinicopathologic and molecular cytogenetic study of 24 cases, emphasizing unusual and diverse histologic features. Am J Surg Pathol 2012;36(9):1395–403.

49. Hahn HP, Fletcher CD. Primary mediastinal liposarcoma: clinicopathologic analysis of 24 cases. Am J Surg Pathol 2007;31(12):1868–74.

50. Wilkinson L, Coucher J, Murphy M, et al. CIC-rearranged sarcoma of the pleura: an unreported primary site, expanding the anatomical distribution of an emerging entity. Pathology 2018;50(4):469–72.

51. Gui H, Sussman RT, Jian B, et al. Primary pulmonary myxoid sarcoma and myxoid angiomatoid fibrous histiocytoma: a unifying continuum with shared and distinct features. Am J Surg Pathol 2020;44(11): 1535–40.

52. Capkova L, Koubkova L, Kodet R. Expression of carbonic anhydrase IX (CAIX) in malignant mesothelioma. An immunohistochemical and immunocytochemical study. Neoplasma 2014;61(2):161–9.

Invasion and Grading of Pulmonary Non-Mucinous Adenocarcinoma

Andre L. Moreira, MD, PhD*, Fang Zhou, MD

KEYWORDS

• Lung adenocarcinoma • Tumor grading • Invasion • Prognosis

Key points

- Quantification of different growth patterns has taken on a prominent role in the assessment of lung adenocarcinoma invasion and grade.
- The current staging system subtracts the lepidic pattern from tumor size.
- The current grading system places an emphasis on the presence of high-grade patterns (solid, micropapillary, complex glands).
- Beware of the many pitfalls in recognizing histologic architectural patterns.
- Consistent and widespread application of these classification systems will help advance our knowledge of lung cancer.

ABSTRACT

Lung adenocarcinoma staging and grading were recently updated to reflect the link between histologic growth patterns and outcomes. The lepidic growth pattern is regarded as "in-situ," whereas all other patterns are regarded as invasive, though with stratification. Solid, micropapillary, and complex glandular patterns are associated with worse prognosis than papillary and acinar patterns. These recent changes have improved prognostic stratification. However, multiple pitfalls exist in measuring invasive size and in classifying lung adenocarcinoma growth patterns. Awareness of these limitations and recommended practices will help the pathology community achieve consistent prognostic performance and potentially contribute to improved patient management.

OVERVIEW

Estimates of tumor prognosis are used to guide disease management. For pulmonary adenocarcinomas, tumor stage and grade are used to designate tumor extent and estimate the risk of recurrence. The American Joint Committee on Cancer (AJCC) uses the tumor, node, and metastasis (TNM) system as the basis of their prognostic stage group classification.[1] In lung cancer, T is defined by both tumor size and extent of local invasion or satellite growth. In pathologic staging (pTNM), tumor size measurement is based on gross examination and may be adjusted based on microscopic findings. For lung adenocarcinoma, like in other tumors, the pT classification is currently based on the invasive component of the tumor. The World Health Organization (WHO) Classification of Thoracic Tumors[2] recognizes the lepidic pattern as in situ, whereas all other growth patterns are considered invasive with metastatic potential. Therefore, in the staging of lung adenocarcinoma, the microscopic measurement of the lepidic component is subtracted from the total tumor size. Although exclusion of the lepidic component has resulted in better prognostic stratification based on historical data, the prospective real-world implications of this practice are currently unknown.[3–8]

Department of Pathology, New York University Grossman School of Medicine, 560 First Avenue, New York, NY 10016, USA
* Corresponding author.
E-mail address: andre.moreira@nyulangone.org

Surgical Pathology 17 (2024) 271–285
https://doi.org/10.1016/j.path.2023.11.009
1875-9181/24/© 2023 Elsevier Inc. All rights reserved.

Tumor grade in lung adenocarcinoma is an adjunct to tumor stage that provides additional prognostic information, in particular for lower stage tumors. In other organs systems such as prostate and mammary carcinoma, tumor grade contributes to therapeutic decision-making. In lung carcinoma, the influence of tumor grade on patient management is presently limited due to lack of clinical trial data. The grading of lung adenocarcinoma depends on the quantification of different growth patterns, which will be described in more detail later.

Distinguishing between lepidic and other growth patterns in lung adenocarcinoma can be difficult, with poor reproducibility in challenging cases, even among expert pulmonary pathologists.[9] There are multiple mimickers of invasive patterns, and there is variability in how pathologists measure invasive size. Attempting to overcome such diagnostic pitfalls is critical to achieving consistent classification and prognostication. In this article, the authors discuss the current understanding of invasion and grading in lung adenocarcinoma, as well as the limitations and controversies relevant to general surgical pathologists.

INVASION AND PATHOLOGIC STAGE

In 2011, the term "bronchioloalveolar carcinoma" was supplanted by the concept of pulmonary "adenocarcinoma in-situ" (AIS), which is defined as a ≤ 3 cm tumor with pure lepidic growth pattern.[10] Lepidic pattern is defined as tumor cells growing along preexisting alveolar walls without invasion into the pulmonary parenchyma. Acinar, papillary, solid, micropapillary, and other variations (collectively termed "complex glandular pattern") are considered invasive patterns, whereas lepidic is the only pattern regarded as in situ (noninvasive). AIS was adopted by the 4th edition of the WHO in 2015.

Several studies pointed out that the lepidic-predominant tumors with small areas of invasion behaved similarly to AIS in survival and recurrence rates.[3,11,12] Thus, the 4th edition of the WHO also included the term "minimally invasive adenocarcinoma" (MIA).[13] MIA is defined as a lepidic-predominant tumor measuring ≤ 3 cm overall that contains ≤ 5 mm of invasive pattern(s). The cutoffs of 3 cm for total tumor size and 0.5 cm for invasive size were defined by consensus and reflect the observations from the original studies that gave rise to the identification of these tumors.[10,11,14–16] The prognosis of the rare pure lepidic adenocarcinomas that measure more than 3 cm is unknown.[17] When AIS or MIA presents as a single pulmonary lesion, it is associated with good prognosis and no recurrence.[3,18–20]

The conceptual acceptance of an in situ form of lung adenocarcinoma subjected lung pathology to the recommendation of the Union for International Cancer Control that only the invasive size should be used for TNM staging. Thus, in 2016, the International Association for the Study of Lung Cancer (IASLC) published a proposal to measure only the invasive patterns in the pathologic staging of nonmucinous lung adenocarcinoma.[6] The proposal also called for AIS to be staged as tumor adenocarcinoma in situ (Tis) and for MIA to be staged as tumor adenocarcinoma minimally invasive (T1mi). This proposal was adopted in the 8th edition of the AJCC pTNM system, which was published in 2017 and went into effect in 2018.[1] Tumors with greater than 5 mm of invasive growth, pleural invasion, lymphovascular invasion (LVI), and/or spread through airspaces are excluded from the AIS and MIA categories and are instead staged as pT1 to pT4 based on their invasive size and extent.[1]

Very few predominantly invasive tumors greater than 3 cm are affected by the subtraction of lepidic component from staging. The types of lung adenocarcinoma that are most often affected by this change are the lepidic-predominant adenocarcinomas confined to the pulmonary parenchyma. Such tumors are often ≤ 3 cm in size without pleural invasion (pT1a–pT1c), lack nodal and distant metastases, and are surgically resected. They are usually associated with high survival and low recurrence rates. Thus, there is limited evidence in the literature regarding whether the subtraction of lepidic component from staging sub-stratifies outcomes in a clinically meaningful way that should guide adjuvant therapy decisions.[5–7,21,22] One study previously published in 2013 showed that among patients staged as prognostic group I based on total tumor size, those with invasive size ≤ 2 cm (n = 449) did not benefit from chemotherapy, whereas those with invasive size greater than 2 cm (n = 154) did benefit from chemotherapy.[5] In another study, published in 2018 in response to the IASLCs proposal to subtract lepidic pattern from staging, restaging of a large historical cohort of stage I to IIA cases (n = 1704) showed that approximately a third (n = 30) of the patients in prognostic stage group IIA (n = 95) were down-staged to IB or IA, and the recurrence rates of the entire cohort became better stratified compared with the staging that was previously based on total tumor size.[7] Although this finding suggested the possibility of avoiding adjuvant therapy for these down-staged patients, adjuvant therapy rates were not assessed in the study. So there is an unresolved question of how many of the down-staged patients had better outcomes because they had already received adjuvant therapy (because they had historically been staged as IIA).[7]

The phenomenon of lepidic-patterned spread of invasive tumors has been described, though uncommonly, in metastatic tumors to the lung, mesotheliomas, and invasive squamous cell carcinomas[23–25]; thus, it is unknown how much of the lepidic components in lung adenocarcinomas truly represent in situ disease.[24] There is currently no way to distinguish invasive from in situ lepidic growth. However, given the indolent nature of AIS and MIA, it is reasonable to presume for now that in the majority of tumors with a significant lepidic component, most if not all of the lepidic pattern represents in situ disease. The real-world implications of subtracting the lepidic component from tumor staging still need to be evaluated in prospective follow-up studies and clinical trials.

GROSS AND MICROSCOPIC MEASUREMENTS OF INVASION

The measurement of tumor size is performed during gross examination. For pathologic staging, the measurement is revised by the pathologist based on microscopy because adjacent benign pathology (eg, organizing pneumonia), and lepidic disease may need to be excluded. It is difficult to differentiate between invasive and lepidic components grossly.[6] Lepidic components can also be mistaken grossly for adjacent normal parenchyma, which is one of the reasons grossly normal parenchyma flanking the tumor should be included in the sampled sections.

Pre-analytical issues that can interfere with gross evaluation of the tumor size include formalin fixation and specimen inflation. Formalin fixation can cause tissue shrinkage.[26,27] Pre- versus post-fixation size variations are greatest in lepidic-predominant tumors,[26–28] which may explain some of the tumor measurement discrepancies between radiology and pathology. Radiographic measurements of the tumor can be larger than gross measurements, especially when they include ground glass areas that often correspond to lepidic components histologically and when the radiologic measurements are taken on maximal inhalation. Another cause of radiology–pathology tumor size discrepancies is the collapse of surgically excised lung parenchyma, which some investigators term "iatrogenic collapse."[7,29] Collapse is also a pitfall in the histologic determination of the size of invasion for pathologic staging, which will be further discussed later in this article.[29] However, grossing protocols are not standardized among laboratories. There is no precise assessment of how fixation, inflation, and parenchymal collapse influence the size estimation of the invasive component.[26–28]

MICROSCOPIC MEASUREMENT OF INVASION

The size of invasion can be measured on histology using a ruler or ocular micrometer. Several factors may influence the microscopic assessment of invasion. Different rules apply depending on whether there is one single focus of invasion or multiple foci of invasion. The most common scenario is the presence of a single focus of invasion: the area is marked microscopically, and the measurement of invasion is taken in the greatest dimension to determine the pT stage. In the second most common scenario, the region of invasion involves multiple slides: in this case, the alternate method is to estimate the percentage of invasive components and then calculate the size of invasion. A similar approach can be used when multiple areas of invasion are seen in a small tumor limited to one slide, although it is unclear if there is any clinical significance to this type of limited invasion.[19,30]

The presence of intralesional scarring presents a challenge for measurements. When the scar is seen in the center of the tumor, the entire area of scar is included in the measurement of invasion, as it is assumed to be a response to the neoplastic process; when the scar is seen at the periphery of the tumor, such as in the case of apical caps, then the scar should not be included in the measurement as it is perceived to be preexisting scar tissue.[6]

DIFFERENTIAL DIAGNOSIS: MIMICKERS OF INVASION

The determination of invasion in low-stage, low-grade tumors has been repeatedly shown to have poor interobserver reproducibility,[9,31–33] whereas there is higher interobserver reproducibility in the identification of invasive pattern-predominant tumors, LVI, and pleural involvement. Most of the inconsistencies in recognizing invasion stem from the distinction of lepidic pattern from papillary[34] and acinar patterns.[35] One of the greatest mimickers of invasion is parenchymal collapse. Surgery-related (iatrogenic) collapse of the alveolar network creates compression-related artifacts. Gland-like structures mimic the acinar pattern of invasion (**Fig. 1**A); folded parenchyma mimics papillary pattern (**Fig. 1**B); and clumped parenchyma causes tumor cell tufting that mimics micropapillary pattern on transection (**Fig. 1**C). True papillary pattern, with complex arborization, is demonstrated in **Fig. 1**D. These effects are even more pronounced when alveolar walls are thickened by

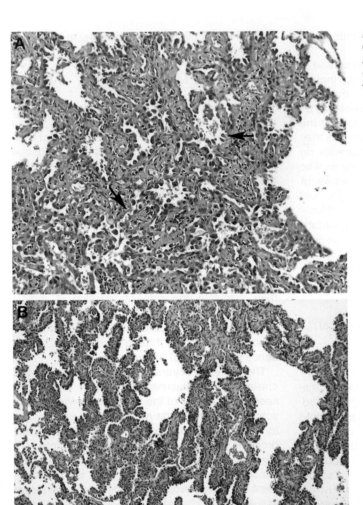

Fig. 1. Mimickers of invasion. (*A*) Collapse of lepidic tumor can mimic acinar pattern of invasion (*arrows*) (20x). (*B*) Folded parenchyma in a lepidic tumor can mimic papillary pattern (10x).

chronic inflammation or fibrosis. Perfusion of the parenchyma by the injection of formalin into the specimen does not always fully abate the artifacts caused by iatrogenic collapse.[29]

Several features have been proposed to differentiate true invasion from parenchymal collapse. Desmoplastic stroma and effacement of the alveolar architecture favor invasive growth.[29] However, desmoplasia is difficult to ascertain on microscopic examination and may not be seen in all invasive patterns. Desmoplasia may be absent even in clearly invasive patterns such as micropapillary and solid growth patterns (**Fig. 2**). In addition, organizing tissue in the healing needle track of a previous biopsy may mimic desmoplastic reaction and entrap alveolar epithelial cells in angular glandular shapes (**Fig. 3**).[36] Knowledge of a previous procedure (core biopsy or fine needle

aspiration biopsy), and the observation of the linear nature of the needle biopsy scar, may prevent its misinterpretation as invasion.

Histologic features that favor collapsed lepidic component over invasion include the following: compressed adjacent benign alveoli; the detection of parallel or "streaming" spaces; and abrupt transition from a tumor monolayer to benign pneumocytes (vs acinar pattern). The detection of parenchymal collapse may be confounded by the presence of intra-alveolar macrophages within the spaces, which can be disentangled from tumor cells by immunohistochemistry showing lack of keratin expression and/or positive staining for macrophage markers within the monocytes. Other histologic features, such as angulated glands without desmoplasia and alveolar septal thickening, have been proposed to favor lepidic pattern[3]; however, all

Fig. 1. (*C*) Clumping of parenchyma can cause tumor cell tufting that mimics micropapillary pattern on transection (*arrows*) (20x). (*D*) True papillary pattern, with complex arborization and fibrovascular core (10x).

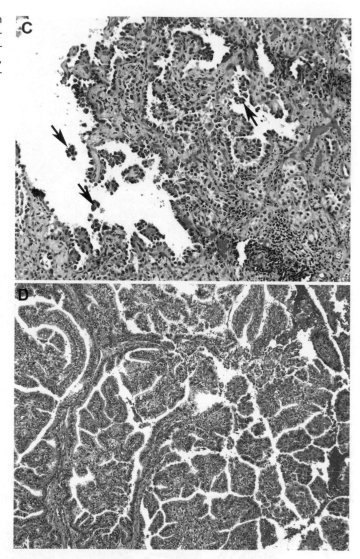

these features can also be seen in invasive patterns[3] and are thus not reliable characteristics in this differential diagnosis.

Nuclear grade is another histologic feature that has been proposed to distinguish between invasive and in situ components. High nuclear grade is more frequently seen in invasive components.[29,37,38] A sharp transition between nuclear grades is suggestive of a shift between lepidic and invasive patterns (**Fig. 4**). However, the presence of a continuum of nuclear grades is unhelpful in the differential diagnosis, because any nuclear grade can be seen in both lepidic and invasive growth patterns. Recently, the presence of extensive epithelial cell proliferation (EEP) has been proposed as a feature favoring invasive disease. In EEP, a tumor architecturally appears to be organized in a lepidic pattern, but the malignant epithelial cells are arranged in two or more layers and

usually have high nuclear grade (**Fig. 5**). High nuclear grade and multilayering should be discerned on high power magnification. EEP has high interobserver reproducibility.[29]

The Elastin stain has been proposed to help in the differential diagnosis of invasive versus in situ patterns. In theory, the detection of a preserved, compressed preexisting elastic framework favors lepidic pattern with parenchymal collapse, whereas the loss of elastic fibers favors invasive growth pattern. Thus, it has been argued that elastin stain has the potential to enhance interobserver reproducibility.[39] However, this stain is technically difficult to perform and interpret. Studies on the topic have so far not found evidence that elastin stain improves interobserver reproducibility in the assessment of invasion.[9,33] Thus, its acceptance and utility in differentiating invasion from lepidic component remain limited.[29]

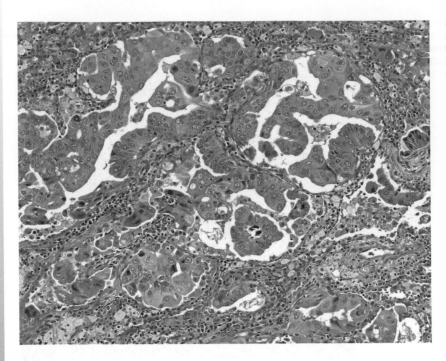

Fig. 2. Desmoplasia is not always present with invasive pattern. Desmoplasia may be absent in clearly invasive patterns (40x).

SUMMARY (INVASION)

The distinction of invasive from lepidic component in small, well-differentiated adenocarcinoma of the lung remains difficult. Because measurement of the invasive component is essential for pathologic staging, what can a pathologist do when presented with this dilemma? The recommendation from the IASLC is that when invasion in a certain area cannot be determined with certainty, the area should be upgraded to invasive, to reflect the practice that is already prevalent among pathologists.[29] Although this recommendation conflicts with the current recommendation from the AJCC that favors downstaging tumors in cases of uncertainty, in small low-grade tumors measuring ≤ 3 cm (which compose the majority of cases affected by this predicament), the IASLC pathology committee's recommendation

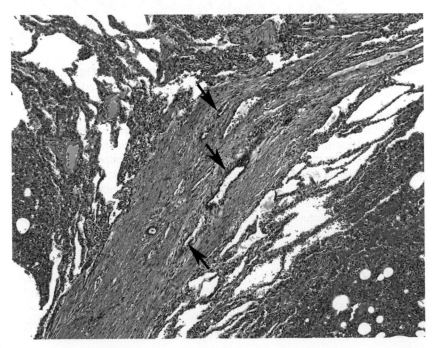

Fig. 3. A healing biopsy site can mimic invasion. Organizing tissue can mimic desmoplasia and entrap pneumocytes in angular glandular patterns (*arrows*). Knowledge of a previous biopsy procedure, and observing the linear shape of the scar, can help to prevent misinterpretation (10x).

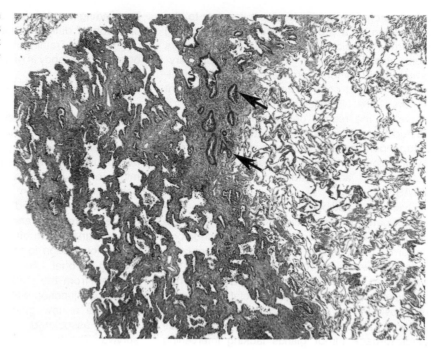

Fig. 4. A sharp transition between nuclear grades is suggestive of a shift from lepidic to invasive patterns (*arrows*) (10x).

does not affect clinical management, as all these tumors are currently treated surgically without systemic therapy.

TUMOR GRADING: BACKGROUND

Because pulmonary adenocarcinomas are often heterogeneous with different combinations of histologic growth patterns, the WHO recommends classification by the predominant pattern, reporting incremental percentages of all the patterns present in a given tumor. The five patterns officially recognized by the WHO are lepidic, acinar, papillary, micropapillary, and solid.[10,40,41] Several studies demonstrated a correlation between the predominant pattern of non-mucinous lung

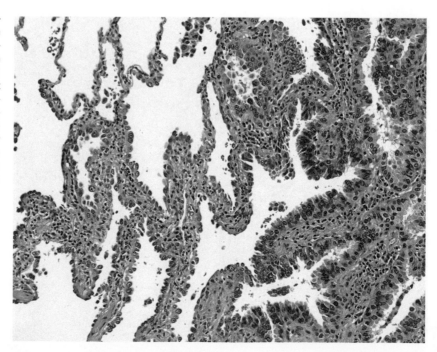

Fig. 5. Extensive epithelial cell proliferation (EEP) favors invasive disease. Despite having a lepidic architectural pattern, the malignant epithelial cells are arranged in two or more layers, and usually have high nuclear grade. EEP is seen on the right side of this figure, whereas in situ disease is seen on the left (20x).

adenocarcinoma and outcomes, leading to the suggestion of a provisional three-tiered grading system in which lepidic-predominant tumors were classified as low grade, acinar/papillary-predominant tumors were classified as intermediate grade, and solid/micropapillary-predominant tumors were classified as high grade.[10,12,41,42] However, the results of additional studies suggested that other histologic features were better independent determinants of recurrence and survival, including minor components of high-grade pattern(s)[43–47] and spread through alveolar spaces (STAS).[48–50]

Over time, it also became apparent that some histologic patterns did not conform to the WHOs five patterns of lung adenocarcinoma.[51] The cribriform pattern is characterized by solid nests of neoplastic cells with sieve-like perforations (Fig. 6). In 2015, it was added to the WHO as a high-grade pattern of the acinar subtype that was associated with poor prognosis.[41,52–55] Other poorly formed glandular patterns have also been described: fused glands (back-to-back tumor glands lacking intervening stroma) (Fig. 7), ribbon-like formations with irregular borders, and single cells infiltrating desmoplastic stroma (Fig. 8).[56] Together, these patterns are commonly referred to as complex glandular patterns (CGPs) and are associated with higher recurrence, with prognosis more similar to solid and micropapillary patterns.[52,57–62] One report suggests that cribriform pattern is associated with poor outcome, whereas fused gland pattern falls between intermediate and high-grade outcomes.[63]

This finding may be due to differences in the interpretation of different CGPs, which is a relatively new concept. Training images may improve pathologists' consistency in recognizing these patterns.[57]

A NEW GRADING SYSTEM

As discussed in the previous section, it became clear that the predominant pattern alone was an insufficient basis for grading pulmonary nonmucinous adenocarcinomas. The pathology committee of the IASLC was thus tasked to create a better grading system.[56] Because the predominant pattern was used in the WHO classification of adenocarcinoma and already showed dependable prognostic stratification, it was maintained as the foundation in the creation of IASLCs new grading model. Several additional variables selected from the medical literature were evaluated in conjunction with the predominant pattern to devise a new grading system that is more strongly associated with recurrence and overall survival. The study was conducted using several data sets originating from different geographic regions, thereby avoiding single institution and investigator biases. The study began with a discovery/training data set, from which different models were created. Two models that showed good performance with respect to outcomes stratification were then validated and tested using new data sets. The data sets used for the discovery and validation steps were composed of prognostic stage group I adenocarcinomas only, and the final

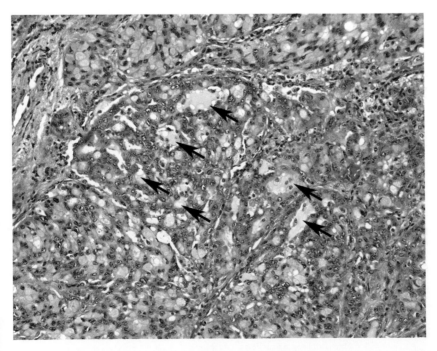

Fig. 6. Cribriform pattern. In this adenocarcinoma with signet ring cell features, solid nests of tumor cells with sieve-like perforations (arrows) are present, which is characteristic of the high-grade cribriform pattern (20x).

Fig. 7. Fused glands pattern. Back-to-back tumor glands are seen without intervening stroma, which is one of the high-grade complex glandular patterns (*arrows*) (20x).

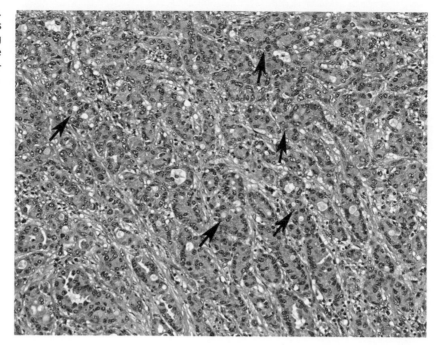

testing of the model was performed on a separate data set containing adenocarcinomas in prognostic stage groups I to III.

The two models that underwent validation and testing were the following: model 1 was composed of the two most predominant (primary and secondary) growth patterns, and model 2 was composed of the predominant pattern plus high-grade pattern(s). The addition of all patterns, whether as weighted percentages or as binary findings, resulted in similar model performance. When other histologic modifiers (STAS, nuclear grade, and mitotic counts) were added to the two models, the results from the discovery/training set suggested that one of the modifiers had a significant impact on model performance. However, when the models were used on the validation data set, the effects of the modifiers could not be reproduced; in the validation data set, a different modifier showed higher impact on model performance. Therefore, the modifiers were not included in the final model. The discrepancy may have arisen due to interobserver variations in these modifiers: there is considerable variation in the definition and interpretation of STAS among investigators[64,65] and poor reproducibility in nuclear grading (kappa = 0.45–0.58).[66,67]

The difference between model 1 and model 2 was not significantly different; therefore, the committee decided to implement model 2 that is composed of the predominant pattern plus high-grade pattern, as the final model, to reflect pathologists' traditional practice of grading tumors based on their worst component. Model 2 required a cutoff value for the high-grade component. Several studies indicated that different percentages of high-grade pattern can influence prognosis. Using statistical methods to determine the best combination of sensitivity and specificity for the test, the IASLC established this cutoff at 20%.

THE PROPOSED GRADING SYSTEM

The IASLC grading system builds on the predominant pattern grading system by upshifting any tumor composed of ≥ 20% high-grade pattern(s) into the poorly differentiated category (grade 3). Grade 1 tumors are lepidic-predominant, and grade 2 tumors are acinar- and/or papillary-predominant tumors; both grades have less than 20% high-grade pattern(s). CGPs are included in the high-grade pattern category alongside the solid and micropapillary patterns. This new IALSC grading system shows improved prognostic stratification compared with the predominant pattern model, and it has been validated by many subsequent studies.[56,59,68–71]

One of the most significant consequences of the IASLC grading system was the upgrade of acinar/papillary-predominant tumors with ≥ 20% of high-grade pattern to the grade 3 category. For example, in the predominant pattern grading system, acinar-predominant tumors composed approximately 40% to 50% of all tumors, but were

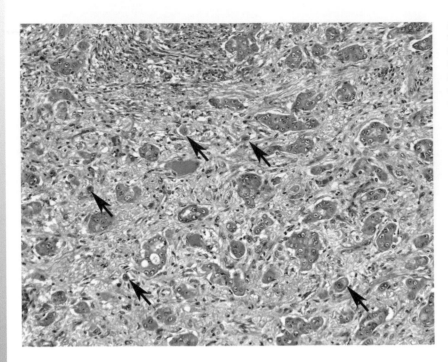

Fig. 8. Single cells infiltrating stroma. Irregular clusters and individual tumor cells (*arrows*) are seen in this high-grade complex glandular pattern (20x).

all classified as intermediate grade despite their wide range of clinical outcomes.[53,56] The use of the IASLC grading system improves the stratification of this heterogeneous group, as reported in recent validation studies.[56,59,68–71]

Numerous histologic features reportedly associated with prognosis on univariate analyses, such as nuclear and cytologic grade, STAS, mitotic count, and necrosis, are actually correlated with each other and/or tumor grade rather than being independent prognostic predictors; they lose significance on multivariate analysis.[56,65,69,71] LVI also correlates with prognosis and is seen with increasing frequency in higher grade tumors and patterns.[69–72] However, LVI was not formally evaluated during the creation of the IASLC grading system, and there are conflicting results in the medical literature on the role of LVI as a modifier in the IASLC grading system.[68,70]

There are conflicting results on the association between tumor grade and molecular profile.[68,69,71,73] However, a recent publication showed a strong association between IASLC grade and programmed death ligand -1 (PD-L1) expression on lung adenocarcinomas, which suggests that the selection of tumor blocks with higher grade histologic patterns for PD-L1 immunohistochemistry may decrease false-negative PD-L1 results.[73]

TUMOR GRADE: PITFALLS

The above-described challenges in the recognition of growth patterns constitute a major pitfall in both

tumor grading and staging. Interobserver reproducibility analyses were included in the IASLCs original publication of the new grading system and subsequent validation studies. The results have shown good reproducibility, with moderate to significant agreement among study participants.[56,59,68] Most of the discrepancies involved the distinction between lepidic and papillary/acinar patterns, which is a well-described occurrence,[9,74,75] and in the quantification of high-grade patterns, especially near the 20% threshold.[56] Training has the potential to improve concordance in pattern recognition.[76] Interestingly, discrepancies in recognizing these patterns have seemingly not affected the overall ability of investigators to grade the tumors in a prognostically meaningful way.

Discrepancies in adenocarcinoma pattern subtyping may persist when using digital pathology and artificial intelligence algorithms, because the lack of perfect agreement, even among expert lung pathologists, compels the extraction of a potentially divergent "ground truth" based on majority human consensus for the training of each computational algorithm.[74]

PROSPECTIVE APPLICATIONS OF GRADING

Some aspects of the IASLCs grading system remain to be expanded. Its applications are currently largely limited to invasive non-mucinous lung adenocarcinomas, yet some investigators have found a correlation between architectural patterns and outcomes in invasive mucinous carcinomas of the lung.[77,78] The utility of grading in biopsy and cytology specimens is also constrained by sampling bias in these architecturally heterogeneous tumors[41,43,79]; although adenocarcinoma patterns may be described, the reporting of a histologic grade or predominant pattern is not currently recommended in small diagnostic samples because their significance is unknown. Finally, the area under the curve (AUC) for the IASLC model was between 0.7 and 0.8 for both overall survival and relapse-free survival in the original IASLC proposal and a validation study, which leaves significant room for improvement.[56,59]

Despite its limitations, the IASLCs grading model is a validated, reproducible system for grading resected non-mucinous adenocarcinomas that can be applied easily by any pathologist. It is included in the current WHO, and it was incorporated into the College of American Pathologists' Lung Cancer Protocol Template in 2021.[80] The inclusion of this grading system in cancer guidelines ensures that this data point is collected consistently in cancer data sets and clinical trials.

Although the improved prognostic stratification of the new grading system is clear, the implications for patient management are still under investigation. The currently ongoing ADAURA2 trial includes tumor grade (including ≥20% high-grade histology) as a histologic parameter and aims to evaluate response to osimertinib in the adjuvant setting for stage IA2-IA3 epithelial growth factor receptor (EGFR)-mutant lung cancer.[81] Recent studies have shown a correlation between higher grade on frozen section and shorter recurrence-free survival,[65] as well as a higher recurrence rate among grade 3 tumors treated by sublobectomy resections compared with lobectomies.[82] However, additional validation studies and prospective trials are needed before grade on frozen is used for patient care decisions.

It is hoped that just like in breast and prostate cancers, the rapid and widespread adoption of this grading system will produce actionable clinical trial results[83] as well as stimulate the formation and refinement of grading systems for other types of lung cancer.

SUMMARY

The staging and grading systems of non-mucinous lung adenocarcinomas have evolved over the past decade to incorporate the mounting evidence that different growth patterns are associated with differing clinical outcomes. The new staging and grading systems undoubtedly offer improved prognostic stratification over previous systems. The introduction of AIS (pTis) and MIA (pT1mi)

have separated out two very indolent prognostic groups among the formerly pT1 tumors, and studies thus far support the improved performance of IASLCs latest grading proposal. Additional prospective studies are still needed to assess the real-world consequences of downstaging and de-escalating treatment based on the subtraction of the lepidic component from staging, as well as whether treatment should be escalated based on higher histologic grade.

These staging and grading systems are both unavoidably affected by how well the growth patterns are recognized by pathologists, because noninvasive patterns contribute to lower stage and grade designations, whereas invasive patterns contribute to higher stage and grade designations. Although interobserver reproducibility in the recognition of these patterns is imperfect, studies have shown that training may improve interobserver concordance. Consistent and widespread inclusion of these new staging and grading systems in clinical trials and routine pathology reports will play a vital role in advancing our understanding of lung cancer.

CLINICS CARE POINTS

- Grading of pulmonary adenocarcinoma improves prognostic stratification.

- Grading for pulmonary adenocarcinoma is a standardized tool to evaluate recurrence and therapy associated response in a heteogeneous tumors.

DISCLOSURE

The authors have nothing to disclose.

REFERENCES

1. Amin MB, American Joint Committee on Cancer., American Cancer Society. AJCC cancer staging manual. Eight edition/editor-in-chief, Mahul B. Amin, MD, FCAP ; editors, Stephen B. Edge, MD, FACS and 16 others ; Donna M. Gress, RHIT, CTR - Technical editor ; Laura R. Meyer, CAPM - Managing editor. ed. American Joint Committee on Cancer, Springer; 2017:xvii, 1024 pages.
2. Board WCoTE, ed. Thoracic tumours. 5th ed. International Agency for Research on Cancer; 2021. https://publications.iarc.fr/595.
3. Yoshizawa A, Motoi N, Riely GJ, et al. Impact of proposed IASLC/ATS/ERS classification of lung adenocarcinoma: prognostic subgroups and implications

for further revision of staging based on analysis of 514 stage I cases. Mod Pathol 2011;24(5):653–64.

4. Warth A, Muley T, Meister M, et al. The novel histologic International Association for the Study of Lung Cancer/American Thoracic Society/European Respiratory Society classification system of lung adenocarcinoma is a stage-independent predictor of survival. J Clin Oncol 2012;30(13):1438–46.

5. Tsutani Y, Miyata Y, Mimae T, et al. The prognostic role of pathologic invasive component size, excluding lepidic growth, in stage I lung adenocarcinoma. J Thorac Cardiovasc Surg 2013;146(3):580–5.

6. Travis WD, Asamura H, Bankier AA, et al. The IASLC Lung Cancer Staging Project: Proposals for Coding T Categories for Subsolid Nodules and Assessment of Tumor Size in Part-Solid Tumors in the Forthcoming Eighth Edition of the TNM Classification of Lung Cancer. J Thorac Oncol 2016;11(8):1204–23.

7. Kameda K, Eguchi T, Lu S, et al. Implications of the Eighth Edition of the TNM Proposal: Invasive Versus Total Tumor Size for the T Descriptor in Pathologic Stage I-IIA Lung Adenocarcinoma. J Thorac Oncol 2018;13(12):1919–29.

8. Amin M. American Joint committee on cancer., American cancer Society. AJCC cancer staging manual. Eighth edition edition. American Joint Committee on Cancer, Springer; 2017.

9. Thunnissen E, Beasley MB, Borczuk AC, et al. Reproducibility of histopathological subtypes and invasion in pulmonary adenocarcinoma. An international interobserver study. Mod Pathol 2012;25(12):1574–83.

10. Travis WD, Brambilla E, Noguchi M, et al. International association for the study of lung cancer/American thoracic society/European respiratory society international multidisciplinary classification of lung adenocarcinoma. J Thorac Oncol 2011;6(2):244–85.

11. Yotsukura M, Asamura H, Motoi N, et al. Long-Term Prognosis of Patients With Resected Adenocarcinoma In Situ and Minimally Invasive Adenocarcinoma of the Lung. J Thorac Oncol 2021;16(8):1312–20.

12. Yoshizawa A, Sumiyoshi S, Sonobe M, et al. Validation of the IASLC/ATS/ERS lung adenocarcinoma classification for prognosis and association with EGFR and KRAS gene mutations: analysis of 440 Japanese patients. J Thorac Oncol 2013;8(1):52–61.

13. Travis WD, Brambilla E, Burke A, et al. WHO classification of tumours of the lung, pleura, thymus and heart. World Health Organization classification of tumours, 4th edition 7 vol. International Agency for Research on Cancer; 2015:412 pages : illustrations.

14. Moreira AL. Bronchioloalveolar Carcinoma and Minimally Invasive Adenocarcinoma. Surg Pathol Clin 2010;3(1):1–26.

15. Dacic S. Minimally invasive adenocarcinomas of the lung. Adv Anat Pathol 2009;16(3):166–71.

16. Yim J, Zhu LC, Chiriboga L, et al. Histologic features are important prognostic indicators in early stages lung adenocarcinomas. Mod Pathol 2007;20(2):233–41.

17. Inafuku K, Yokose T, Ito H, et al. Should Pathologically Noninvasive Lung Adenocarcinoma Larger Than 3 cm Be Classified as T1a? Ann Thorac Surg 2019;108(6):1678–84.

18. Okada M. Subtyping lung adenocarcinoma according to the novel 2011 IASLC/ATS/ERS classification: correlation with patient prognosis. Thorac Surg Clin 2013;23(2):179–86.

19. Kadota K, Villena-Vargas J, Yoshizawa A, et al. Prognostic significance of adenocarcinoma in situ, minimally invasive adenocarcinoma, and nonmucinous lepidic predominant invasive adenocarcinoma of the lung in patients with stage I disease. Am J Surg Pathol 2014;38(4):448–60.

20. Behera M, Owonikoko TK, Gal AA, et al. Lung Adenocarcinoma Staging Using the 2011 IASLC/ATS/ERS Classification: A Pooled Analysis of Adenocarcinoma In Situ and Minimally Invasive Adenocarcinoma. Clin Lung Cancer 2016;17(5):e57–64.

21. Okubo Y, Kashima J, Teishikata T, et al. Prognostic Impact of the Histologic Lepidic Component in Pathologic Stage IA Adenocarcinoma. J Thorac Oncol 2022;17(1):67–75.

22. Kinoshita F, Shimokawa M, Takenaka T, et al. Prognostic impact of noninvasive areas in resected pathological stage IA lung adenocarcinoma. Thorac Cancer 2023. https://doi.org/10.1111/1759-7714.14910.

23. USCAP 112th Annual Meeting Abstracts. Lab Invest 2023;103(3):S1.

24. Guerrieri C, Lindner M, Sesti J, et al. Pulmonary squamous cell carcinoma with a lepidic-pagetoid growth pattern. Pathologica 2022;114(4):304–11.

25. RanYue W, ChunYan W, Likun H, et al. Diffuse intrapulmonary mesothelioma mimicking pulmonary lepidic adenocarcinoma: a rare case report and review of the literature. Diagn Pathol 2023;18(1):64.

26. Hsu PK, Huang HC, Hsieh CC, et al. Effect of formalin fixation on tumor size determination in stage I non-small cell lung cancer. Ann Thorac Surg 2007;84(6):1825–9.

27. Park HS, Lee S, Haam S, et al. Effect of formalin fixation and tumour size in small-sized non-small-cell lung cancer: a prospective, single-centre study. Histopathology 2017;71(3):437–45.

28. Isaka T, Yokose T, Ito H, et al. Comparison between CT tumor size and pathological tumor size in frozen section examinations of lung adenocarcinoma. Lung Cancer 2014;85(1):40–6.

29. Thunnissen E, Beasley MB, Borczuk A, et al. Defining Morphologic Features of Invasion in

Pulmonary Nonmucinous Adenocarcinoma With Lepidic Growth: A Proposal by the International Association for the Study of Lung Cancer Pathology Committee. J Thorac Oncol 2023;18(4):447–62.

30. Anderson KR, Onken A, Heidinger BH, et al. Pathologic T Descriptor of Nonmucinous Lung Adenocarcinomas Now Based on Invasive Tumor Size: How Should Pathologists Measure Invasion? Am J Clin Pathol 2018;150(6):499–506.

31. Bian T, Jiang D, Feng J, et al. Lepidic component at tumor margin: an independent prognostic factor in invasive lung adenocarcinoma. Hum Pathol 2019; 83:106–14.

32. Jeon HW, Kim YD, Sim SB, et al. Prognostic impact according to the proportion of the lepidic subtype in stage IA acinar-predominant lung adenocarcinoma. Thorac Cancer 2021;12(14):2072–7.

33. Shih AR, Uruga H, Bozkurtlar E, et al. Problems in the reproducibility of classification of small lung adenocarcinoma: an international interobserver study. Histopathology 2019;75(5):649–59.

34. Thunnissen E, Belien JA, Kerr KM, et al. In compressed lung tissue microscopic sections of adenocarcinoma in situ may mimic papillary adenocarcinoma. Arch Pathol Lab Med 2013;137(12):1792–7.

35. Blaauwgeers JLG, Filipello F, Lissenberg-Witte B, et al. Understanding the Morphology of Non-Mucinous Adenocarcinoma in Situ (AIS) of the Lung in Iatrogenic Collapse with the Use of CK7 and Elastin Staining [Abstract]. Abstract. Lab Invest 2023;103(3):S1594. https://doi.org/10.1016/j.labinv.2023.100101. Supplement.

36. Doxtader EE, Mukhopadhyay S, Katzenstein AL. Biopsy-site changes in lung adenocarcinoma with prior core needle biopsy: a potential pitfall in the assessment of stromal invasion. Am J Surg Pathol 2013;37(3):443–6.

37. von der Thusen JH, Tham YS, Pattenden H, et al. Prognostic significance of predominant histologic pattern and nuclear grade in resected adenocarcinoma of the lung: potential parameters for a grading system. J Thorac Oncol 2013;8(1):37–44.

38. Borczuk AC. Updates in grading and invasion assessment in lung adenocarcinoma. Mod Pathol 2022;35(Suppl 1):28–35.

39. Thunnissen E, Motoi N, Minami Y, et al. Elastin in pulmonary pathology: relevance in tumours with a lepidic or papillary appearance. A comprehensive understanding from a morphological viewpoint. Histopathology 2022;80(3):457–67.

40. World Health O, Travis WD, World Health O, International Agency for Research on C, International Academy of P, International Association for the Study of Lung C. Pathology and genetics of tumours of the lung, pleura, thymus and heart. World Health Organization classification of tumours 7. IARC Press; 2004:344 pages : illustrations (chiefly color), 1 color map.

41. Travis WD, Brambilla E, Nicholson AG, et al. The 2015 World Health Organization Classification of Lung Tumors: Impact of Genetic, Clinical and Radiologic Advances Since the 2004 Classification. J Thorac Oncol 2015;10(9):1243–60.

42. Motoi N, Szoke J, Riely GJ, et al. Lung adenocarcinoma: modification of the 2004 WHO mixed subtype to include the major histologic subtype suggests correlations between papillary and micropapillary adenocarcinoma subtypes, EGFR mutations and gene expression analysis. Am J Surg Pathol 2008; 32(6):810–27.

43. Sica G, Yoshizawa A, Sima CS, et al. A grading system of lung adenocarcinomas based on histologic pattern is predictive of disease recurrence in stage I tumors. Am J Surg Pathol 2010;34(8):1155–62.

44. Zhao Y, Wang R, Shen X, et al. Minor Components of Micropapillary and Solid Subtypes in Lung Adenocarcinoma are Predictors of Lymph Node Metastasis and Poor Prognosis. Ann Surg Oncol 2016;23(6):2099–105.

45. Chang C, Sun X, Zhao W, et al. Minor components of micropapillary and solid subtypes in lung invasive adenocarcinoma (</= 3 cm): PET/CT findings and correlations with lymph node metastasis. Radiol Med 2020;125(3):257–64.

46. Li J, You W, Zheng D, et al. A comprehensive evaluation of clinicopathologic characteristics, molecular features and prognosis in lung adenocarcinoma with solid component. J Cancer Res Clin Oncol 2018;144(4):725–34.

47. Nitadori J, Bograd AJ, Kadota K, et al. Impact of micropapillary histologic subtype in selecting limited resection vs lobectomy for lung adenocarcinoma of 2cm or smaller. J Natl Cancer Inst 2013;105(16):1212–20.

48. Chen D, Mao Y, Wen J, et al. Tumor Spread Through Air Spaces in Non-Small Cell Lung Cancer: A Systematic Review and Meta-Analysis. Ann Thorac Surg 2019;108(3):945–54.

49. Liu H, Yin Q, Yang G, et al. Prognostic Impact of Tumor Spread Through Air Spaces in Non-small Cell Lung Cancers: a Meta-Analysis Including 3564 Patients. Pathol Oncol Res 2019;25(4):1303–10.

50. Warth A, Muley T, Kossakowski CA, et al. Prognostic Impact of Intra-alveolar Tumor Spread in Pulmonary Adenocarcinoma. Am J Surg Pathol 2015;39(6):793–801.

51. Branca G, Ieni A, Barresi V, et al. An Updated Review of Cribriform Carcinomas with Emphasis on Histopathological Diagnosis and Prognostic Significance. Onco Rev 2017;11(1):317.

52. Moreira AL, Joubert P, Downey RJ, et al. Cribriform and fused glands are patterns of high-grade pulmonary adenocarcinoma. Hum Pathol 2014;45(2):213–20.

53. Kadota K, Yeh YC, Sima CS, et al. The cribriform pattern identifies a subset of acinar predominant

tumors with poor prognosis in patients with stage I lung adenocarcinoma: a conceptual proposal to classify cribriform predominant tumors as a distinct histologic subtype. Mod Pathol 2014;27(5):690–700.

54. Warth A, Muley T, Kossakowski C, et al. Prognostic impact and clinicopathological correlations of the cribriform pattern in pulmonary adenocarcinoma. J Thorac Oncol 2015;10(4):638–44.

55. Kadota K, Kushida Y, Kagawa S, et al. Cribriform Subtype is an Independent Predictor of Recurrence and Survival After Adjustment for the Eighth Edition of TNM Staging System in Patients With Resected Lung Adenocarcinoma. J Thorac Oncol 2019; 14(2):245–54.

56. Moreira AL, Ocampo PSS, Xia Y, et al. A Grading System for Invasive Pulmonary Adenocarcinoma: A Proposal From the International Association for the Study of Lung Cancer Pathology Committee. J Thorac Oncol 2020;15(10):1599–610.

57. Wang C, Durra HY, Huang Y, et al. Interobserver reproducibility study of the histological patterns of primary lung adenocarcinoma with emphasis on a more complex glandular pattern distinct from the typical acinar pattern. Int J Surg Pathol 2014;22(2): 149–55.

58. Rokutan-Kurata M, Yoshizawa A, Nakajima N, et al. Discohesive growth pattern (Disco-p) as an unfavorable prognostic factor in lung adenocarcinoma: an analysis of 1062 Japanese patients with resected lung adenocarcinoma. Mod Pathol 2020;33(9): 1722–31.

59. Rokutan-Kurata M, Yoshizawa A, Ueno K, et al. Validation Study of the International Association for the Study of Lung Cancer Histologic Grading System of Invasive Lung Adenocarcinoma. J Thorac Oncol 2021;16(10):1753–8.

60. Bai J, Deng C, Zheng Q, et al. Comprehensive analysis of mutational profile and prognostic significance of complex glandular pattern in lung adenocarcinoma. Transl Lung Cancer Res 2022;11(7): 1337–47.

61. Hydbring P. Complex glandular pattern as an independent predictor of survival probability in lung adenocarcinoma. Transl Lung Cancer Res 2022; 11(9):1739–41.

62. Ding Q, Chen D, Shen S, et al. Clinical profiles and intraoperative identification of complex glands in stage I lung adenocarcinoma. Eur J Cardio Thorac Surg 2023;(3):63.

63. Bosse Y, Gagne A, Althakfi W, et al. Prognostic value of complex glandular patterns in invasive pulmonary adenocarcinomas. Hum Pathol 2022;128:56–68.

64. Thunnissen E, Blaauwgeers HJ, de Cuba EM, et al. Ex Vivo Artifacts and Histopathologic Pitfalls in the Lung. Arch Pathol Lab Med 2016;140(3):212–20.

65. Zhou F, Villalba JA, Sayo TMS, et al. Assessment of the feasibility of frozen sections for the detection of

spread through air spaces (STAS) in pulmonary adenocarcinoma. Mod Pathol 2022;35(2):210–7.

66. Nakazato Y, Maeshima AM, Ishikawa Y, et al. Interobserver agreement in the nuclear grading of primary pulmonary adenocarcinoma. J Thorac Oncol 2013;8(6):736–43.

67. Nakazato Y, Minami Y, Kobayashi H, et al. Nuclear grading of primary pulmonary adenocarcinomas: correlation between nuclear size and prognosis. Cancer 2010;116(8):2011–9.

68. Deng C, Zheng Q, Zhang Y, et al. Validation of the Novel International Association for the Study of Lung Cancer Grading System for Invasive Pulmonary Adenocarcinoma and Association With Common Driver Mutations. J Thorac Oncol 2021;16(10): 1684–93.

69. Fujikawa R, Muraoka Y, Kashima J, et al. Clinicopathologic and Genotypic Features of Lung Adenocarcinoma Characterized by the International Association for the Study of Lung Cancer Grading System. J Thorac Oncol 2022;17(5):700–7.

70. Kagimoto A, Tsutani Y, Kambara T, et al. Utility of Newly Proposed Grading System From International Association for the Study of Lung Cancer for Invasive Lung Adenocarcinoma. JTO Clin Res Rep 2021;2(2):100126.

71. Woo W, Cha YJ, Kim BJ, et al. Validation Study of New IASLC Histology Grading System in Stage I Non-Mucinous Adenocarcinoma Comparing With Minimally Invasive Adenocarcinoma. Clin Lung Cancer 2022;23(7):e435–42.

72. Kosaka T, Shimizu K, Nakazawa S, et al. Clinicopathological features of small-sized peripheral squamous cell lung cancer. Mol Clin Oncol 2020;12(1): 69–74.

73. Argyropoulos K, Basu A, Park K, et al. Correlation of Programmed Death-Ligand 1 Expression With Lung Adenocarcinoma Histologic and Molecular Subgroups in Primary and Metastatic Sites. Mod Pathol 2023;36(9):100245.

74. Lami K, Bychkov A, Matsumoto K, et al. Overcoming the Interobserver Variability in Lung Adenocarcinoma Subtyping: A Clustering Approach to Establish a Ground Truth for Downstream Applications. Arch Pathol Lab Med 2023;147(8):885–95.

75. Warth A, Stenzinger A, von Brunneck AC, et al. Interobserver variability in the application of the novel IASLC/ATS/ERS classification for pulmonary adenocarcinomas. Eur Respir J 2012;40(5):1221–7.

76. Warth A, Cortis J, Fink L, et al. Training increases concordance in classifying pulmonary adenocarcinomas according to the novel IASLC/ATS/ERS classification. Virchows Arch 2012;461(2):185–93.

77. Chang WC, Zhang YZ, Lim E, et al. Prognostic Impact of Histopathologic Features in Pulmonary Invasive Mucinous Adenocarcinomas. Am J Clin Pathol 2020;154(1):88–102.

78. Lin G, Li H, Kuang J, et al. Acinar-predominant pattern correlates with poorer prognosis in invasive mucinous adenocarcinoma of the lung. Am J Clin Pathol 2018;149(5):373–8.

79. Rodriguez EF, Dacic S, Pantanowitz L, et al. Cytopathology of pulmonary adenocarcinoma with a single histological pattern using the proposed International Association for the Study of Lung Cancer/American Thoracic Society/European Respiratory Society (IASLC/ATS/ERS) classification. Cancer Cytopathol 2015;123(5):306–17.

80. Cancer Protocol Templates. College of American Pathologists https://www.cap.org/protocols-and-guide lines/cancer-reporting-tools/cancer-protocol-templates. Accessed October 17, 2023.

81. Tsutani Y, Goldman JW, Dacic S, et al. Adjuvant Osimertinib vs. Placebo in Completely Resected Stage IA2-IA3 EGFR-Mutated NSCLC: ADAURA2. Clin Lung Cancer 2023;24(4):376–80.

82. Wang K, Liu X, Ding Y, et al. A pretreatment prediction model of grade 3 tumors classed by the IASLC grading system in lung adenocarcinoma. BMC Pulm Med 2023;23(1):377.

83. Nicholson AG, Moreira AL, Mino-Kenudson M, et al. Grading in Lung Adenocarcinoma: Another New Normal. J Thorac Oncol 2021;16(10):1601–4.

Pathologic Response Evaluation in Neoadjuvant-Treated Lung Cancer

Sanja Dacic, MD, PhD

KEYWORDS

• Pathologic response • Neoadjuvant • Lung cancer • Resection

Key points

- Pathologic response may serve as a surrogate marker of outcome in patients with lung cancer treated with neoadjuvant therapy.
- The tumor bed includes viable tumor, stroma, and necrosis which should be assessed in 10% increments for 100% of the total tumor bed.
- The tumor bed is the area where the original pretreatment tumor was located.
- Major pathologic response is defined as $\leq$ 10% of viable tumor at the primary tumor site.
- Pathologic complete response refers to no viable tumor at the primary tumor and in the lymph nodes.

ABSTRACT

Major pathologic response (MPR) and pathologic complete response (pCR) are increasingly being used in non-small cell lung carcinoma neoadjuvant clinical trials as an early endpoint of survival. MPR for all histologic types of lung cancer is $\leq$ 10% of viable tumor, while pCR requires no viable tumor. The International Association for the Study of Lung Cancer multidisciplinary recommendation for the assessment of response in surgically resected lung carcinomas after neoadjuvant therapy was the first attempt to standardize grossing processing and microscopic evaluation.

INTRODUCTION

Pathologic response has been proposed as an early clinical trial endpoint for disease-free and overall survival in neoadjuvant clinical trials for many tumor types.[1-3] Similarly, pathologic response has become a surrogate of outcomes following neoadjuvant chemotherapy and, most recently, neoadjuvant immunotherapy clinical trials in non-small cell lung carcinoma (NSCLC).[4-12] The efficacy of the treatment can be assessed by major pathologic response (MPR) and pathologic complete response (pCR). MPR is defined as $\leq$10% viable tumor at the primary tumor site for all histologic subtypes of NSCLC, while pCR refers to 0% viable tumor at both primary tumor site and lymph nodes. Until recently, only few studies have described gross and microscopic assessments of the lung resection specimens after neoadjuvant therapies.[4,13-15] Numerous histologic criteria have been reviewed and reported, and the major 3 features include necrosis, stroma, and viable tumor.[11,13,15-17] The percent of viable tumor has consistently been shown to be the only prognostically significant histologic indicator.[13,17] It was also noticed that the same histologic changes attributed to treatment effect can be seen in resection specimens without a

Department of Pathology Yale School of Medicine, 200 So Frontage Street, EP2-607, New Haven, CT 06510, USA
E-mail address: sanja.dacic@yale.edu

Surgical Pathology 17 (2024) 287–293
https://doi.org/10.1016/j.path.2023.11.010
1875-9181/24/© 2023 Elsevier Inc. All rights reserved.

surgpath.theclinics.com

history of neoadjuvant treatment, and therefore it is essential for the pathologists to be aware of the treatment history. In contrast to breast carcinoma, there was no standardized approach to gross processing and microscopic examination of lung resection specimens treated with different types of neoadjuvant therapies.[18] The International Association for the Study of Lung Cancer (IASLC) recently published multidisciplinary guidelines for a standardized approach for gross processing and microscopic pathologic assessment of response to all neoadjuvant therapies (chemotherapy, immunotherapy, and targeted therapies) in surgically resected NSCLC.[19] This was the first attempt to standardize thoracic pathology practices. There is still a lack of consensus for estimating the percentages of each tumor bed component microscopically. In most studies, a semiquantitative or "eyeball" approach was applied.[4,13,17] Other studies used average of total percentage of viable tumor across all histologic slides of the tumor bed.[5,20] Most recently, weighted approach using the MPR calculator tool has been developed.[20,21] This approach takes into account the proportion of the tumor bed sampled on each slide. Although it is uncertain which approach best predicts the outcomes, the IASLC reproducibility study showed no difference between weighted and average approaches suggesting that simpler and more practical approaches should be adopted into clinical practice.[20]

In addition to the IASLC scoring proposal, immune-related pathologic response criteria (irPRC) have been proposed for all tumor types including lung treated with immune checkpoint inhibitors.[22,23] This scoring system defines the tumor bed as the sum of the residual viable tumor, necrosis, and regression bed. The regression bed is defined as proliferative fibrosis with neovascularization and evidence of immune activation and cell death. The intratumoral stroma is counted as viable tumor. Even though there are some differences between the 2 scoring systems, namely definitions of regression bed and stroma, there are also similarities particularly in the assessment of viable tumor. Therefore, it would be expected that these 2 scoring systems do not show significant differences in the assessment of MPR and particularly pCR.

Examination of the lymph nodes in lung resection specimens after neoadjuvant therapy is a critical step in the assessment of complete pathologic complete response (cPR). Data on the assessment of response in lymph nodes are limited and earlier proposals stated that lymph nodes should be assessed in the same way as primary tumors.[24,25] The IASLC recommendation for lymph nodes include the same histologic criteria as for the primary tumor including viable tumor, stroma, and necrosis. Studies have shown that patients with negative lymph nodes have a better survival than those with positive lymph nodes even if primary tumor shows MPR.[24] However, there is still no consensus on cutoff to define pathologic response in lymph nodes.

In addition to traditional histologic assessment of pathologic response, machine learning and deep learning algorithms have been developed with an intent to provide a more accurate and reproducible pathologic response assessment.[26] Tissue or blood biomarker analyses have been also used in clinical trials particularly in immuno-oncology.[27–29]

GROSS FEATURES

The first step in the gross examination of the surgically resected lung specimen after neoadjuvant therapy is to identify the tumor bed. The tumor bed is area where the original pretreatment tumor was located. There are different gross presentations of the tumor bed (Fig. 1). In cases with little or no response, the common gross presentation is similar to that of untreated tumors such as easily identifiable pleural retraction or palpable tumor mass (see Fig. 1A). In cases with pCR or MPR, it may be difficult to identify a lesion. Those cases frequently show a small delicate scar (see Fig. 1B). In those cases, it is essential to ask the surgeon to mark the original tumor location. It is also essential to review pretreatment and the most recent computed tomography (CT) scans of the chest to identify the tumor in the gross resection specimen. Although specimens should be fixed for 6 to 48 hours, the size of tumor bed should be measured on the fresh, unfixed specimen. The tumor bed ≤ 3 cm should be entirely submitted for microscopic examination. If the tumor bed is larger than 3 cm, the largest cross section should be entirely submitted with additional sections per 1 cm. Another proposal for large tumors was to submit at least 50% of the tumor bed. If the initial microscopic examination suggests a cPR, the entire tumor bed should be submitted for microscopic examination. Histologic sections at the periphery of the tumor bed should include the border of the tumor with at least 1 cm of the surrounding nonneoplastic lung parenchyma to define the edge of the tumor. The gross descriptions should contain an estimate of the percentage of necrosis. This is particularly important for the large necrotic cavitary tumors for which the microscopic assessment of necrosis may be

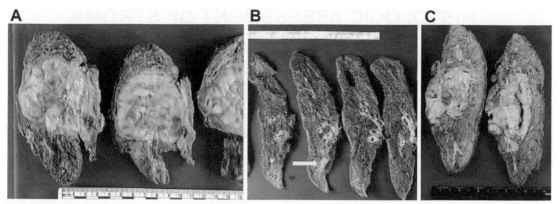

Fig. 1. Gross appearance of the tumor bed. (*A*) Lung and chest wall. The pretreatment squamous cell carcinoma was invading the chest wall. The posttreatment resection showed the tumor bed with yellow areas of necrosis, firm fibrosis, and possible viable tumor. On a gross examination, the impression was that the tumor was invading the chest wall. However, histologic sections showed no viable tumor in the chest wall. (*B*) Complete pathologic response. A small subpleural scar with no microscopic evidence of viable tumor. (*C*) Squamous cell carcinoma with extensive necrosis with cavitation. Gross estimate of the percentage of necrosis is essential as microscopic sections may underestimate how much necrosis is present in the tumor bed.

inaccurate and correlation between gross and microscopic findings is essential (see **Fig.** 1C).

Dense fibrosis or organizing pneumonia can appear white or tan on gross examination and is difficult to distinguish from viable tumor. In those cases, the presence of adjacent organizing pneumonia and/or interstitial fibrosis and inflammation may preclude a reliable assessment of the tumor bed size on gross examination alone.

Lymph nodes should be submitted entirely. If the lymph node metastasis measures greater than 2 cm, the lymph node can be bisected and the central section through the tumor can be submitted. However, individual laboratories may follow their internal guidelines for lymph node sampling including sampling of the entire lymph nodes regardless of their size.

MICROSCOPIC FEATURES

Microscopic examination of the tumor bed includes the assessment of viable tumor, stroma, and necrosis in 10% increments for 100% total of the tumor bed, unless the amount is less than 5% (**Fig.** 2). The stroma includes fibrosis and inflammation (**Fig.** 3). The fibrosis can be dense collagenized, fibroelastic, or myxoid. The inflammation can be chronic with lymphocytes, plasma cells, and lymphoid aggregates. Neutrophils, histiocytes, multinucleated giant cells, and xanthogranulomatous reaction can also be seen. The xanthogranulomatous reaction shows foamy macrophages and foreign body multinucleated giant cells associated with the cholesterol cleft. Necrosis can consist of a completely necrotic tissue and could be

HISTOLOGIC COMPONENTS OF TUMOR BED

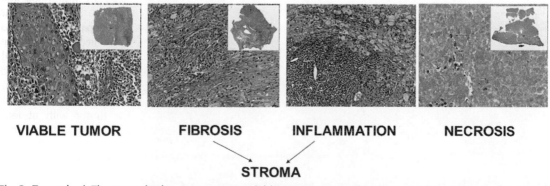

| VIABLE TUMOR | FIBROSIS | INFLAMMATION | NECROSIS |

STROMA

Fig. 2. Tumor bed. The tumor bed components are viable tumor, stroma (fibrosis and inflammation), and necrosis. Each component should be estimated in 10% increments for 100% total.

HISTOLOGIC ASSESSMENT OF STROMA

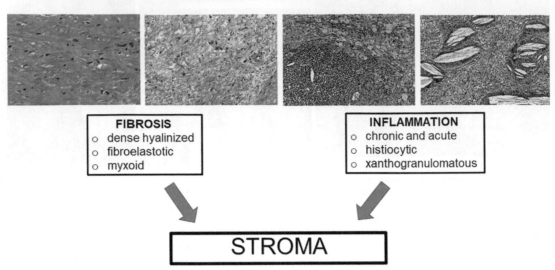

FIBROSIS
o dense hyalinized
o fibroelastotic
o myxoid

INFLAMMATION
o chronic and acute
o histiocytic
o xanthogranulomatous

STROMA

Fig. 3. Stroma. The stroma is composed of fibrosis and inflammation. Fibrosis can be dense hyalinized, fibroelastotic, and myxoid. Inflammation can be chronic, acute, histiocytic, and xanthogranulomatous. These changes can be also observed in treatment-naïve lung carcinoma resections.

admixed with neutrophils and other inflammatory cells. Keratin pearls can be seen in the areas of necrosis and they should not be counted as a viable tumor. Fibrovascular cores of a papillary adenocarcinoma and alveolated septae of lepidic adenocarcinoma should be counted as viable tumor rather than stroma. Colloid adenocarcinoma frequently present as abundant extracellular mucin pools with rare viable tumor cells, both of which should be considered viable tumor.

DIFFERENTIAL DIAGNOSIS

In contrast to breast cancer and melanoma, the assessment of the tumor bed can be very challenging in the lung. Frequently, the adjacent nonneoplastic lung shows marked reactive changes such as prominent type II pneumocyte atypia that is difficult to differentiate from lepidic adenocarcinoma, and there are no immunohistochemical markers that distinguish between the 2. The second common issue is the presence of other reactive changes such as organizing pneumonia and marked inflammation that can interfere with the tumor bed measurement and visual assessment (**Fig. 4**). In those cases, the best approach is to identify nonneoplastic intact lung alveolar septa which are not components of the tumor bed. Fibroelastotic scars can be seen in the lung in the absence of neoadjuvant therapy, most frequently

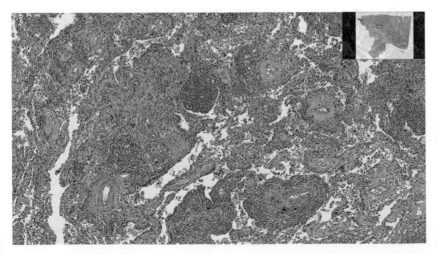

Fig. 4. Background lung. Lung parenchyma adjacent to the tumor bed (insert) showing organizing pneumonia, chronic inflammation, and prominent blood vessels with perivascular lymphocytic inflammation.

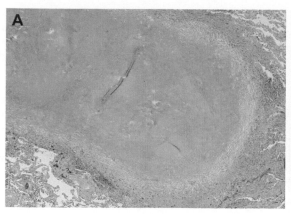 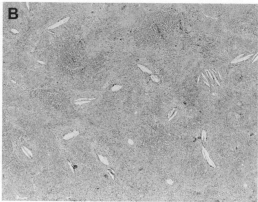

Fig. 5. Necrotizing granuloma. (*A*) Infection caused necrotizing granuloma presenting as a round nodule surrounded by histiocytic aggregates outside of the tumor bed. (*B*) Giant cells and cholesterol clefts in the tumor bed stroma.

in association with adenocarcinoma. Apical caps associated with infarcts have the same morphologic appearance as fibroelastosis associated with neoadjuvant treatment. Elastic fiber-rich fibrosis is a feature of pleuroparenchymal fibroelastosis which can occur following chemotherapy and transplantation of the bone marrow or lung.

Vascular changes including inflammation mimicking vasculitis or medial fibrotic thickening with obliteration and recanalization can be seen in treatment-naïve lungs. In some cases, a small cluster of viable tumor cells can be difficult to differentiate from histiocytic reactions. In such cases, immunostains for keratin and macrophages may be helpful.

Postobstructive cicatricial organizing pneumonia can be difficult to distinguish from the tumor bed, particularly for central tumors. In such cases, correlation with pretreatment CT studies can be helpful.

Necrotizing granulomas caused by infection should be distinguished from a separate tumor nodule (**Fig. 5**A–B). Infectious granulomas show central necrosis surrounded by prominent foreign body giant cell reaction occasionally forming granulomas. These granulomas and giant cells tend to be circumferential around necrosis. In contrast, granulomas and giant cells related to treatment are usually randomly distributed included in the center of necrosis. Granulomas and anthracosilicotic nodules are frequently found in the lymph nodes and should be distinguished from a histiocytic reaction to treatment. Identification of carbon pigment and polarizable silica particles should be helpful to make that distinction.

PRACTICAL APPLICATIONS

The pathologic stage of surgically resected NSCLC after neoadjuvant therapy should be included in the pathology report. In cases with no response, a grossly measured size of the identified tumor mass should be used for the post–neoadjuvant therapy pathological tumor (ypT) stage. If the tumor showed a response resulting in multiple foci of viable carcinoma admixed with stroma and necrosis, the tumor size should be calculated by multiplying the percentage of the viable tumor times the maximum dimension of the tumor bed. For tumors extending into adjacent structures such as the chest wall (pT3) prior to neoadjuvant therapy, the ypT stage should be determined only by the extent of viable tumor spread after therapy. For lepidic tumors, both total size and invasive size should be documented, but the pathological tumor (pT) stage is determined by invasive size. In neoadjuvant settings, 2 adjustments for ypT should be made for invasive size and for the percent viable tumor.

If there is no viable tumor at the primary site but lymph nodes are positive, the staging should be ypT0 yp N1-3 depending on the involved lymph node station. Those cases are considered to show MPR but not pCR.

SUMMARY

The pathologic response to neoadjuvant treatment in surgically resected NSCLC should be evaluated using appropriately fixed and sampled specimens. Microscopic assessment of MPR should be standardized and uniform in the clinical trials and in daily clinical practice. More work is required to determine the assessment of pathologic response in lymph nodes. Surgical pathology reports should be standardized to include at least the percentage of viable tumor and pathologic stage.

CLINICS CARE POINTS

- Changes related to treatment can be observed in treatment-naïve carcinomas.

- Knowledge about neoadjuvant treatment is essential for adequate specimen processing, histologic assessment, and pathologic staging.

- Gross measurements of the tumor bed may not be accurate due to secondary changes in the background nonneoplastic lung parenchyma.

- Tumor beds ≤ 3 cm should be entirely submitted.

- If the tumor bed is larger than 3 cm, the largest cross section should be entirely submitted with additional sections per 1 cm.

- If the initial sampling of greater than 3 cm tumor bed suggests pCR, the entire tumor bed should be submitted for microscopic evaluation.

DISCLOSURE

Dr S. Dacic reports personal fees from Astra Zeneca and Genentech, outside the submitted work.

REFERENCES

1. Thomas JSJ, Provenzano E, Hiller L, et al. Central pathology review with two-stage quality assurance for pathological response after neoadjuvant chemotherapy in the ARTemis Trial. Mod Pathol 2017;30(8): 1069–77.

2. Yau C, Osdoit M, van der Noordaa M, et al. Residual cancer burden after neoadjuvant chemotherapy and long-term survival outcomes in breast cancer: a multicentre pooled analysis of 5161 patients. Lancet Oncol 2022;23(1):149–60.

3. Menzies AM, Amaria RN, Rozeman EA, et al. Pathological response and survival with neoadjuvant therapy in melanoma: a pooled analysis from the International Neoadjuvant Melanoma Consortium (INMC). Nat Med 2021;27(2):301–9.

4. Junker K, Thomas M, Schulmann K, et al. Tumour regression in non-small-cell lung cancer following neoadjuvant therapy. Histological assessment. J Cancer Res Clin Oncol 1997;123(9):469–77.

5. Pataer A, Kalhor N, Correa AM, et al. Histopathologic response criteria predict survival of patients with resected lung cancer after neoadjuvant chemotherapy. J Thorac Oncol 2012;7(5):825–32.

6. Cascone T, Leung CH, Weissferdt A, et al. Neoadjuvant chemotherapy plus nivolumab with or without ipilimumab in operable non-small cell lung cancer: the phase 2 platform NEOSTAR trial. Nat Med 2023;29(3):593–604.

7. Cascone T, William WN Jr, Weissferdt A, et al. Neoadjuvant nivolumab or nivolumab plus ipilimumab in operable non-small cell lung cancer: the phase 2 randomized NEOSTAR trial. Nat Med 2021;27(3): 504–14.

8. Shu CA, Gainor JF, Awad MM, et al. Neoadjuvant atezolizumab and chemotherapy in patients with resectable non-small-cell lung cancer: an open-label, multicentre, single-arm, phase 2 trial. Lancet Oncol 2020;21(6):786–95.

9. Lee JM, Kim AW, Marjanski T, et al. Important Surgical and Clinical End Points in Neoadjuvant Immunotherapy Trials in Resectable NSCLC. JTO Clin Res Rep 2021;2(10):100221.

10. Provencio M, Nadal E, Insa A, et al. Neoadjuvant chemotherapy and nivolumab in resectable non-small-cell lung cancer (NADIM): an open-label, multicentre, single-arm, phase 2 trial. Lancet Oncol 2020;21(11):1413–22.

11. Hellmann MD, Chaft JE, William WN Jr, et al. Pathological response after neoadjuvant chemotherapy in resectable non-small-cell lung cancers: proposal for the use of major pathological response as a surrogate endpoint. Lancet Oncol 2014;15(1): e42–50.

12. Heymach JV, Mitsudomi T, Harpole D, et al. Design and Rationale for a Phase III, Double-Blind, Placebo-Controlled Study of Neoadjuvant Durvalumab + Chemotherapy Followed by Adjuvant Durvalumab for the Treatment of Patients With Resectable Stages II and III non-small-cell Lung Cancer: The AEGEAN Trial. Clin Lung Cancer 2022;23(3):e247–51.

13. Qu Y, Emoto K, Eguchi T, et al. Pathologic Assessment After Neoadjuvant Chemotherapy for NSCLC: Importance and Implications of Distinguishing Adenocarcinoma From Squamous Cell Carcinoma. J Thorac Oncol 2019;14(3):482–93.

14. Pataer A, Weissferdt A, Correa AM, et al. Major Pathologic Response and Prognostic Score Predict Survival in Patients With Lung Cancer Receiving Neoadjuvant Chemotherapy. JTO Clin Res Rep 2022;3(11):100420.

15. Blaauwgeers JL, Kappers I, Klomp HM, et al. Complete pathological response is predictive for clinical outcome after tri-modality therapy for carcinomas of the superior pulmonary sulcus. Virchows Arch 2013; 462(5):547–56.

16. Junker K, Langner K, Klinke F, et al. Grading of tumor regression in non-small cell lung cancer : morphology and prognosis. Chest 2001;120(5):1584–91.

17. Weissferdt A, Pataer A, Vaporciyan AA, et al. Agreement on Major Pathological Response in NSCLC

Patients Receiving Neoadjuvant Chemotherapy. Clin Lung Cancer 2020;21(4):341–8.

18. Sahoo S, Krings G, Chen YY, et al. Standardizing Pathologic Evaluation of Breast Carcinoma After Neoadjuvant Chemotherapy. Arch Pathol Lab Med 2022;147(5):591–603.

19. Travis WD, Dacic S, Wistuba I, et al. IASLC Multidisciplinary Recommendations for Pathologic Assessment of Lung Cancer Resection Specimens After Neoadjuvant Therapy. J Thorac Oncol 2020;15(5):709–40.

20. Dacic S, Travis W, Redman M, et al. International Association for the Study of Lung Cancer Study of Reproducibility in Assessment of Pathologic Response in Resected Lung Cancers After Neoadjuvant Therapy. J Thorac Oncol 2023;18(10):1290–302.

21. Saqi A, Leslie KO, Moreira AL, et al. Assessing Pathologic Response in Resected Lung Cancers: Current Standards, Proposal for a Novel Pathologic Response Calculator Tool, and Challenges in Practice. JTO Clin Res Rep 2022;3(5):100310.

22. Cottrell TR, Thompson ED, Forde PM, et al. Pathologic features of response to neoadjuvant anti-PD-1 in resected non-small-cell lung carcinoma: a proposal for quantitative immune-related pathologic response criteria (irPRC). Ann Oncol 2018;29(8):1853–60.

23. Stein JE, Lipson EJ, Cottrell TR, et al. Pan-Tumor Pathologic Scoring of Response to PD-(L)1 Blockade. Clin Cancer Res 2020;26(3):545–51.

24. Pataer A, Weissferdt A, Vaporciyan AA, et al. Evaluation of Pathologic Response in Lymph Nodes of Patients With Lung Cancer Receiving Neoadjuvant Chemotherapy. J Thorac Oncol 2021;16(8):1289–97.

25. Zens P, Bello C, Scherz A, et al. A prognostic score for non-small cell lung cancer resected after neoadjuvant therapy in comparison with the tumor-node-metastases classification and major pathological response. Mod Pathol 2021;34(7):1333–44.

26. Dacic S, Travis WD, Giltnane JM, et al. Artificial intelligence (AI) -powered pathologic response (PathR) assessment of resection specimens after neoadjuvant atezolizumab in patients with non-small cell lung cancer: Results from LCMC3 study. J Clin Oncol 2021;39:106.

27. Forde PM, Spicer J, Lu S, et al. Neoadjuvant Nivolumab plus Chemotherapy in Resectable Lung Cancer. N Engl J Med 2022;386(21):1973–85.

28. Goldberg SB, Narayan A, Kole AJ, et al. Early Assessment of Lung Cancer Immunotherapy Response via Circulating Tumor DNA. Clin Cancer Res 2018;24(8):1872–80.

29. Gandara DR, Paul SM, Kowanetz M, et al. Blood-based tumor mutational burden as a predictor of clinical benefit in non-small-cell lung cancer patients treated with atezolizumab. Nat Med 2018;24(9):1441–8.

Microsatellite Instability, Mismatch Repair, and Tumor Mutation Burden in Lung Cancer

Oana C. Rosca, MD[a,b,*], Oana E. Vele, MD[a,c]

KEYWORDS

- Lung cancer • Immune checkpoint inhibitors • Immunotherapy • Biomarkers
- Microsatellite instability/mismatch repair deficiency • Tumor mutation burden

Key points

- Immune checkpoint inhibitors (ICIs) are among the most significant developments in cancer therapeutic modalities and changed the landscape of lung cancer management.
- New biomarkers such as microsatellite instability/mismatch repair deficiency and tumor mutation burden were developed to predict response to ICIs.
- Existing biomarkers require further refinement in their assessment.
- Search of ideal biomarkers to predict response to ICIs continues.
- Complementary use of the existing and novel immune biomarkers could improve selection of patients potentially benefiting from ICIs.

ABSTRACT

Since US Food and Drug Administration approval of programmed death ligand 1 (PD-L1) as the first companion diagnostic for immune checkpoint inhibitors (ICIs) in non-small cell lung cancer, many patients have experienced increased overall survival. To improve selection of ICI responders versus nonresponders, microsatellite instability/mismatch repair deficiency (MSI/MMR) and tumor mutation burden (TMB) came into play. Clinical data show PD-L1, MSI/MMR, and TMB are independent predictive immunotherapy biomarkers. Harmonization of testing methodologies, optimization of assay design, and results analysis are ongoing. Future algorithms to determine immunotherapy eligibility might involve complementary use of current and novel biomarkers. Artificial intelligence could facilitate algorithm implementation to convert complex genetic data into recommendations for specific ICIs.

BACKGROUND

As cancer became a worldwide leading killer, lung cancer emerged and remains, despite treatment breakthroughs, the most common cause of death, surpassing female breast, prostate, colorectal, and pancreas malignancies.[1]

Furthermore, recent delays in diagnosis and access to therapy were caused by coronavirus disease

[a] Molecular Pathologist/Cytopathologist, Donald and Barbara Zucker School of Medicine at Hofstra/Northwell;
[b] Department of Pathology and Laboratory Medicine, 2200 Northern Boulevard, Suite 104, Greenvale, NY 11548, USA; [c] Department of Pathology and Laboratory Medicine, Lenox Hill Hospital, New York, NY 10075, USA
* Corresponding author: 2200 Northern Boulevard, Suite 104, Greenvale, NY 11548, USA
E-mail address: orafael@northwell.edu
Twitter: @OanaCRosca (O.C.R.)

Surgical Pathology 17 (2024) 295–305
https://doi.org/10.1016/j.path.2023.11.011
1875-9181/24/© 2023 Elsevier Inc. All rights reserved.

2019 (COVID-19), with a shift toward higher stage at diagnosis, prompting the medical community to constantly modify guidelines and evaluate different therapeutic approaches.[2,3] Recent developments in non-small cell lung cancer (NSCLC) precision medicine led to major improvements in disease management. Among the most significant developments in therapeutic modalities are immune checkpoint inhibitors (ICIs), approved by the US Food and Drug Administration (FDA) for use in advanced or metastatic NSCLC as first and later lines of treatment, as monotherapies or in combination with other therapeutic strategies.

Malignant cells can overexpress specific ligands on their surface, which bind to inhibitory receptors on the surface of effector T-cells, deactivating their antitumor activity. This escape mechanism of cancer cells can be disrupted by ICIs. Their main targets are programmed cell death 1 (PD-1), programmed death ligand 1 (PD-L1), cytotoxic T-lymphocyte-associated antigen 4 (CTLA-4), and lymphocyte-activation gene 3 (LAG-3).

An increased load of tumor neoantigens creates an environment for the immune cells to be primed to act if the interaction between tumor cell PD-L1 and the T-cell PD-1 is blocked. Acquired gene alterations in the antigen presentation pathway further tune the impact of the immunogenic neoantigen load on the immune checkpoint blockade by adjusting the ability of T-cells to present peptides to the immune system. Highly mutated tumors bear neoantigens that make them more susceptible to the activated immune system, correlating with response to ICIs.[4] The efficacy of ICIs depends on the natural immune response to either private or public neoantigens. A neoantigen is a mutated peptide that is presented by a human leukocyte antigen (HLA) on the cell surface and can be recognized by the immune system. The private neoantigens emerge from non-recurrent driver or passenger mutations, which might not be present in all cells. The public neoantigens emerge from recurrent driver mutations shared by many patients. Successfully targeting them has encountered many challenges, as most of the driver mutations do not lead to neoantigens presented by common HLAs. The binding affinity of the neoantigen and HLA affects the presentation capability to the immune system. Public neoantigen and HLA type combined screening could be used to select optimal immunotherapy.[5,6]

Lung tumors arise from accumulation of mutations acquired through defects in DNA repair pathways and/or by exposure to environmental factors such as tobacco smoke, ultraviolet light and DNA-damaging therapies.[7] Up to 95% of NSCLC can express PD-L1 with implicit poor prognosis; therefore immunotherapy can be a powerful tool in the armamentarium against lung cancer.[8]

Immuno-oncology has revolutionized cancer therapy and since the first FDA approved PD-1 inhibitors in 2014, the ICI list expanded rapidly. Various studies showed that anti-PD-1/PD-L1 therapies alone or in conjunction with chemoradiotherapy can improve median overall survival (OS) and could have synergistic effects in NSCLC when combined with targeted agents such as tyrosine kinase inhibitors (TKIs).[9]

The focus of this article is on the state of microsatellite instability/mismatch repair deficiency (MSI/MMR) and tumor mutation burden (TMB) as determinants of response to PD-1 pathway blockade in lung cancer with a brief mention of PD-L1 immunohistochemistry (IHC).

Approved ICIs are usually paired with companion diagnostic IHCs and can be used based on defined percentage of tumor membranous immunoreactivity (eg, 1% for pembrolizumab or 50% for ceplimimab).[10] Although there are inconsistencies among studies on the interchangeability of antibodies and there is no standardized threshold for PD-L1 reactivity, patients with NSCLC can experience longer progression-free survival (PFS) and OS after treatment with ICIs compared to chemotherapy.[11]

To harmonize the PD-L1 testing, the Blueprint PD-L1 IHC assay comparison project was conducted (2017–2018).[12,13] A 2021 review by Prince and colleagues concluded that 28-8-, 22C3-, and SP263-based assays show strong analytical concordance for the assessment of PD-L1 expression in lung cancer.[14]

Tumor proportion score (TPS) or combined positive score (CPS) is employed in interpretations of PD-L1 IHC depending on tumor type. TPS score, currently used for NSCLC, represents the percentage of PD-L1 reactive tumor cells out of the total of tumor cells. Conversely, CPS is calculated by the number of PD-L1 reactive tumor cells, lymphocytes, and macrophages divided by the total number of viable tumor cells multiplied by 100. A minimum of 100 viable cells is usually required for an accurate TPS analysis.

Interestingly, PD-L1-negative IHC is not necessarily a predictor for lack of ICIs benefit, perhaps because of intrinsic tumor heterogeneity or maybe assay imperfections including lack of ideal sensitivity and specificity. Similarly, PD-L1-positive IHC does not correlate entirely with patients' response to therapy, which can widely vary from complete resolution to no benefits. In some settings, PD-L1 expression seems to be more of a prognostic rather than predictive biomarker.[15] Although IHC scoring is inherently difficult to measure objectively, the advantage is the short turnaround time and reduced sample requirements.[16–18] Small biopsies and cytology samples demonstrated similar PD-L1 status compared with corresponding surgical specimens, despite tumor heterogeneity; however, differences have been proven between the original PD-L1 expression and subsequent metastases, usually a change from positive to negative status. ICIs or platinum chemotherapy also appear to affect the PD-L1 status.[10] Additionally, some solid tumors treated with ICIs show initial pseudoprogression before clinically measurable response.[19,20]

Efficacy of ICIs seems to be reduced in tumors with driver mutations and in association with previous use of steroids. ICIs might not always have the desired outcome and despite their benefit, can have adverse effects (fatigue, diarrhea, itching, rash and pneumonitis), which can lead to death if not recognized and treated in a timely manner. Moreover, ICI therapy can be costly; therefore patient selection must be optimized through the use of relevant biomarkers.[11,21]

In comparison to the PD-1 pathway targeting drugs, use of CTLA-4 antibodies was limited by lower efficacy and more frequent adverse effects.[11,22]

LAG-3-blocking antibody was FDA approved in 2022 for treatment of melanoma. Studies are underway to explore it as a promising target in other cancers.[23]

MICROSATELLITE INSTABILITY/MISMATCH REPAIR DEFICIENCY

The MSI/MMR and more recently TMB were approved by FDA as predictive biomarkers to determine eligibility for therapy with ICIs in patients with solid tumors including NSCLC. MSI status and TMB value are now included routinely in the tumor multigene next-generation sequencing (NGS) reports regardless of the type of cancer. Their use in clinical practice emerged in the context of the noted variability of responses to immunotherapy in tumors selected based on the PD-L1-expression.

Microsatellites (MSs) are short repetitive DNA sequences (1–6 bp) accounting for about 3% of the human genome and are prone to errors during DNA replication or repair.[24] They are also known as short tandem repeats (STRs) or simple sequence repeats (SSRs) and are altered by DNA polymerase slippage during replication. The MMR system maintains the genomic integrity and is involved in prevention of tumorigenesis. It includes various enzymes with 4 genes playing a critical role in the MMR status assessment: *MLH1* (mutL homologue 1), *PMS2* (postmeiotic segregation increased 2),

MSH2 (mutS homologue 2), and *MSH6* (mutS homologue 6). They can be detected by IHC. Lack of protein expression or dysfunctional proteins generate defective MMR (dMMR) status.

MSI is caused by deficiency of the MMR system and can present as microsatellite instability high (MSI-H) or microsatellite instability low (MSI-L). In other words, MSI is a marker of dMMR characterized by hypermutable cells. It is an actionable phenotype that can predict tumor response to ICIs, and MSI-H/dMMR tumors frequently benefit from immunotherapy.

Clinical trials proved that the biology of MSI status was similar across tumor types, which prompted the FDA to approve pembrolizumab in 2017 as the first tumor-agnostic biomarker with indications for ICIs, regardless of tumor site or histology.[25–28]

Based on clinical evidence, microsatellite stable (MSS) tumors are significantly less likely than MSI-H tumors to respond to anti-PD-1 ICIs.[29–31]

Defects in MMR can either be inherited or acquired. MSI is commonly associated with Lynch syndrome, a hereditary condition that increases the risk of developing certain tumors such as colorectal cancer. However, MSI-H is generally infrequent in lung tumors, with previous studies reporting less than 1% prevalence in lung squamous cell carcinoma (SqCC) and adenocarcinoma (ADC).

Reported incidence of MSI-H in lung small cell carcinoma (SCC) has been limited and conflicting.[32–35] SCC is characterized by a high TMB and evades the immune system.[10] ICIs appear to have little influence in OS of patients with SCC. However, several studies noted a small subset of SCC patients can benefit and even have sustained response when treated with PD-L1 monotherapy or combined with CTLA-4 blockade. These patients could belong to the inflamed SCC subtype that may be more susceptible to immunotherapy.[36,37] Additional investigational studies are looking into identifying which subtypes of SCC can benefit from and maintain response to ICIs.[38,39]

Cigarette smoking is linked to about 80% of lung cancer deaths, and the number may be higher in SCC.[40] NSCLC mutations related to smoking contribute to neoantigen formation and subsequent recruitment of effector T-cells.[41] Cigarette smoking can also influence the NSCLC evolution, pathology, molecular features, treatment benefits, and overall outcomes.[42]

MICROSATELLITE INSTABILITY/MISMATCH REPAIR TESTING METHODOLOGY

Various methods can be employed for detection of MSI status in patients diagnosed with cancer: IHC and molecular assays. A 1997 National Cancer Institute (NCI) consensus meeting recommended testing a core panel of 5 markers to determine the status of MSI and to be used as reference for future research in the field. The Bethesda panel consists of 2 single nucleotide repeat loci (BAT25 and BAT26) and 3 multi-nucleotide repeat loci (D2S123, D5S346 and D17S250).[43] A second recommended panel with higher sensitivity and specificity uses 5 poly-A mononucleotide repeats: BAT25, BAT26, NR21, NR24, and NR27.[44]

MSI tumor testing has been routinely performed by polymerase chain reaction (PCR) and capillary electrophoresis. Commercial assays can analyze paired normal and tumor tissues to determine MSI at the minimum standard 5 NCI-recommended loci. Many laboratories are now using various panels, and positive results are usually reported as MSI-H (instability in 2 or more markers) or MSI-L (1 marker is unstable).

MMR proteins (MLH1, MSH2, MSH6 and PMS2) are ubiquitously expressed in cell nuclei, and IHC can be employed as a rapid and inexpensive tool to assess them. Despite only providing results on the MMR proteins, IHC has broad availability and accuracy up to 95%. Preanalytical issue such as tissue fixation can lead to false-negative results. The 4 proteins form heterodimers: MLH1-PMS2 and MSH2-MSH6, respectively. Therefore, mutations in the MMR genes result in degradation of the heterodimers and subsequent loss of both obligatory and secondary proteins. MLH1 mutations lead to IHC loss of both MLH1 and PMS2. Similarly, MSH2 mutations lead to IHC loss of both MSH2 and MSH6. On the other hand, when mutations occur in PMS2 or MSH6, other MMR proteins, such as PMS1 or MSH3, can compensate, and the heterodimers can remain stable; therefore, there is no IHC loss of MLH1 and MSH2, respectively. In summary, the PMS2 antibody detects all cases with either MLH1 or PMS2 alterations, while the MSH6 antibody detects all cases with either MSH2 or MSH6 alterations. Aberrant staining patterns (cytoplasmic, dot-like or perinuclear staining) may occasionally be seen. Presence of normal tissue as an internal positive control helps with interpretation. Various mutations in any of the MMR genes can yield defective proteins that are antigenically intact, with no impact on the normal IHC expression pattern. MSI can be used when doubting IHC results. Notably, tumor heterogeneity can also influence MMR IHC, especially in small specimens such as biopsies.[44]

NGS using various bioinformatic approaches and algorithms can assess MSI by interrogating numerous microsatellites and genes, exceeding 90% accuracy. Additionally, NGS panels can provide information, not only on MSI and TMB, but also on targetable genetic alterations. Moreover, NGS testing can be employed if there is a discordance between MSI (PCR) and MMR (IHC).[27,45,46]

MANTIS, MSISensor, mSINGS, and MSIseq are among modalities of detecting MSI by computational tools combined with NGS data.[47–50]

A different methodology is the SmMIP assay, which shows high sensitivity, and, unlike PCR, does not require paired tumor-germline analysis.[51]

TUMOR MUTATION BURDEN

TMB, also referred to as neoantigen burden or mutation load, estimates the acquired somatic mutations accumulated in cancer cell genome, when compared with the germline. It is usually reported as mutations per megabase (muts/Mb). The TMB value and the MSI/MMR status are assessing the same biological phenomenon using different approaches, each with its own limitations.

High TMB produces more novel proteins (neoantigens) in the tumor cells, further stimulating the immune response. Therefore, patients with the highest number of clonal neoantigens are the most likely to respond to treatment. Various studies assessed TMB as a predictor of the efficacy of ICIs, including in lung cancer.[52,53] A retrospective analysis of NSCLC patients treated with pembrolizumab determined that a high TMB based on nonsynonymous mutations detected by whole-exome sequencing (WES) correlated with a robust clinical benefit and PFS. In a 2019 paper, Chan and colleagues illustrated the timeline for developing immunotherapy biomarkers.[54]

TUMOR MUTATION BURDEN TESTING METHODOLOGY

To calculate TMB, the number of somatic mutations detected and confirmed by bioinformatics pipeline is divided by the size of the sequence targeted in the analysis. The final value is a variable dependent on the testing methodology (WES versus targeted gene panels), types of mutations included (synonymous versus nonsynonymous), the bioinformatics filters (eg, artifacts and germline variants), and database used.[55] For an accurate estimation, it was suggested to normalize the TMB value relative to sample tumor purity. This can be achieved by increasing sequencing depth and dividing variant allele frequency (VAF) by purity and increasing the threshold.[56] The variation in sequencing depth and tumor purity could lead to a significant overestimation of the TMB, particularly in samples with numerous somatic mutations at low VAF. Analyzing the mutant allele frequency spectrum could facilitate accurate TMB estimation in these samples.[57]

The mutation types considered for TMB assessment can vary. Mutations producing neo-antigens were initially considered to be captured in the analysis. Acquired mutations that confer a selective tumor growth advantage are referred as drivers, versus passenger mutations that do not affect the tumor growth. Genetic alterations include non-synonymous and synonymous mutations, insertions, deletions, copy number gains and losses, and chromosomal translocations. Non-synonymous alterations, most of which are point mutations, change the encoded amino acid (missense mutations). Synonymous mutations do not alter amino acid coding (silent mutations) but could impact protein levels and functionality by altering mRNA splicing, stability, and translation efficiency. Silent mutations, representing 6% to 8% of all driver mutations in cancer, occur mainly in oncogenes and in 1 tumor suppressor gene (TP53).[58] Insertions or deletions disrupt the reading frame (frameshift), leading to a multitude of neoantigens of high immunogenic potency, more likely to induce a strong antitumor immune response. These are common in the MMR-deficient tumors. The contribution to the neoantigenic load of the chromosomal translocation and post-translational modifications of non-mutated proteins is not captured routinely in the TMB measurement.[54]

Friends of Cancer Research and Quality Assurance Initiative Pathology outlined guidelines for TMB assessment, recommending a VAF cut-off of 5% and not considering synonymous variants.[59] However, including all types of mutations increases the accuracy of TMB estimation.[4] Of note, the tumor indel burden, made of frameshift small insertions and deletions, which could produce a large quantity of highly immunogenic neoantigens, was reported with prognostic impact in different cancer types. It was found to lack a significant impact on OS in lung SqCC and ADC.[60]

TMB has a wide range within tumor types, from 0.001 muts/Mb to more than 400 muts/Mb,[61] especially noted in NSCLCs with 10 times more somatic mutations in the smoker compared with never-smoker mutational signature.[62] There is a strong dose-effect correlation between smoking and TMB in advanced lung ADC.[63] Furthermore, the wide range of TMB within smokers and never-smokers in NSCLC could be explained by previously reported deleterious mutations in genes essential for DNA repair and replication.[59,64,65]

Although TMB was originally estimated by whole genome or WES, it was more recently determined

that targeted gene panels can accurately assess it in a timely and cost-effective manner, mitigating the need of development of a new dedicated assay.[53] NGS, although not readily available in some practices and still an expensive test, is desirable for integrated reporting.[27] Assay complexity and need of highly trained staff and bioinformatics pipelines are some challenges of the NGS testing.[66]

The exome's size of 30 to 35 Mb is capture protocol-dependent. It represents approximately 1% of the human genome and includes approximately 180,000 exons.[67] WES requires high sequencing capacity, larger amounts of high-quality DNA, and higher tumor cell content than most current clinical methodologies. Although initially used as an investigational tool on fresh frozen tissue for projects like The Cancer Genome Atlas, WES can now use formalin-fixed tissue for clinical purposes. This progress has been made possible by bioinformatics tools, capable to filter out formalin-induced sequencing artifacts. Furthermore, bioinformatics tools are used as alternative to the standard analysis of matched tumor and germline (blood or tissue) samples for subtraction of germline variants. This approach reduces the false-positive mutation calls. A limitation is the possible ancestry bias in the germline variant databases for ancestries that are not adequately represented. In addition, filtering out the clonal hematopoiesis-derived variants in the tumor requires matched blood sample analysis. Lung cancer samples, often small, benefit from the development of targeted gene panels (300–500 genes, at least 1 Mb) for clinical use at lower cost and shorter turnaround time. To reduce the overestimation of the TMB by NGS cancer panels, the recurrent driver gene mutations, which characterize the tumor, are excluded from the TMB count.[53]

Factors affecting the estimation of TMB with NGS panels include tumor cell content and intratumor heterogeneity, types of mutations counted, specimen type-dependent DNA quality, sequencing strategy (WES versus targeted genes panel), and bioinformatics that filter out artifacts. The design of the targeted panel and the read depth impact TMB accuracy. A size of 1.5 to 3 Mb is adequate for a good approximation of the TMB. Panels below 1 Mb are not accurate, particularly when proximal to the cut off for the immunotherapy eligibility.[68-70]

Alcohol-based cytologic samples with adequate tumor cellularity and DNA yield can be a source of higher-quality DNA for TMB estimation than histologic specimens that are subject to formalin-fixation induced artifacts. Formalin can result in the C > T artifact, by deamination of cytosine, followed by incorporation of adenine instead of thymine during PCR. This artifact can lead to overestimation of TMB in some samples with greater than 5% allele frequency.[53,71]

The observation that a high TMB would predict responsiveness to ICIs prompted the need to further define the TMB cut-off that would clinically distinguish responders from nonresponders. Subsequently, a value of 10 muts/Mb was first established.[72] A quest for optimal TMB cut-off values across tumor types was carried through numerous clinical trials.[73] Various cut-offs were reported, from ≥10 muts/Mb to >20 muts/Mb. Higher cut-off values have better specificity and less sensitivity.[74] A more recent study found that in NSCLC a cut-off above 19.0 muts/Mb correlates better with OS.[75]

For liquid biopsy, TMB cut-off corresponding to the tissue 10 muts/Mb is increased to 16 muts/Mb.[76]

TMB was reported more likely to be at least 10 muts/Mb in metastases compared with primary tumors in both lung SqCC and ADC and highest in brain metastases from lung ADC.[77] Lower TMB estimates were reported in lymph nodes metastasis, which might reflect lower tumor cell content and/or less subclonal diversity when compared with the primary tumor with multiple intermixed distinct subclones.[78]

Current data show that standardization of panel-based TMB estimation is still needed. Both sensitivity and positive predictive value could be improved by using bioinformatics in conjunction with a comprehensive sequencing database to minimize calling of false-negative alterations.[54,59,79]

TUMOR MUTATION BURDEN AND HUMAN LEUKOCYTE ANTIGEN

It was hypothesized that HLA-class I genotype could predict cancer response to ICIs, possibly increasing survival.[80] Loss of heterozygosity (LOH) of HLA in tumors is an immune escape mechanism and leads to subclonal expansion. Tumors with HLA LOH show a higher TMB, which can be corrected with bioinformatics and computational tools. The algorithms involve eliminating the mutations that encode neoantigens that will not bind to the preserved HLA allele. Therefore, TMB-based survival prediction could be improved by incorporating the LOH of HLA into the TMB assessment.[10,53,81]

CURRENT NATIONAL COMPREHENSIVE CANCER NETWORK GUIDELINES INSIGHT

TMB by itself is an imperfect biomarker. Some patients with low TMB respond to ICIs, while others with high levels are nonresponders.[82]

TMB does not appear to correlate consistently with the neoantigen load. Lack of standardization of TMB measurements across laboratories and inconsistencies in TMB estimation (technical problems, cut-off delineation) prompted NCCN in 2020 to remove TMB as a biomarker to determine eligibility for ICIs in advanced NSCLC. Further work is needed to refine the clinical use of TMB as a predictive biomarker for response to ICIs.[18,27,53,82,83]

MUTATIONS IN NON-SMALL CELL LUNG CANCER AND IMMUNE CHECKPOINT INHIBITORS

Various studies analyzed the simultaneous presence of MSI and molecular alterations in lung cancer.

TMB is lower in lung ADCs with targetable mutations from patients who never smoked than tumors in smokers. Tumors with driver mutations lack CD8+ tumor-infiltrating lymphocytes (TILs) and are regarded as cold, therefore do not respond to ICIs. High TMB, absence of activating alterations, smoking. and HLA status correlate with response to immunotherapy.[84]

In general, cancers with known targetable mutations are conducive to respective robust therapeutic approaches rather than to immunotherapy. Knowing the molecular profile before treatment initiation plays a significant role, as TKIs used after ICIs or a combination of them can heighten immune-related toxicity without additional benefit. Used in combination with chemotherapy, ICIs seem to benefit patients previously treated with targeted therapies.[84] Moreover, mutational signatures can overcome limitations of morphology and IHC in tumor classification. They can potentially indicate the tumor origin based on alterations related to causative environmental mutagens as ultraviolet light and tobacco.[27,66]

EGFR, *ALK,* and *ROS1* genetic alterations predict a lack of benefit from ICIs mainly because of low TMB, while response in *BRAF* V600 E and *MET* exon 14 skipping mutations can be variable. *KRAS* is the most common driver alteration in lung ADC regardless of smoking status. ICIs showed benefit in *KRAS*-mutated tumors, and although concurrent alterations such as *STK11* or *KEAP1* can negatively impact the response, their status does not seem to dictate the choice of immunotherapy. Conflicting data are available on *SMARCA4* mutations; however, concurrent *KRAS/SMARCA4* alterations appear to confer a poor prognosis after ICIs. Tumors with *RET* fusions show limited efficacy to ICIs compared with targeted therapy and chemotherapy; however, the benefit of chemotherapy-immunotherapy is uncertain. Retrospective studies showed various efficacity (from 7.4% to 27.3%) of immunotherapy in HER2-mutant tumors. HER2 (ERBB2) has higher mutation frequency in EGFR-mutant MSI-H lung ADC. There are currently insufficient data for ICIs in tumors with other drivers such as NTRK1/2/3.[10,41,84,85]

Chalmers and colleagues showed that MMR genes and DNA polymerases ε (POLE) and delta 1 (POLD1) cause hypermutant cancers.[4,86,87] POLE mutational signatures can contribute to high TMB independent of MSI status.[44,73]

More data are needed to accurately interpret the complex genetic landscape in conjunction with TMB and response to immunotherapy. ICIs have limitations, adverse effects, and substantial cost and have shown limited median survival gain. However, in patients without a targetable driver alteration, ICIs are among the first-line recommended therapeutic alternatives (alone or in combination with chemotherapy), if there are no clinical contraindications.[88]

In patients with advanced disease who are not amenable to biopsy or cancer resection, liquid biopsy could provide insight into tumor genetic profile with opportunities to follow-up markers and subsequent therapeutic and prognostic implications.[44,53]

MICROSATELLITE INSTABILITY/MISMATCH REPAIR DEFICIENCY, TUMOR MUTATION BURDEN, AND PROGRAMMED DEATH LIGAND 1 RELATIONSHIP

The relationship among MSI/MMR, TMB, and PD-L1 was addressed by various studies. A recent study on NSCLC found that 14.1% of cases were high TMB, but only 0.6% were MSI-H.[89] In another study, high TMB and MSI-H were found in 0.5% of NSCLC cases, TMB-high and PD-L1 positivity in 7.7%, MSI-H and PD-L1 positivity in 0.4%, and positivity in all 3 markers in 0.3% of cases.[90] Tian and colleagues also reported TMB was higher in MSI-H lung cancer. In contrast, no significant difference in PD-L1 expression was seen for MSI-H and MSS tumors. The most common mutated genes associated with MSI-H were TP53, EGFR, LRP1B, BRCA2, and NOTCH1.[85] Luchini and colleagues found that PD-1/PD-L1 can be expressed even in MSI-negative and/or TMB-low cases. They also concluded that it is possible to have a TMB-high in absence of MSI, while MSI-H with TMB-low is rare.[44] Chalmers and colleagues studied over 62,000 samples and showed that 83% of tumors with MSI-H also showed high TMB; however,

only 16% of tumors with high TMB were MSI-H.[4] NSCLC patients with high TMB showed improved PFS after a combination of ICIs regardless of PD-L1 expression.[73]

Overall, TMB, MSI/MMR, and PD-L1 expression in NSCLC show incomplete overlap, suggesting that these are independent predictive markers for selecting ICIs for monotherapy and combination therapy. Used together, they may increase precision in selecting patients likely to benefit from ICIs.[4,53,73,91–93] Relationships among MSI/MMR, TMB, and PD-L1 expression are still being evaluated. as they are complex and may differ based on tumor type and location.[4,44]

SUMMARY AND FUTURE AVENUES

Future algorithms for identifying patients who can benefit from ICIs will most probably entail complementary assessments of tumor and immune cells, including TMB, various genetic alterations, PD-L1 expression, HLA genotype, T-cell receptor repertoire, and gene expression immune signatures.[54]

The complex interactions between tumor and immune cells can be assessed by gene expression profile (GEP) of the tumor and the microenvironment. As such, interferon (IFN)-γ inflamed signature correlated with response to ICIs. Higher GEP scores predicted better response to ICIs in various clinical trials. Newer biomarkers will likely play a role in future assessment of response to immune checkpoint blockade.

TILs and the microbiome could potentially influence the complex interactions among MSI/MMR, TMB, and PD-L1, but the intricate mechanism among these variables is yet to be fully understood.[41,44,53] TILs might increase response to ICIs, improving NSCLC survival.[80] The relationship between gut microbiome and the immune system was regarded as a potential predictor of ICIs effectiveness, because antibiotic therapy has negatively impacted response to ICIs. Furthermore, proton pump inhibitors and histamine-2-receptor antagonists alter the gut microbiome.[80,94]

A 2021 retrospective study pointed to DNA methylation pattern (EPIMMUNE methylation signature) as a predictor of differentiating between ICIs responders versus nonresponders in NSCLS. The EPIMMUNE signature was associated with improved outcome after ICIs therapy.[95]

Oncolytic viruses may have the potential to be used as a treatment in various tumors, as a standalone or combination therapy with ICIs or chemotherapy. Developing novel therapeutic combinations could potentially improve outcomes in patients with lung cancer.[96]

Starving cancer cells might lead to novel tumor alterations, which can stimulate the immune system or enhance the effects of chemotherapy.[97] Subjecting a combination of biomarkers and clinical information to machine learning could also improve assessment in response and outcomes to treatment with ICIs.[80]

The theragnostic and prognostic value of biomarkers in lung cancer may vary in conjunction with other factors such as unique patient characteristics, the presence of other genetic alterations, or the specifics of the chosen immunotherapy. As the field of cancer research is evolving, additional research can provide more insight for the clinical significance of MSI/MMR and TMB in lung tumors and find new avenues to predict response to immunotherapy.

DISCLOSURE

The Authors have nothing to disclose.

REFERENCES

1. Siegel RL, Miller KD, Wagle NS, et al. Cancer statistics, 2023. CA Cancer J Clin 2023;73(1):17–48.
2. Moubarak S, Merheb D, Basbous L, et al. COVID-19 and lung cancer: update on the latest screening, diagnosis, management and challenges. J Int Med Res 2022;50(9), 3000605221125047.
3. Cantini L, Mentrasti G, Russo GL, et al. Evaluation of COVID-19 impact on DELAYing diagnostic-therapeutic pathways of lung cancer patients in Italy (COVID-DELAY study): fewer cases and higher stages from a real-world scenario. ESMO Open 2022;7(2):100406. Erratum in: ESMO Open. 2022 Apr 1;7(2):100471.
4. Chalmers ZR, Connelly CF, Fabrizio D, et al. Analysis of 100,000 human cancer genomes reveals the landscape of tumor mutational burden. Genome Med 2017;9(1):34.
5. Pearlman AH, Hwang MS, Konig MF, et al. Targeting public neoantigens for cancer immunotherapy. Nat Cancer 2021;2(5):487–97. Epub 2021 May 17. Erratum in: Nat Cancer. 2021 Aug;2(8):865-867.
6. Havel JJ, Chowell D, Chan TA. The evolving landscape of biomarkers for checkpoint inhibitor immunotherapy. Nat Rev Cancer 2019;19(3):133–50.
7. Vogelstein B, Papadopoulos N, Velculescu VE, et al. Cancer genome landscapes. Science 2013; 339(6127):1546–58.
8. Chen DS, Irving BA, Hodi FS. Molecular pathways: next-generation immunotherapy–inhibiting programmed death-ligand 1 and programmed death-1. Clin Cancer Res 2012;18(24):6580–7.
9. de Jong D, Das JP, Ma H, et al. Novel targets, novel treatments: the changing landscape of

non-small cell lung cancer. Cancers 2023;15(10): 2855.
10. Sholl LM. Biomarkers of response to checkpoint inhibitors beyond PD-L1 in lung cancer. Mod Pathol 2022;35(Suppl 1):66–74.
11. Li H, van der Merwe PA, Sivakumar S. Biomarkers of response to PD-1 pathway blockade. Br J Cancer 2022;126(12):1663–75.
12. Hirsch FR, McElhinny A, Stanforth D, et al. PD-L1 immunohistochemistry assays for lung cancer: results from phase 1 of the blueprint PD-L1 IHC assay comparison project. J Thorac Oncol 2017;12(2): 208–22.
13. Tsao MS, Kerr KM, Kockx M, et al. PD-L1 immunohistochemistry comparability study in real-life clinical samples: results of blueprint phase 2 project. J Thorac Oncol 2018;13(9):1302–11.
14. Prince EA, Sanzari JK, Pandya D, et al. Analytical concordance of PD-L1 assays utilizing antibodies from FDA-approved diagnostics in advanced cancers: a systematic literature review. JCO Precis Oncol 2021;5:953–73.
15. Chang E, Pelosof L, Lemery S, et al. Systematic review of PD-1/PD-L1 inhibitors in oncology: from personalized medicine to public health. Oncol 2021;26(10):e1786–99.
16. Troncone G, Gridelli C. The reproducibility of PD-L1 scoring in lung cancer: can the pathologists do better? Transl Lung Cancer Res 2017;6(Suppl 1):S74–7.
17. Rimm DL, Han G, Taube JM, et al. A prospective, multi-institutional, pathologist-based assessment of 4 immunohistochemistry assays for PD-L1 expression in non-small cell lung cancer. JAMA Oncol 2017;3(8):1051–8.
18. Ettinger DS, Wood DE, Aisner DL, et al. NCCN guidelines insights: non-small cell lung cancer, version 2.2021. J Natl Compr Canc Netw 2021; 19(3):254–66.
19. FDA regulatory science in action. Impact story: determining the clinical benefit of treatment beyond progression with immune checkpoint inhibitors. Available at: https://www.fda.gov/drugs/regulatory-science-action/impact-story-determining-clinical-benefit-treatment-beyond-progression-immune-checkpoint-inhibitors Accessed, August 19, 2023.
20. Chiou VL, Burotto M. Pseudoprogression and immune-related response in solid tumors. J Clin Oncol 2015;33(31):3541–3.
21. Khoja L, Day D, Wei-Wu Chen T, et al. Tumour- and class-specific patterns of immune-related adverse events of immune checkpoint inhibitors: a systematic review. Ann Oncol 2017;28(10):2377–85.
22. El Osta B, Hu F, Sadek R, et al. Not all immune-checkpoint inhibitors are created equal: meta-analysis and systematic review of immune-related adverse events in cancer trials. Crit Rev Oncol Hematol 2017;119:1–12.

23. Available at: https://www.fda.gov/drugs/resources-information-approved-drugs/fda-approves-opdualag-unresectable-or-metastatic-melanoma Accessed, August 13, 2023.

24. Lander ES, Linton LM, Birren B, et al. International human genome sequencing consortium. Initial sequencing and analysis of the human genome. Nature 2001;409(6822):860–921 . Erratum in: Nature 2001 Aug 2;412(6846):565. Erratum in: Nature 2001 Jun 7;411(6838):720. Szustakowki, J [corrected to Szustakowski, J]. PMID: 11237011.

25. Lemery S, Keegan P, Pazdur R. First FDA approval agnostic of cancer site - when a biomarker defines the indication. N Engl J Med 2017;377(15):1409–12.

26. Marcus L, Lemery SJ, Keegan P, et al. FDA approval summary: pembrolizumab for the treatment of microsatellite instability-high solid tumors. Clin Cancer Res 2019;25(13):3753–8.

27. Parilla M, Ritterhouse LL. Beyond the variants: mutational patterns in next-generation sequencing data for cancer precision medicine. Front Cell Dev Biol 2020;8:370.

28. Available at: https://www.fda.gov/drugs/resources-information-approved-drugs/fda-grants-accelerated-approval-pembrolizumab-first-tissuesite-agnostic-in dication Accessed, August 13, 2023.

29. Gatalica Z, Snyder C, Maney T, et al. Programmed cell death 1 (PD-1) and its ligand (PD-L1) in common cancers and their correlation with molecular cancer type. Cancer Epidemiol Biomarkers Prev 2014;23(12):2965–70.

30. Kroemer G, Galluzzi L, Zitvogel L, et al. Colorectal cancer: the first neoplasia found to be under immunosurveillance and the last one to respond to immunotherapy? OncoImmunology 2015;4(7):e1058597.

31. Lal N, Beggs AD, Willcox BE, et al. An immunogenomic stratification of colorectal cancer: Implications for development of targeted immunotherapy. OncoImmunology 2015;4(3):e976052.

32. Pylkkänen L, Karjalainen A, Anttila S, et al. No evidence of microsatellite instability but frequent loss of heterozygosity in primary resected lung cancer. Environ Mol Mutagen 1997;30(2):217–23.

33. Gonzalez R, Silva JM, Sanchez A, et al. Microsatellite alterations and TP53 mutations in plasma DNA of small-cell lung cancer patients: follow-up study and prognostic significance. Ann Oncol 2000; 11(9):1097–104.

34. Chen XQ, Stroun M, Magnenat JL, et al. Microsatellite alterations in plasma DNA of small cell lung cancer patients. Nat Med 1996;2(9):1033–5.

35. Merlo A, Mabry M, Gabrielson E, et al. Frequent microsatellite instability in primary small cell lung cancer. Cancer Res 1994;54(8):2098–101.

36. Frese KK, Simpson KL, Dive C. Small cell lung cancer enters the era of precision medicine. Cancer Cell 2021;39(3):297–9.

37. Gay CM, Stewart CA, Park EM, et al. Patterns of transcription factor programs and immune pathway activation define four major subtypes of SCLC with distinct therapeutic vulnerabilities. Cancer Cell 2021;39(3):346–60.e7.

38. Poirier JT, George J, Owonikoko TK, et al. New approaches to SCLC therapy: from the laboratory to the clinic. J Thorac Oncol 2020;15(4):520–40.

39. Travis WD, Dacic S, Wistuba I, et al. IASLC multidisciplinary recommendations for pathologic assessment of lung cancer resection specimens after neoadjuvant therapy. J Thorac Oncol 2020;15(5): 709–40.

40. Available at: https://www.cancer.org/content/dam/CRC/PDF/Public/8709.00.pdf Accessed July 9, 2023.

41. Taube JM, Galon J, Sholl LM, et al. Implications of the tumor immune microenvironment for staging and therapeutics. Mod Pathol 2018;31(2): 214–34.

42. Tseng JS, Chiang CJ, Chen KC, et al. Association of smoking with patient characteristics and outcomes in small cell lung carcinoma, 2011-2018. JAMA Netw Open 2022;5(3):e224830. Erratum in: JAMA Netw Open. 2022 Jun 1;5(6):e2221124.

43. Boland CR, Thibodeau SN, Hamilton SR, et al. A National Cancer Institute workshop on microsatellite instability for cancer detection and familial predisposition: development of international criteria for the determination of microsatellite instability in colorectal cancer. Cancer Res 1998;58(22):5248–57.

44. Luchini C, Bibeau F, Ligtenberg MJL, et al. ESMO recommendations on microsatellite instability testing for immunotherapy in cancer, and its relationship with PD-1/PD-L1 expression and tumour mutational burden: a systematic review-based approach. Ann Oncol 2019;30(8):1232–43.

45. Yang RK, Chen H, Roy-Chowdhuri S, et al. Clinical testing for mismatch repair in neoplasms using multiple laboratory methods. Cancers 2022;14(19):4550.

46. Li K, Luo H, Huang L, et al. Microsatellite instability: a review of what the oncologist should know. Cancer Cell Int 2020;20:16.

47. Kautto EA, Bonneville R, Miya J, et al. Performance evaluation for rapid detection of pan-cancer microsatellite instability with MANTIS. Oncotarget 2017; 8(5):7452–63.

48. Huang MN, McPherson JR, Cutcutache I, et al. MSIseq: software for assessing microsatellite instability from catalogs of somatic mutations. Sci Rep 2015; 5:13321.

49. Salipante SJ, Scroggins SM, Hampel HL, et al. Microsatellite instability detection by next generation sequencing. Clin Chem 2014;60(9):1192–9.

50. Niu B, Ye K, Zhang Q, et al. MSIsensor: microsatellite instability detection using paired tumor-normal sequence data. Bioinformatics 2014;30(7):1015–6.

51. Waalkes A, Smith N, Penewit K, et al. Accurate pan-cancer molecular diagnosis of microsatellite instability by single-molecule molecular inversion probe capture and high-throughput sequencing. Clin Chem 2018;64(6):950–8.

52. Zhao P, Li L, Jiang X, et al. Mismatch repair deficiency/microsatellite instability-high as a predictor for anti-PD-1/PD-L1 immunotherapy efficacy. J Hematol Oncol 2019;12(1):54.

53. Sholl LM, Hirsch FR, Hwang D, et al. The promises and challenges of tumor mutation burden as an immunotherapy biomarker: a perspective from the international association for the study of lung cancer pathology committee. J Thorac Oncol 2020 Sep;15(9):1409–24.

54. Chan TA, Yarchoan M, Jaffee E, et al. Development of tumor mutation burden as an immunotherapy biomarker: utility for the oncology clinic. Ann Oncol 2019;30(1):44–56.

55. Sha D, Jin Z, Budczies J, et al. Tumor mutational burden as a predictive biomarker in solid tumors. Cancer Discov 2020 Dec;10(12):1808–25.

56. Fernandez EM, Eng K, Beg S, et al. Cancer-specific thresholds adjust for whole exome sequencing-based tumor mutational burden distribution. JCO Precis Oncol 2019;3:00400. PO.18.

57. Makrooni MA, O'Sullivan B, Seoighe C. Bias and inconsistency in the estimation of tumour mutation burden. BMC Cancer 2022;22(1):840.

58. Supek F, Miñana B, Valcárcel J, et al. Synonymous mutations frequently act as driver mutations in human cancers. Cell 2014;156(6):1324–35.

59. Meri-Abad M, Moreno-Manuel A, García SG, et al. Clinical and technical insights of tumour mutational burden in non-small cell lung cancer. Crit Rev Oncol Hematol 2023;182:103891.

60. Wu HX, Wang ZX, Zhao Q, et al. Tumor mutational and indel burden: a systematic pan-cancer evaluation as prognostic biomarkers. Ann Transl Med 2019;7(22):640.

61. Alexandrov LB, Nik-Zainal S, Wedge DC, et al. Signatures of mutational processes in human cancer. Nature 2013;500(7463):415–21. Erratum in: Nature. 2013 Oct 10;502(7470):258. Imielinsk, Marcin [corrected to Imielinski, Marcin]. PMID: 23945592; PMCID: PMC3776390.

62. Govindan R, Ding L, Griffith M, et al. Genomic landscape of non-small cell lung cancer in smokers and never-smokers. Cell 2012;150(6):1121–34.

63. Wang X, Ricciuti B, Nguyen T, et al. Association between smoking history and tumor mutation burden in advanced non-small cell lung cancer. Cancer Res 2021;81(9):2566–73.

64. Rizvi NA, Hellmann MD, Snyder A, et al. Cancer immunology. mutational landscape determines sensitivity to PD-1 blockade in non-small cell lung cancer. Science 2015;348(6230):124–8.

65. Sharma Y, Miladi M, Dukare S, et al. A pan-cancer analysis of synonymous mutations. Nat Commun 2019;10(1):2569.

66. Willard N, Sholl L, Aisner D. Panel sequencing for targeted therapy selection in solid tumors. Clin Lab Med 2022;42(3):309–23.

67. Ng SB, Turner EH, Robertson PD, et al. Targeted capture and massively parallel sequencing of 12 human exomes. Nature 2009;461(7261):272–6.

68. Allgäuer M, Budczies J, Christopoulos P, et al. Implementing tumor mutational burden (TMB) analysis in routine diagnostics-a primer for molecular pathologists and clinicians. Transl Lung Cancer Res 2018;7(6):703–15.

69. Budczies J, Allgäuer M, Litchfield K, et al. Optimizing panel-based tumor mutational burden (TMB) measurement. Ann Oncol 2019;30(9):1496–506.

70. Buchhalter I, Rempel E, Endris V, et al. Size matters: dissecting key parameters for panel-based tumor mutational burden analysis. Int J Cancer 2019;144(4):848–58.

71. Alborelli I, Bratic Hench I, Chijioke O, et al. Robust assessment of tumor mutational burden in cytological specimens from lung cancer patients. Lung Cancer 2020;149:84–9.

72. Marabelle A, Fakih M, Lopez J, et al. Association of tumour mutational burden with outcomes in patients with advanced solid tumours treated with pembrolizumab: prospective biomarker analysis of the multicohort, open-label, phase 2 KEYNOTE-158 study. Lancet Oncol 2020;21(10):1353–65.

73. Ritterhouse LL. Tumor mutational burden. Cancer Cytopathol 2019;127(12):735–6.

74. Palmeri M, Mehnert J, Silk AW, et al. Real-world application of tumor mutational burden-high (TMB-high) and microsatellite instability (MSI) confirms their utility as immunotherapy biomarkers. ESMO Open 2022;7(1):100336.

75. Ricciuti B, Wang X, Alessi JV, et al. Association of high tumor mutation burden in non-small cell lung cancers with increased immune infiltration and improved clinical outcomes of PD-L1 blockade across PD-L1 expression levels. JAMA Oncol 2022;8(8):1160–8. Erratum in: JAMA Oncol. 2022 Nov 1;8(11):1702.

76. Gandara DR, Paul SM, Kowanetz M, et al. Blood-based tumor mutational burden as a predictor of clinical benefit in non-small-cell lung cancer patients treated with atezolizumab. Nat Med 2018;24(9):1441–8.

77. Stein MK, Pandey M, Xiu J, et al. Tumor mutational burden is site specific in non-small-cell lung cancer and is highest in lung adenocarcinoma brain metastases. JCO Precis Oncol 2019;3:1–13.

78. Kazdal D, Endris V, Allgäuer M, et al. Spatial and temporal heterogeneity of panel-based tumor

mutational burden in pulmonary adenocarcinoma: separating biology from technical artifacts. J Thorac Oncol 2019;14(11):1935–47.

79. Garofalo A, Sholl L, Reardon B, et al. The impact of tumor profiling approaches and genomic data strategies for cancer precision medicine. Genome Med 2016;8(1):79.

80. Ritterhouse LL, Gogakos T. Molecular biomarkers of response to cancer immunotherapy. Clin Lab Med 2022;42(3):469–84.

81. Shim JH, Kim HS, Cha H, et al. HLA-corrected tumor mutation burden and homologous recombination deficiency for the prediction of response to PD-(L)1 blockade in advanced non-small-cell lung cancer patients. Ann Oncol 2020;31(7):902–11.

82. Sesma A, Pardo J, Cruellas M, et al. From tumor mutational burden to blood t cell receptor: looking for the best predictive biomarker in lung cancer treated with immunotherapy. Cancers 2020;12(10):2974.

83. NCCN clinical practice guidelines in oncology: non-small cell lung cancer version 3.2023. Available at: nccn.org. Accessed July 8, 2023.

84. Calles A, Riess JW, Brahmer JR. Checkpoint blockade in lung cancer with driver mutation: choose the road wisely. Am Soc Clin Oncol Educ Book 2020;40:372–84.

85. Tian J, Wang H, Lu C, et al. Genomic characteristics and prognosis of lung cancer patients with MSI-H: A cohort study. Lung Cancer 2023;181:107255.

86. Heitzer E, Tomlinson I. Replicative DNA polymerase mutations in cancer. Curr Opin Genet Dev 2014; 24(100):107–13.

87. Roberts SA, Gordenin DA. Hypermutation in human cancer genomes: footprints and mechanisms. Nat Rev Cancer 2014;14(12):786–800. Erratum in: Nat Rev Cancer. 2015 Nov;15(11):694.

88. Grant MJ, Herbst RS, Goldberg SB. Selecting the optimal immunotherapy regimen in driver-negative metastatic NSCLC. Nat Rev Clin Oncol 2021; 18(10):625–44.

89. Vanderwalde A, Spetzler D, Xiao N, et al. Microsatellite instability status determined by next-generation sequencing and compared with PD-L1 and tumor mutational burden in 11,348 patients. Cancer Med 2018;7(3):746–56. Erratum in: Cancer Med. 2018 Jun;7(6):2792.

90. Usuda K, Niida Y, Iwai S, et al. Higher tumor mutation burden and higher pd-l1 activity predicts the efficacy of immune checkpoint inhibitor treatment in a patient with four lung cancers. a case report. Front Oncol 2020;10:689.

91. Rizvi H, Sanchez-Vega F, La K, et al. Molecular determinants of response to anti-programmed cell death (PD)-1 and anti-programmed death-ligand 1 (PD-L1) blockade in patients with non-small-cell lung cancer profiled with targeted next-generation sequencing. J Clin Oncol 2018;36(7):633–41. Epub 2018 Jan 16. Erratum in: J Clin Oncol. 2018 Jun 1;36(16):1645.

92. Yarchoan M, Albacker LA, Hopkins AC, et al. PD-L1 expression and tumor mutational burden are independent biomarkers in most cancers. JCI Insight 2019;4(6):e126908.

93. Hellmann MD, Nathanson T, Rizvi H, et al. Genomic features of response to combination immunotherapy in patients with advanced non-small-cell lung cancer. Cancer Cell 2018;33(5):843–52.e4.

94. Li N, Wan Z, Lu D, et al. Long-term benefit of immunotherapy in a patient with squamous lung cancer exhibiting mismatch repair deficient/high microsatellite instability/high tumor mutational burden: a case report and literature review. Front Immunol 2023; 13:1088683.

95. Heller G. DNA methylation as predictive marker of response to immunotherapy? memo 2021;14:150–3.

96. Li Z, Feiyue Z, Gaofeng L, et al. Lung cancer and oncolytic virotherapy–enemy's enemy. Transl Oncol 2023;27:101563.

97. Hida K, Maishi N, Matsuda A, et al. Beyond starving cancer: anti-angiogenic therapy. J Med Ultrason 2023. https://doi.org/10.1007/s10396-023-01310-1.

Molecular Testing in Lung Cancer
Recommendations and Update

Alain C. Borczuk, MD

KEYWORDS

• Molecular testing • Tissue stewardship • Lung • Adenocarcinoma

---

Key points

- Combining liquid-based molecular testing (cell-free DNA) with tissue-based testing yields highest success rates at detecting targetable alterations.

- The success of testing on cytologic and tissue samples requires careful tissue stewardship protocols.

- Test selection can guide success, and understanding of testing panels can help match samples with best available testing.

- Current molecular testing includes a panel of Kirsten rat sarcoma proto-oncogene; epidermal growth factor receptor (EGFR) (including exon 20); anaplastic lymphoma kinase (ALK); ROS proto-oncogene 1, receptor tyrosine kinase; B-Raf proto-oncogene, serine/threonine kinase; neurotrophic receptor tyrosine kinase 1/2/3; RET; erb-b2 receptor tyrosine kinase 2; and MET ex14 in advanced disease along with programmed death-ligand 1 (PD-L1) testing and EGFR and ALK in earlier-stage disease.

ABSTRACT

Adoption of molecular testing in lung cancer is increasing. Molecular testing for staging and prediction of response for targeted therapy remain the main indications, and although utilization of blood-based testing for tumor is growing, the use of the diagnostic cytology and tissue specimens is equally important. The pathologist needs to optimize reflex testing, incorporate stage-based algorithms, and understand types of tests for timely and complete assessment in the majority of cases. When tissue is limited, testing should capture the most frequent alterations to maximize the yield of what are largely mutually exclusive alterations, avoiding the need for repeat biopsy.

improved response rate of tyrosine kinase inhibitors over chemotherapy in a subset of adenocarcinomas[1]—to what is now a wide spectrum of molecular alterations with targeted medications (Table 1). Although these alterations are making inroads into lung cancer classification and have been used as part of staging of multiple lung nodules, they most commonly serve a predictive role for treatment response and improved survival with specific medication. These medications either directly impact the oncogenic effect of the mutated gene or, alternatively, impact a pathway activated by a particular gene mutation. In some instances, the molecular test serves to guide treatment choices with other agents; for example, patients with tumors with mutations in EGFR are far less likely to respond to immunotherapy.

OVERVIEW

During the course of nearly 20 years, molecular testing in lung cancer has evolved from what was initially focused on a single target—epidermal growth factor receptor (EGFR) for the promise of

TISSUE STEWARDSHIP

For the surgical pathologist, this expansion in knowledge has occurred in a relatively short amount of time and across many different tumor types. The types of testing that we use to

---

Anatomic Pathology, Northwell Health, 2200 Northern Boulevard Suite 104, Greenvale, NY 11548, USA
E-mail address: aborczuk@northwell.edu

Surgical Pathology 17 (2024) 307–320
https://doi.org/10.1016/j.path.2023.11.012
1875-9181/24/© 2023 Elsevier Inc. All rights reserved.

Table 1
Summary of the molecular alterations and their current matching with drugs that target their activity

Alteration	First-Line Therapy	Subsequent Therapy
EGFR mutation (exon18, 19, 21)	Osimertinib Afatinib Erlotinib Gefitinib Dacomitinib	T790 M mutation Osimertinib
EGFR mutation (exon 20 ins/dup)		Amivantamab-vmjw Mobocertinib
KRAS-G12C		Sotorasib Adagrasib
ALK translocation	Alectinib Brigatinib Ceritinib Crizotinib Lorlatinib	Alectinib Brigatinib Ceritinib Lorlatinib
ROS1 translocation	Ceritinib Crizotinib Entrectinib	Lorlatinib Entrectinib
BRAF V600	Dabrafenib + trametinib Dabrafenib Vemurafenib	Dabrafenib + trametinib
NTRK translocation	Entrectinib Larotrectinib	Entrectinib Larotrectinib
RET translocation	Selpercatinib Pralsetinib Cabocantinib	Selpercatinib Pralsetinib Cabocantinib
MET exon 14 skipping	Capmatinib Crizotinib Tepotinib	Capmatinib Crizotinib Tepotinib
ERBB2 insertion		Fam-trastuzumab deruxtecan-nxki Ado-trastuzumab emtansine

Abbreviations: ERBB2, Erb-B2 receptor tyrosine kinase 2; ins/dup, insertions and duplications.

interrogate some of these alterations vary based on test availability and the value of certain types of assays as surrogates for the molecular alteration. As this knowledge base is superimposed on the needs for primary diagnosis, which include traditional hematoxylin and eosin sections, special stains, and ancillary techniques such as immunohistochemistry, the management of a new diagnosis of lung cancer involves a series of decisions which begin with determination of malignancy, then move on to classification and subclassification of that malignancy, and then to a set of molecular tests. In an era where sample sizes have become smaller, often as little as an endobronchial ultrasound-guided lymph node aspirate, pathologists and pathology laboratories must incorporate workflows that take into consideration a process that preserves tissue for all these potential needs. This concept of tissue stewardship may also extend to consideration of clinical trial eligibility.

In many instances, this approach is incorporated into the workflow of the laboratory to include all samples of a particular type that have a high frequency of malignancy. Even after malignancy is ascertained, considerations such as stage may not yet be known and therefore the sample needs to be ready for a future request. Protocols that do not inadvertently exhaust tissue during processing are central to tissue stewardship. Such technical approaches include separating cores into different blocks rather than combining all cores into one block, cutting unstained sections up front to avoid frequent return to the same block (which can cause tissue loss through repeated facing of the block), and combining workflows that use the block for different purposes such as unstained slides, special stains, and ancillary tests such as immunohistochemistry. Active management by the pathologist to limit the use of immunohistochemistry to those most relevant to the diagnosis and to carefully assess the first set of slides for which blocks can be optimized for molecular testing versus which blocks are sufficient for immunohistochemistry. Some considerations in this space include the number of cells needed to additionally assess immunohistochemistry versus the percent of tumor cells needed for a successful molecular test.[2] In some specific instances such as FISH testing or PD-L1 immunohistochemistry, a minimum number of cells is needed for a successful test to assure proper sensitivity and specificity.

With the above in mind, test selection becomes of some consideration as well. Certain tests have been incorporated into desired criteria in the World Health Organization (WHO) lung cancer classification; these might include immunohistochemistry for NUT midline carcinoma family member 1 (NUT), which is a surrogate for NUT translocation, or loss of BRG1 immunohistochemistry as a surrogate for SMARCA4 loss in a SMARCA4-deficient thoracic tumor or carcinoma. The implication of this subclassification as a desired but not required element is weighed against the potential need for a wider molecular panel. The pathologist must ask—does this subclassification supersede molecular testing in a small sample? In other scenarios, the combination of a biopsy or biopsies alongside a resected nodule or lymph node metastasis may require multiple molecular tests to guide staging. Is the requested testing part of predictive molecular testing along existing guidelines such as National Comprehensive Cancer Network (NCCN) or College of American Pathologists (CAP)/International Association for the Study of Lung Cancer (IASLC)/ AMP? If a sample is of limited cellularity, should a targeted panel be performed which might be technically successful but would not include all targets, or an attempt for a more inclusive panel with a risk of failure? Is it best to request a different sample, either as liquid biopsy or new tissue biopsy?

USE OF MOLECULAR TESTS IN THE DIAGNOSIS OF LUNG CANCER

The WHO lung cancer classification is predicated on a principle that the classification should be useful internationally and across many different practice settings. Therefore, it is primarily focused on morphology with only a handful of diagnoses requiring an ancillary test, usually immunohistochemistry. That being said molecular alterations are at the underpinning of certain diagnostic categories, such as aforementioned NUT carcinoma or SMARCA4-deficient tumors. When the differential includes fetal-type adenocarcinoma, we again use a nuclear immunohistochemistry pattern for

B-catenin as a surrogate for B-catenin mutation. In solitary fibrous tumor, immunohistochemistry for STAT6 serves as a surrogate for NAB3::STAT6 fusion. Similar surrogate approaches may be at our disposal for inflammatory myofibroblastic tumor (IMT) such as immunohistochemistry (IHC) for anaplastic lymphoma kinase (ALK) or calmodulin-binding transcription activator 1 in epithelioid hemangioendothelioma; however, the increasingly complex set of fusions associated with malignant spindle cell tumors place this immunohistochemistry approach in opposition to a tissue stewardship approach, as it may be more efficient to use an RNA-based fusion panel to encompass a wider differential. In addition, even one tumor type may have a wider spectrum of alterations, for example, ALK, ROS, and neurotrophic receptor tyrosine kinase (NTRK) fusions associated with IMT neoplasms This is a challenge given a longer turnaround time for these molecular fusion tests as compared with IHC; however, this decision needs to be made relatively early in the algorithm to allow additional time for test results. Not every laboratory has in-house access to some of these surrogate immunohistochemistry markers, and therefore, send out testing may have a longer turn-around time, even for immunohistochemistry. Therefore, a consideration of tissue stewardship includes proper laboratory processing but also early recognition of potential tumor variants with judicious use of IHC, FISH testing, or molecular fusion testing.

USE OF MOLECULAR TESTS IN STAGING

Although the American Joint Committee on Cancer (AJCC) 8th edition focuses on comprehensive histologic assessment, radiologic and pathologic correlation for ground-glass lesion with non-mucinous lepidic histology (adenocarcinoma in situ [AIS], minimally invasive adenocarcinoma [MIA], and lepidic predminant adenocarcinoma [LPA]), molecular testing is increasingly used in this setting. Although some of the original studies focused on comparative genomic hybridization approaches, there is an evolving use of targeted gene mutation panels and larger next-generation sequencing (NGS) panels. It has been most useful in adenocarcinoma that can have features that strongly suggest primary such as non-mucinous lepidic patterns when paired with a second adenocarcinoma that lacks lepidic pattern or has a histologic feature in common with the invasive component of the first tumor. Scenarios for molecular testing can also include two adenocarcinomas with overlapping common patterns such as acinar pattern and in tumors where arguments can be made histologically for both similarity and difference. This approach may also be helpful in squamous carcinomas, but with more limited data.

The basic principle in these settings is to use oncogene alterations in the tumor that are either sufficiently rare that they would not likely occur in both tumors by chance or represent somatic alterations in tumor suppressor genes[3,4] that would be unlikely to occur in two different tumors as evidence of metastatic tumor. Mutations that cause oncogenic activation of a protein usually occur in hotspots. Therefore, the finding of a common EGFR mutation in two tumors may not be sufficient evidence for metastasis, whereas finding a rare (<1%) frequency mutation in two tumors is stronger evidence. In contrast, loss of function mutation in tumor suppressor genes is usually quite varied (not hotspot), and therefore, the finding of the same somatic mutation, for example, in TP53, is also a strong evidence of the same origin. Alternatively, two distinct driver alterations in the two tumors indicate separate primaries, as could two distinct tumor-suppressor gene mutations. Pitfalls not only include an oncogenic driver that occurs at high frequency but also a secondary alteration seen in one tumor but not the other. This could be associated with tumor progression rather than indication of a second primary. Another pitfall is that neither tumor has a specific alteration, a problem that occurs more often with smaller testing panels. It is also important in this setting to distinguish alterations that are somatic from those that are potentially germline; germline alterations will be present in every sample from the patient independent of whether the tumors are independent primaries or multiple nodules of the same tumor. Consideration of mutation variant allele frequency as compared with tumor cellularity becomes critical to distinguish somatic from germline alterations.

The experience in this arena indicates that the impression of independent primaries can be supported by different driver alterations or different somatic mutations in tumor suppressor genes, and multiple nodules of the same origin have the same uncommon driver or the same somatic alteration in a tumor suppressor gene. It is important to note that the original studies used comparative genomic hybridization and showed very compelling evidence that specific patterns of deletion across the genome could serve as a basis for what might be a fingerprint for a particular tumor. Overall, the combination of morphology and molecular testing can be used in this setting, and these approaches are more robust in adenocarcinoma that has a wider variety of driver alterations then in squamous carcinoma. It is notable that in squamous cell carcinoma, the limitation of morphology in distinguishing multiple primaries

from metastases is more profound, and as a result, molecular testing in this setting may evolve as being of even greater importance.

In the staging setting, an evolving use of molecular testing provides additional information for the likelihood of metastasis or the likelihood of persistent disease during the course of therapy. For example, studies have demonstrated a benefit to adjuvant therapy with early-stage lung cancer including stage 2a and possibly stage 1B. In a patient with a particularly aggressive histology but node-negative disease, the finding of the specific molecular alteration in the blood as circulating DNA or as circulating tumor cells when compared with the primary tumor may become a strong impetus for additional therapy. Such molecular staging is a future direction for molecular testing.[5] Another emerging area for liquid biopsies is the monitoring of disease during the course of therapy to evaluate therapeutic success as well as initiation of new therapy; there may also be a role in for liquid biopsy to make treatment decisions when stage-based decisions remain unclear. For example, the finding of circulating tumor cells or cell-free DNA matching alterations in the primary tumor could serve as further evidence for the need for adjuvant therapy after resection. This remains an important role for liquid biopsy for which there is no current recommendation.[6]

USE OF MOLECULAR TESTS IN THERAPEUTIC PREDICTION

Molecular testing in lung cancer for the purposes of prediction has grown, and the algorithms around use of molecular testing in this arena critical to understand. Lung cancer remains a common malignancy that presents at high stage, is the most common cause of cancer-related mortality, and for which adenocarcinoma is the most common subtype. Numerous FDA-approved agents are available matched to particular alterations, and adenocarcinomas are the most likely to harbor these alterations.[7,8]

DECISIONS AROUND TESTING

Many testing considerations enter the discussion of predictive marker testing. Because this decision-making occurs at the time of diagnosis of new malignancy, an understanding of the guidelines is critical. Testing for molecular alterations span from surrogate test by immunohistochemistry, FISH-based tests for amplifications and fusions, DNA-based tests for mutations best used for point mutations, insertions and deletions, DNA-based test for fusions, and RNA-based tests for fusions and splice variants. Overall, immuno-histochemistry and FISH-based tests need fewer slides and lower tumor cell percentage, but test only for single analytes. Some single-target assays also have relatively low tissue input needs (poly-merase chain reaction-based) with increasing tis-sue utilization for molecular tests that interrogate multiple targets using NGS. Depending on the tis-sue area and tumor cell percentage, 10 to 20 slides may be needed. Among NGS tests, there are amplicon-based and hybrid capture assays[9] with different tissue input needs but with different sen-sitivities and specificities. Overall, amplicon-based assays require less input but may not allow for a full range of detection; one principle of targeted amplicon-based tests is that they can only detect what is in their panel—excellent sensitivity when on the panel, but no detection when not on the panel.

RNA-based tests may provide enhanced detec-tion of fusions and splice variants by the lack of in-trons in RNA. For some tests such as anchored multiplex polymerase chain reaction (mPCR), fusion detection includes identification of the target gene and its fusion partner and can identify tumors with novel fusions with the target gene. Us-ing an RNA-based anchored mPCR approach may be ideal when the fusion partner is relevant, or when there are numerous fusion partners (along-side novel fusions) with a particular target gene. For example, this can be an important consider-ation with alterations such as RET fusion in which there are already identified greater than 50 distinct partners.

However, testing both DNA for point mutations, insertions and deletions and RNA for fusions, while feasible from one tissue submission, may require more tumor tissue. Therefore, an understanding of the assays being used for the molecular testing requested is important as it determines the sensi-tivity and specificity of the assay for particular ana-lytes and also the amount of tissue input and tumor cellularity needed to achieve that sensitivity and specificity.[10–12]

It is also important to understand the situation for which testing is being requested. For example, in stage 1B to IIIA lung cancer, immunotherapy[13] and targeted therapy for EGFR[14] may be indicated in patients after surgical resection. In this setting, immunohistochemistry for ALK and molecular testing for EGFR may guide targeted therapy as well as immunotherapy, with the understanding that certain immunotherapy agents are not recom-mended for patients with EGFR and ALK muta-tions. In this setting, and depending on the amount of tissue available, a rapid test for EGFR combined with immunohistochemistry for ALK

can guide therapy with a very short turnaround time without waiting for a full NGS panel. Such an approach brings back into the algorithm a sin-gle gene type test which can be low-cost, rapid, and with low DNA input. Depending on the stage and clinical situation, a NGS test could be per-formed either simultaneously or in sequence depending on the urgency of that additional infor-mation.[15] In advanced disease, the pathologist must look at the individual case to decide whether tissue adequacy allows for a full panel (eg, including RNA-based fusion detection to include rare alterations) or whether a smaller and less sen-sitive panel would be sufficient. Such a decision could also be a way to stretch two separate spec-imens both of which are insufficient for a full NGS panel but for which individual testing could be done on the two separate specimens using a more targeted approach.[16]

To expand on this, although the NCCN guide-lines clearly support NGS-based platforms in mo-lecular testing for lung cancer, individual decisions may be based on the availability of tissue in a particular sample. A combination of immunohisto-chemistry for ALK and PD-L1, combined with a targeted 15-gene panel detects variants in more than 70% of patients using only 20 ng of DNA. To put this in perspective, this is a marked in-crease over single gene testing for EGFR but falls short of a full panel that could include rarer muta-tions and RNA fusions. On the other side of this discussion would be a need for a larger amount of DNA as well as an equal amount of RNA to achieve a larger panel and potentially a testing fail-ure. Because many of the alterations found in lung cancer are mutually exclusive (eg, a driver alter-ation such EGFR or Kirsten rat sarcoma proto-oncogene [KRAS]), the identification of a driver alteration in a targeted panel using limited tissue can avoid a repeat biopsy.[17]

In terms of the success of testing on tissue, fail-ure rates are often linked to inadequate tissue cellularity and inadequate amount of DNA or RNA input. In one study using 50 ng of nucleic acid and 20% tumor cellularity as a cutoff, a suc-cess rate of 87.5% was achieved in non-small cell lung cancer. Overall, very few cases fail for purely technical reasons with that screening approach. In this study, it was unclear whether cases that failed based on tissue input would have yielded a result with smaller amount of tumor, or alternatively whether a different assay (as in the prior 20 ng example) would have yielded a target in a subset of those cases, avoiding repeat biopsy or liquid biopsy.[18]

The issue of reflex testing[19] has also been examined, that is, testing based on pathologist request at diagnosis. While subject to issues around reimbursement and designation of requesting physician, reflex testing is expeditious and is therefore initiated at the time of diagnosis along with PD-L1 immunohistochemistry. To avoid unnecessary utilization, reflex testing guidelines must be set and for the local institution, best discussed in a multidisciplinary setting.

The testing of cell-free DNA or liquid biopsy has emerged as an important tool in molecular testing. It is clear that the combination of liquid biopsy with tissue biopsy can combine specificity of a molecular result with the tissue-based diagnosis at the time of initial diagnosis. It is possible to perform molecular testing on the tissue for cases in which the liquid assay is not informative. There are alterations found through liquid biopsy that reflect alterations in the peripheral blood as part of clonal hematopoiesis and it is important to repeat tissue-based testing when these liquid-based tests are non-informative. Studies examining liquid biopsy overall show excellent performance if the above caveats are considered. Concern remains with differences in assays and interlaboratory discrepancy, leading to recommendations around performing both liquid-based and tissue-based assays when possible.[6,20,21] Therefore, liquid biopsy can be used in the initial identification of an alteration to reduce turnaround time to therapy, and in the absence of an alteration, tissue testing can be initiated. It can also be particularly helpful in settings in which the tissue is sufficient for diagnosis and for PD-L1 testing but not for a full panel of molecular tests.

TEST ADOPTION

The adoption of molecular testing is also an ongoing concern and reflects multifactorial cause. Among those concerns include lack of physician request, cost, patient decisions not to pursue therapy, limited tissue samples, and access to medical care. Access to more extensive NGS tests may be influenced by health care setting, and therefore, adoption of testing is a critical issue to further examined.[22] The increased use of liquid biopsy has increased the rate of success of molecular testing, especially in settings in which tissue samples were too limited. It is clear that there is a higher probability of receiving a systemic therapy if molecular testing has been requested.[23] Interestingly, although molecular testing has increased in lung cancer when studied during the last decade, utilization of targeted therapies may not have followed this testing.[24] One consistent feature among studies is that reliance on one platform is the least desirable and that having access to multiple platforms that include liquid biopsy, single gene assays, immunohistochemistry, FISH, and NGS increases adoption and decreases time to treatment.[25,26] Having this information available before first-line treatment decisions leads to improved outcome.[27,28]

CURRENT PREDICTIVE TESTING: TARGET MOLECULAR ALTERATIONS

A summary of the molecular alterations and their current matching with drugs that target their activity is shown in Table 1. For pathologists, this includes EGFR, ALK, NTRK, ROS, B-Raf proto-oncogene, serine/threonine kinase (BRAF), KRAS, RET, MET, and erb-b2 receptor tyrosine kinase 2 (ERBB2).

As we discuss each alteration as a general group based on the gene target, specific testing considerations will be noted as well as stage, histology, frequency, and specific associations. Overall, the histology and specific associations should not be used as guidance for testing; the frequency of the alteration may determine a choice of test in a low tissue situation. These guidelines apply to non-small cell, non-squamous carcinomas as required testing primarily in the metastatic setting, and for squamous cell carcinoma in the metastatic setting, suggested testing. The reason for this difference in recommendation is that most of the alterations are not seen in squamous cell carcinoma routinely, but when present in squamous cell carcinoma can be targetable. In addition, especially in the diagnosis of small samples, the histologic squamous cell carcinoma can be part of a larger tumor which is adenosquamous and as likely to harbor targetable alterations as adenocarcinoma.

Epidermal Growth Factor Receptor

The most common alterations in EGFR are exon 19 deletions and point mutations in exon 21, specifically L858 R mutations.[29] In addition to stage 4 metastatic disease, testing for EGFR is needed to guide immunotherapy as well as targeted therapy in stage IB–IIIA disease.[14,30] In addition to the above alterations, point mutations L861Q, G719X, and S768I are also considered targetable. The identification of T790 M mutations generally indicates prior targeted therapy; however, the finding of this alteration in a previously untreated patient should raise a concern for germline T790 M mutation and referral for genetic testing. In this setting, repeat testing after therapy is a strong consideration not only for emerging mutations but also for changes in histology such as small cell or squamous carcinoma, as these may necessitate a change in therapeutic approach.[31–33]

These traditional EGFR alterations can be captured by single gene DNA assays including rapid real-time PCR assays but also have been incorporated into targeted multi-gene PCR assays as well as NGS panels. This allows for decisions around rapid turnaround time as well as quantity of tissue in the sample. Because these alterations encompass 20% to 25% of adenocarcinomas, EGFR testing is particularly important. Most sample types will be sufficient for this testing including small biopsies and cytology cell blocks[34] as well as smears. It is also of note that bone biopsies are testable as long as decalcification with acid-based decalcifiers are avoided; appropriate agents can include ethylenediaminetetraacetic acid (EDTA) decalcification or the preparation of samples that do not require decalcification through sample separation into different blocks or tissue scrapes. FISH testing for amplification is not suggested, and although mutation specific immunohistochemistry is available, its role is unclear given the wide variety of test options for EGFR.[35]

As previously noted, testing for non-small cell non-squamous cancer should be reflex in stages above 1B, to include decisions around targeted therapy and immunotherapy, and in high-stage disease for consideration of primary therapy. Squamous cancer should be tested by request and this is suggested not only in patients who are non-smokers for which non-squamous tumors are more common, but potentially in all squamous cell carcinomas.

Epidermal Growth Factor Receptor Exon 20 Insertion

As targeting of these specific EGFR alterations is increasingly successful,[36,37] it is notable that current PCR-based tests may not focus on alterations of exon 20 and may not completely detect the variety of exon 20 insertions. Here again, NGS approaches may be preferred.[38]

Although mutations in exon 20 were historically associated with lack of response, it has become apparent that certain alterations in exon 20, specifically a set of insertion mutations and duplications, may be matched with medications that target them.[39,40] Although many of these alterations occur at position 763 and 764, there are sufficient variety of alterations that warrant NGS type testing to fully capture the range of targets.

Anaplastic Lymphoma Kinase

The most common targetable alteration involving ALK[41] is a paracentric inversion in chromosome 2 resulting in a fusion of EML4::ALK.[42] Less frequent but also targetable fusions have also been reported. Original descriptions of this alteration were tumors with cribriform histology (Fig. 1A) and signet ring features, but although this alone should not guide testing its association, it can be helpful in expediting IHC testing. These patients are generally younger and light or never-smokers; this alteration occurs in less than 5% of lung adenocarcinomas. Immunohistochemistry is an approved approach but must use clones and methodologies of sensitive detection such as clone 5A4 and D5F3. Using these clones and with education around some pitfalls of interpretation, a very high sensitivity and specificity can be achieved using immunohistochemistry.[43] ALK-mutated tumors result in poor response to immunotherapy so testing may be important in tumors of stages 1B to IIIA to guide decisions around adjuvant immunotherapy. There are promising data that ALK alterations may be targetable in early lung cancer in the adjuvant setting for stage IIA to IIIA tumors (Phase III NCT03456076), so rapid testing in the postsurgical adjuvant setting may have wider future indications. The detection of ALK fusions by DNA-based and RNA NGS-based fusion assays has been used successfully. FISH testing using break-apart probes is also an acceptable test.

Although acquired alterations may occur with targeted therapy including point mutations in ALK, retesting is not always performed as change of therapy may be selected independent of the specific alteration.[44]

Neurotrophic Receptor Tyrosine Kinase

Alterations in NTRK can involve one of three genes and multiple fusion partners. As a result, some assays may fail to detect NTRK based on primer design or bioinformatics failure.[45,46] Point mutations are not targetable alterations.

This is a rare alteration in lung cancer,[47] less than 1% of cases, and given its rarity, testing could be extended to all histologic subtypes to capture all cases (Fig. 1B). There have been proposed immunohistochemistry approaches for prescreening cases for testing, and this should be subject to concerns around tissue stewardship in small samples. FISH testing is also not the most efficient approach as multiple probes need to be applied. NGS with examination of RNA fusions remains the best approach for detection of this fusion in advanced lung cancer.[48,49]

ROS Proto-Oncogene 1, Receptor Tyrosine Kinase

Testing for ROS proto-oncogene 1, receptor tyrosine kinase (ROS1) is also recommended in advanced stage non-small cell carcinoma for decisions around targeted first-line therapy[50] with multiple fusion partners, including CD74, EZR,

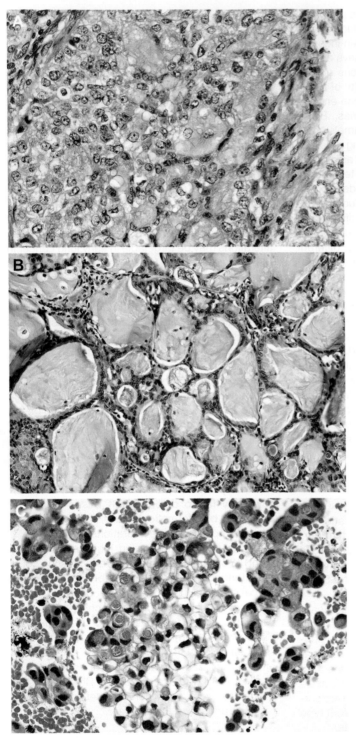

Fig. 1. Histologic patterns with molecular correlations. (*A*) Cribriform patterns with and without intraluminal mucin can be seen with fusion-associated adenocarcinoma, with this case harboring ALK fusion. (*B*) NTRK fusion tumors do not have specific histology, with this example showing cribriform pattern. (*C*) Signet ring feature can be seen with ROS1 fusions, although are also seen in ALK and RET fusion.

SLC34A2, CCDC6, and FIG reported. These alterations represent 1% to 2% of lung adenocarcinomas and are much less frequently described in squamous cell carcinoma. The histology of ROS1 tumors (Fig. 1C) may be similar to that of ALK, with similar demographics. Immunohistochemistry for ROS1 has been proposed as a screening test, but its lack of specificity limits its utility. Therefore, considerations of tissue stewardship should guide the use of immunohistochemistry for ROS1. More appropriate are RNA-based tests that can detect the multiple fusion partners. DNA-based fusion

Fig. 1. (D) Most invasive mucinous adenocarcinoma is KRAS mutated. This tumor has also been associated with NRG1 fusion. (E) RET fusion adenocarcinoma does not have a specific histology pattern but again cribriform histology can be encountered. (F) MET exon 14 skipping tumors may more commonly have spindle or giant cells (shown here). Giant cells can be multinucleated and show emperipolesis.

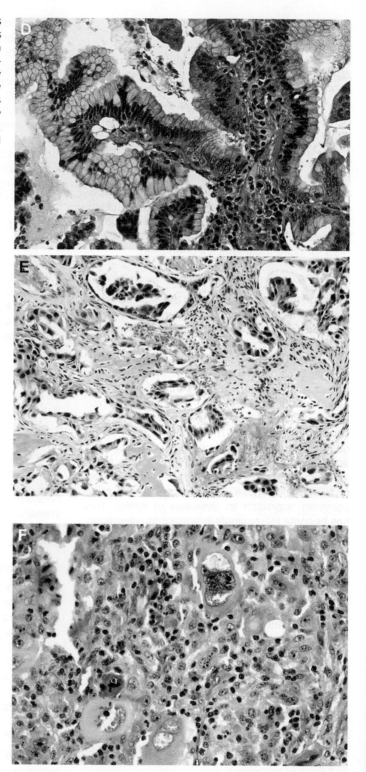

tests as well as single-target break-apart probe FISH can also be performed.

Although alterations may occur after targeted therapy, subsequent therapy may be suggested by disease progression without retesting.[51]

Although ROS1 is a targetable alteration, targeted therapies may fail in particular metastatic sites such as brain and reflects why treatment decisions remain complex even in the setting of a molecular alteration.[52]

B-Raf Proto-Oncogene, Serine/Threonine Kinase

Although there are a variety of mutations in BRAF identified in lung cancer,[53] the alterations in BRAF V600 position are those currently targetable[54,55] and represent a little over half of the BRAF alteration seen in lung cancer. With this range of mutations in mind, this alteration represents 1% to 2% of lung adenocarcinomas. BRAF V600e may be seen in cigarette smokers. Although there are mutation-specific immunohistochemistry available, there are pitfalls in interpretation especially in mucinous tumors that may limit utility. Rapid single-gene testing is available for BRAF, but overall DNA-based tests including panels of NGS for point mutations are often used.

Kirsten Rat Sarcoma Proto-Oncogene, GTPase

Although this alteration remains the most common single gene alteration seen in lung adenocarcinoma composing more than 25% of cases,[56] testing of KRAS was most commonly used, until recently, for its mutually exclusive relationship with other alterations, allowing for molecular classification as a KRAS-mutated tumor and ending need for additional tests. In this regard, point mutations primarily in codon 12 and 13 and less commonly in codon 61, allowed for a variety of rapid single gene assays used in lung cancer and adenocarcinomas of other organs such as colon or pancreas. However, DNA-based tests as part of NGS panels have emerged as being a more common approach to detection of KRAS. This has become increasingly important as alterations. This has become increasingly important as KRAS-G12C mutations, which represent a large proportion of lung adenocarcinoma-related mutations, have become targetable with agents used in subsequent therapy after initial therapy.[57,58]

KRAS mutations, especially transversion mutations (eg, guanine to thymine), are seen in patients who are current or former smokers; transition mutations (eg, cytosine to thymine) can be encountered in never smokers. Although any adenocarcinoma histology can harbor KRAS mutation, a large proportion of invasive mucinous adenocarcinomas harbor KRAS mutation (**Fig.** 1D) and KRAS mutation has also been described in a large proportion of solid pattern adenocarcinomas.

Ret Proto-Oncogene

Mutations in RET are uncommon in lung adenocarcinoma (**Fig.** 1E), about 1% to 2%, and are seen in young, never smokers. They are characterized by a wide variety of different fusion partners. It has been noted specifically that FISH testing may not

be sufficient to detect these alterations reliably. RNA fusion testing with methodologies that can identify the fusion partner is the best approach. RET testing is indicated in advanced disease and the decision for initial therapy in that setting.

In addition to being an indication for targeted therapies,[59,60] the presence of RET fusion may be a negative predictor of immunotherapy outcome, reflecting more aggressive disease. Fusion partner may in fact predict outcome as well. It is also interesting that the choice of chemotherapy with pemetrexed may be influenced by the presence of a RET fusion.[61]

MET Proto-Oncogene, Receptor Tyrosine Kinase

Alterations in MET proto-oncogene (MET) that are currently targetable[62] include a variety of mutations in both exons and introns that result in a splice variant known as MET exon 14 skipping.[63,64] The elimination of exon 14 results in loss of a key signal for protein degradation, allowing for persistent and oncogenic signaling. Although these mutations can be detected at the DNA level through sequencing of the exons and introns in this region, RNA-based testing looking for the fusion transcript emerges as the most sensitive and specific.

METex14 represents 3% to 4% of adenocarcinomas but can be seen in other tumor types including less commonly encountered pleomorphic, spindle and giant cell carcinomas (**Fig.** 1F)[65] but not carcinosarcomas or pulmonary blastomas. Although other tests for MET include immunohistochemistry and FISH testing for amplification, these tests cannot be used in place of a direct test for METex14 skipping.

Erb-b2 Receptor Tyrosine Kinase 2

ERBB2 mutations occur in about 3% of lung cancers[66] specifically non-squamous, non-small cell carcinoma, mainly adenocarcinomas. These alterations are insertions and duplications in exon 20 and do not include cases screened by immunohistochemistry for HER2 or FISH for amplification. The alterations in this gene are complex, and therefore, here again the most reliable approach represents NGS using a DNA-based test.

EMERGING PREDICTIVE MARKERS

Neuregulin 1

This protein interacts with ERBB3 and can activate pathways involving ERBB2. Fusion of neuregulin 1 (NRG1) with a variety of partners occurs in a variety of solid tumors including lung carcinoma, most commonly in invasive mucinous adenocarcinoma.[67–69] This is a rare alteration and likely occurs in less than 0.5% of lung cancer. However, some success has been seen with afatinib, and there is an ongoing study with a monoclonal antibody to ERBB3 (seribantumab) in tumors with this rare fusion.

Kelch-like ECH-Associated Protein 1

At the current time, targeting this alteration, seen primarily in adenocarcinoma, is not part of guidelines, but as a part of targetable pathways of glutamine metabolism, this alteration may become increasingly of interest. It may also predict resistance to immunotherapy.[70]

MET Amplification

Although MET amplification can be seen as an acquired alteration after EGFR targeting[71] and can be seen in tumors with METex14, its role as a biomarker for prediction of therapeutic response as a single alteration is less clear. However, increased response rate to crizotinib has been reported.[72]

SUMMARY

The need for molecular testing in lung cancer is increasing, and although large NGS panels are becoming the recommended approach for advanced disease in both initial and subsequent therapy, molecular testing is also needed in early-stage disease and for optimal immunotherapy treatment planning. The use of liquid biopsy for advanced stage disease allows access to testing for a larger proportion of patients, but continued use of tissue testing is likely for its overall sensitivity, especially in early-stage disease. Existing panels will likely grow to include additional targetable alteration, and in the future, use of molecular testing in staging and assessment of treatment response will expand.

CLINICS CARE POINTS

- Maximize the use of tissue samples in advanced stage patients—this may be the only tissue sample obtained. Use immunohistochemistry judiciously and use tissue preserving protocols.

- Some samples may be usable for a limited testing panel. Limited panels can capture the majority of alterations and avoid rebiopsy.

- Remember that testing now extends to early-stage patients but may not require a full testing panel.

DISCLOSURE

The author has nothing to disclose.

REFERENCES

1. Fukuoka M, Wu YL, Thongprasert S, et al. Biomarker analyses and final overall survival results from a phase III, randomized, open-label, first-line study of gefitinib versus carboplatin/paclitaxel in clinically selected patients with advanced non-small-cell lung cancer in Asia (IPASS). J Clin Oncol 2011;29:2866–74.
2. Penault-Llorca F, Kerr KM, Garrido P, et al. Expert opinion on NSCLC small specimen biomarker testing - Part 1: Tissue collection and management. Virchows Arch 2022;481:335–50.
3. Asmar R, Sonett JR, Singh G, et al. Use of Oncogenic Driver Mutations in Staging of Multiple Primary Lung Carcinomas: A Single-Center Experience. J Thorac Oncol 2017;12:1524–35.
4. Chang JC, Alex D, Bott M, et al. Comprehensive Next-Generation Sequencing Unambiguously Distinguishes Separate Primary Lung Carcinomas From Intrapulmonary Metastases: Comparison with Standard Histopathologic Approach. Clin Cancer Res 2019;25:7113–25.
5. Zhong R, Gao R, Fu W, et al. Accuracy of minimal residual disease detection by circulating tumor DNA profiling in lung cancer: a meta-analysis. BMC Med 2023;21:180.
6. Pascual J, Attard G, Bidard FC, et al. ESMO recommendations on the use of circulating tumour DNA assays for patients with cancer: a report from the ESMO Precision Medicine Working Group. Ann Oncol 2022;33:750–68.
7. Jennings LJ, Arcila ME, Corless C, et al. Guidelines for Validation of Next-Generation Sequencing-Based Oncology Panels: A Joint Consensus Recommendation of the Association for Molecular Pathology and College of American Pathologists. J Mol Diagn 2017;19:341–65.
8. Aziz N, Zhao Q, Bry L, et al. College of American Pathologists' laboratory standards for next-generation sequencing clinical tests. Arch Pathol Lab Med 2015;139:481–93.
9. Drilon A, Wang L, Arcila ME, et al. Broad, Hybrid Capture-Based Next-Generation Sequencing Identifies Actionable Genomic Alterations in Lung Adenocarcinomas Otherwise Negative for Such Alterations by Other Genomic Testing Approaches. Clin Cancer Res 2015;21:3631–9.
10. Bruno R, Fontanini G. Next Generation Sequencing for Gene Fusion Analysis in Lung Cancer: A Literature Review. Diagnostics 2020;10.
11. Lindeman NI, Cagle PT, Aisner DL, et al. Updated Molecular Testing Guideline for the Selection of Lung Cancer Patients for Treatment With Targeted Tyrosine Kinase Inhibitors: Guideline From the College of

American Pathologists, the International Association for the Study of Lung Cancer, and the Association for Molecular Pathology. Arch Pathol Lab Med 2018;142: 321–46.

12. Penault-Llorca F, Kerr KM, Garrido P, et al. Expert opinion on NSCLC small specimen biomarker testing - Part 2: Analysis, reporting, and quality assessment. Virchows Arch 2022;481:351–66.

13. O'Brien M, Paz-Ares L, Marreaud S, et al. Pembrolizumab versus placebo as adjuvant therapy for completely resected stage IB-IIIA non-small-cell lung cancer (PEARLS/KEYNOTE-091): an interim analysis of a randomised, triple-blind, phase 3 trial. Lancet Oncol 2022;23:1274–86.

14. Herbst RS, Wu YL, John T, et al. Adjuvant Osimertinib for Resected EGFR-Mutated Stage IB-IIIA Non-Small-Cell Lung Cancer: Updated Results From the Phase III Randomized ADAURA Trial. J Clin Oncol 2023;41:1830–40.

15. Hanbazazh M, Morlote D, Mackinnon AC, et al. Utility of Single-Gene Testing in Cancer Specimens. Clin Lab Med 2022;42:385–94.

16. Pecciarini L, Brunetto E, Grassini G, et al. Gene Fusion Detection in NSCLC Routine Clinical Practice: Targeted-NGS or FISH? Cells 2023;12.

17. Kuang S, Fung AS, Perdrizet KA, et al. Upfront Next Generation Sequencing in Non-Small Cell Lung Cancer. Curr Oncol 2022;29:4428–37.

18. Latham K, Dong F. The success rates of clinical cancer next-generation sequencing based on pathologic diagnosis: Experience from a single academic laboratory. Am J Clin Pathol 2023; 160(5):533–9.

19. Gosney JR, Paz-Ares L, Janne P, et al. Pathologist-initiated reflex testing for biomarkers in non-small-cell lung cancer: expert consensus on the rationale and considerations for implementation. ESMO Open 2023;8:101587.

20. Barthelemy D, Lescuyer G, Geiguer F, et al. Paired Comparison of Routine Molecular Screening of Patient Samples with Advanced Non-Small Cell Lung Cancer in Circulating Cell-Free DNA Using Three Targeted Assays. Cancers 2023;15.

21. Linder MW, Huggett JF, Baluchova K, et al. Results from an IFCC global survey on laboratory practices for the analysis of circulating tumor DNA. Clin Chim Acta 2023;547:117398.

22. Burns L, Jani C, Radwan A, et al. Implementation Challenges and Disparities in Molecular Testing for Patients With Stage IV NSCLC: Perspectives from an Urban Safety-Net Hospital. Clin Lung Cancer 2023;24:e69–77.

23. Osazuwa-Peters OL, Wilson LE, Check DK, et al. Factors Associated With Receipt of Molecular Testing and its Impact on Time to Initial Systemic Therapy in Metastatic Non-Small Cell Lung Cancer. Clin Lung Cancer 2023;24:305–12.

24. Roberts TJ, Kehl KL, Brooks GA, et al. Practice-Level Variation in Molecular Testing and Use of Targeted Therapy for Patients With Non-Small Cell Lung Cancer and Colorectal Cancer. JAMA Netw Open 2023;6:e2310809.

25. Maity AP, Gangireddy M, Degen KC, et al. Impact of Simultaneous Circulating Tumor DNA and Tissue Genotyping in the Workup of Stage IV Lung Adenocarcinoma on Quality of Care in an Academic Community Medical Center. JCO Oncol Pract 2023;19: 620–5.

26. Yan JT, Jin Y, Lo E, et al. Real-World Biomarker Test Utilization and Subsequent Treatment in Patients with Early-Stage Non-small Cell Lung Cancer in the United States, 2011-2021. Oncol Ther 2023;11: 343–60.

27. Aggarwal C, Marmarelis ME, Hwang WT, et al. Association Between Availability of Molecular Genotyping Results and Overall Survival in Patients With Advanced Nonsquamous Non-Small-Cell Lung Cancer. JCO Precis Oncol 2023;7:e2300191.

28. Arriola E, Bernabe R, Campelo RG, et al. Cost-Effectiveness of Next-Generation Sequencing Versus Single-Gene Testing for the Molecular Diagnosis of Patients With Metastatic Non-Small-Cell Lung Cancer From the Perspective of Spanish Reference Centers. JCO Precis Oncol 2023;7:e2200546.

29. Siegelin MD, Borczuk AC. Epidermal growth factor receptor mutations in lung adenocarcinoma. Lab Invest 2014;94:129–37.

30. Tsao MS, Sakurada A, Cutz JC, et al. Erlotinib in lung cancer - molecular and clinical predictors of outcome. N Engl J Med 2005;353:133–44.

31. Marcoux N, Gettinger SN, O'Kane G, et al. EGFR-Mutant Adenocarcinomas That Transform to Small-Cell Lung Cancer and Other Neuroendocrine Carcinomas: Clinical Outcomes. J Clin Oncol 2019; 37:278–85.

32. Oxnard GR. Strategies for overcoming acquired resistance to epidermal growth factor receptor: targeted therapies in lung cancer. Arch Pathol Lab Med 2012;136:1205–9.

33. Schoenfeld AJ, Chan JM, Kubota D, et al. Tumor Analyses Reveal Squamous Transformation and Off-Target Alterations As Early Resistance Mechanisms to First-line Osimertinib in EGFR-Mutant Lung Cancer. Clin Cancer Res 2020;26:2654–63.

34. VanderLaan PA, Roy-Chowdhuri S, Griffith CC, et al. Molecular testing of cytology specimens: overview of assay selection with focus on lung, salivary gland, and thyroid testing. J Am Soc Cytopathol 2022;11: 403–14.

35. Hirsch FR, Bunn PA Jr. EGFR testing in lung cancer is ready for prime time. Lancet Oncol 2009;10: 432–3.

36. Riely GJ, Neal JW, Camidge DR, et al. Activity and Safety of Mobocertinib (TAK-788) in Previously

Treated Non-Small Cell Lung Cancer with EGFR Exon 20 Insertion Mutations from a Phase I/II Trial. Cancer Discov 2021;11:1688–99.

37. Zhou C, Ramalingam SS, Kim TM, et al. Treatment Outcomes and Safety of Mobocertinib in Platinum-Pretreated Patients With EGFR Exon 20 Insertion-Positive Metastatic Non-Small Cell Lung Cancer: A Phase 1/2 Open-label Nonrandomized Clinical Trial. JAMA Oncol 2021;7:e214761.

38. Ou SI, Hong JL, Christopoulos P, et al. Distribution and Detectability of EGFR Exon 20 Insertion Variants in NSCLC. J Thorac Oncol 2023;18:744–54.

39. Arcila ME, Nafa K, Chaft JE, et al. EGFR exon 20 insertion mutations in lung adenocarcinomas: prevalence, molecular heterogeneity, and clinicopathologic characteristics. Mol Cancer Therapeut 2013;12:220–9.

40. Riess JW, Gandara DR, Frampton GM, et al. Diverse EGFR Exon 20 Insertions and Co-Occurring Molecular Alterations Identified by Comprehensive Genomic Profiling of NSCLC. J Thorac Oncol 2018;13:1560–8.

41. Solomon BJ, Mok T, Kim DW, et al. First-line crizotinib versus chemotherapy in ALK-positive lung cancer. N Engl J Med 2014;371:2167–77.

42. Kwak EL, Bang YJ, Camidge DR, et al. Anaplastic lymphoma kinase inhibition in non-small-cell lung cancer. N Engl J Med 2010;363:1693–703.

43. Ali G, Proietti A, Pelliccioni S, et al. ALK rearrangement in a large series of consecutive non-small cell lung cancers: comparison between a new immunohistochemical approach and fluorescence in situ hybridization for the screening of patients eligible for crizotinib treatment. Arch Pathol Lab Med 2014;138:1449–58.

44. Shaw AT, Bauer TM, de Marinis F, et al. First-Line Lorlatinib or Crizotinib in Advanced ALK-Positive Lung Cancer. N Engl J Med 2020;383:2018–29.

45. Stockley TL, Lo B, Box A, et al. CANTRK: A Canadian Ring Study to Optimize Detection of NTRK Gene Fusions by Next-Generation RNA Sequencing. J Mol Diagn 2023;25:168–74.

46. Stockley TL, Lo B, Box A, et al. Consensus Recommendations to Optimize the Detection and Reporting of NTRK Gene Fusions by RNA-Based Next-Generation Sequencing. Curr Oncol 2023;30:3989–97.

47. Gatalica Z, Xiu J, Swensen J, et al. Molecular characterization of cancers with NTRK gene fusions. Mod Pathol 2019;32:147–53.

48. Farago AF, Taylor MS, Doebele RC, et al. Clinicopathologic Features of Non-Small-Cell Lung Cancer Harboring an NTRK Gene Fusion. JCO Precis Oncol 2018;2018.

49. Doebele RC, Drilon A, Paz-Ares L, et al. Entrectinib in patients with advanced or metastatic NTRK fusion-positive solid tumours: integrated analysis of three phase 1-2 trials. Lancet Oncol 2020;21:271–82.

50. Shaw AT, Ou SH, Bang YJ, et al. Crizotinib in ROS1-rearranged non-small-cell lung cancer. N Engl J Med 2014;371:1963–71.

51. Shaw AT, Solomon BJ, Chiari R, et al. Lorlatinib in advanced ROS1-positive non-small-cell lung cancer: a multicentre, open-label, single-arm, phase 1-2 trial. Lancet Oncol 2019;20:1691–701.

52. Ten Berge D, Damhuis RAM, Aerts J, et al. Real-world treatment patterns and survival of patients with ROS1 rearranged stage IV non-squamous NSCLC in the Netherlands. Lung Cancer 2023;181:107253.

53. Davies H, Bignell GR, Cox C, et al. Mutations of the BRAF gene in human cancer. Nature 2002;417:949–54.

54. Planchard D, Besse B, Groen HJM, et al. Dabrafenib plus trametinib in patients with previously treated BRAF(V600E)-mutant metastatic non-small cell lung cancer: an open-label, multicentre phase 2 trial. Lancet Oncol 2016;17:984–93.

55. Gautschi O, Milia J, Cabarrou B, et al. Targeted Therapy for Patients with BRAF-Mutant Lung Cancer: Results from the European EURAF Cohort. J Thorac Oncol 2015;10:1451–7.

56. Sholl LM, Aisner DL, Varella-Garcia M, et al. Multi-institutional Oncogenic Driver Mutation Analysis in Lung Adenocarcinoma: The Lung Cancer Mutation Consortium Experience. J Thorac Oncol 2015;10:768–77.

57. Janne PA, Riely GJ, Gadgeel SM, et al. Adagrasib in Non-Small-Cell Lung Cancer Harboring a KRAS(G12C) Mutation. N Engl J Med 2022;387:120–31.

58. Skoulidis F, Li BT, Dy GK, et al. Sotorasib for Lung Cancers with KRAS p.G12C Mutation. N Engl J Med 2021;384:2371–81.

59. Michels S, Scheel AH, Scheffler M, et al. Clinicopathological Characteristics of RET Rearranged Lung Cancer in European Patients. J Thorac Oncol 2016;11:122–7.

60. Yoh K, Seto T, Satouchi M, et al. Final survival results for the LURET phase II study of vandetanib in previously treated patients with RET-rearranged advanced non-small cell lung cancer. Lung Cancer 2021;155:40–5.

61. Novello S, Califano R, Reinmuth N, et al. RET Fusion-Positive Non-small Cell Lung Cancer: The Evolving Treatment Landscape. Oncol 2023;28:402–13.

62. Drilon A, Clark JW, Weiss J, et al. Antitumor activity of crizotinib in lung cancers harboring a MET exon 14 alteration. Nat Med 2020;26:47–51.

63. Lee M, Jain P, Wang F, et al. MET alterations and their impact on the future of non-small cell lung cancer (NSCLC) targeted therapies. Expert Opin Ther Targets 2021;25:249–68.

64. Awad MM, Oxnard GR, Jackman DM, et al. MET Exon 14 Mutations in Non-Small-Cell Lung Cancer Are Associated With Advanced Age and Stage-Dependent MET Genomic Amplification and c-Met Overexpression. J Clin Oncol 2016;34:721–30.

65. Liu X, Jia Y, Stoopler MB, et al. Next-Generation Sequencing of Pulmonary Sarcomatoid Carcinoma Reveals High Frequency of Actionable MET Gene Mutations. J Clin Oncol 2016;34:794–802.

66. Pillai RN, Behera M, Berry LD, et al. HER2 mutations in lung adenocarcinomas: A report from the Lung Cancer Mutation Consortium. Cancer 2017;123: 4099–105.

67. Drilon A, Duruisseaux M, Han JY, et al. Clinicopathologic Features and Response to Therapy of NRG1 Fusion-Driven Lung Cancers: The eNRGy1 Global Multicenter Registry. J Clin Oncol 2021;39: 2791–802.

68. Werr L, Plenker D, Dammert MA, et al. CD74-NRG1 Fusions Are Oncogenic In Vivo and Induce Therapeutically Tractable ERBB2:ERBB3 Heterodimerization. Mol Cancer Therapeut 2022;21:821–30.

69. Odintsov I, Lui AJW, Sisso WJ, et al. The Anti-HER3 mAb Seribantumab Effectively Inhibits Growth of Patient-Derived and Isogenic Cell Line and Xenograft Models with Oncogenic NRG1 Fusions. Clin Cancer Res 2021;27:3154–66.

70. Ricciuti B, Arbour KC, Lin JJ, et al. Diminished Efficacy of Programmed Death-(Ligand)1 Inhibition in STK11- and KEAP1-Mutant Lung Adenocarcinoma Is Affected by KRAS Mutation Status. J Thorac Oncol 2022;17:399–410.

71. Wang W, Wang H, Lu P, et al. Crizotinib with or without an EGFR-TKI in treating EGFR-mutant NSCLC patients with acquired MET amplification after failure of EGFR-TKI therapy: a multicenter retrospective study. J Transl Med 2019;17:52.

72. Camidge DR, Otterson GA, Clark JW, et al. Crizotinib in Patients With MET-Amplified NSCLC. J Thorac Oncol 2021;16:1017–29.

Applications of Artificial Intelligence in Lung Pathology

Douglas J. Hartman, MD

KEYWORDS

• Artificial intelligence • Lung pathology • Machine learning • Digital pathology

Key points

- Artificial intelligence tools are being developed to be used in clinical cases.
- Artificial intelligence tools for lung pathology include immunostains, special stains, hematoxylin and eosin stains, and novel features not currently used.
- Development and regulatory frameworks are needed to achieve the full potential.

ABSTRACT

Artificial intelligence/machine learning tools are being created for use in pathology. Some examples related to lung pathology include acid-fast stain evaluation, programmed death ligand-1 (PDL-1) interpretation, evaluating histologic patterns of non–small-cell lung carcinoma, evaluating histologic features in mesothelioma associated with adverse outcomes, predicting response to anti-PDL-1 therapy from hematoxylin and eosin–stained slides, evaluation of tumor microenvironment, evaluating patterns of interstitial lung disease, nondestructive methods for tissue evaluation, and others. There are still some frameworks (regulatory, workflow, and payment) that need to be established for these tools to be integrated into pathology.

INTRODUCTION

Recent years have seen an explosion in the interest and application of artificial intelligence/machine learning (AI/ML). This has impacts in nearly every aspect of society, but medicine has equally been involved with the expectation that the use of AI/ML will improve patient care, reduce burnout, and produce efficiencies.[1–4] The same trend has been seen within pathology. This technology can be applied to new molecular methods in order to analyze vast amounts of data or to combine subtle/small changes with other features. It also can be used to combine many data points present across care teams (anatomic pathology information, radiology features, laboratory values, clinical symptoms, and so forth) in order to influence/advise clinical care. To focus on pathology-specific use cases, AI/ML can be applied for text-based analysis, image-based analysis, and molecular analysis. For text-based analysis, this technology is essentially a more advanced form of natural language processing—a technology that has been around for some time but has not really been adopted for advancing clinical care. Given the remarkable advances in molecular testing, use of AI/ML to digest and interpret the results of the testing is necessary in order to make use of the expansive panels and data points that can be technically derived. In order to reasonably narrow the topic, this article will focus on image-based AI/ML. This area has seen a lot of investment interest from venture capitalists since it could represent a replacement for expert pathologists.[3] However, in the author's opinion, this technology will augment the pathology work that is currently being done by pathologists—similar to how other advances in technology (histochemistry, electron microscopy, immunohistochemistry, or molecular testing) have supplemented the work of pathologists. A similar

University of Pittsburgh Medical Center, 200 Lothrop Street C-620, Pittsburgh, PA 15213, USA
E-mail address: hartmandj@upmc.edu

Surgical Pathology 17 (2024) 321–328
https://doi.org/10.1016/j.path.2023.11.013
1875-9181/24/© 2023 Elsevier Inc. All rights reserved.

surgpath.theclinics.com

"augmented" workflow has been suggested for using AI/ML in radiology and pathology workflows.[5,6]

DEFINITIONS

Many terms are used within the AI/ML space that, although they might be technically different, essentially replicate the same process. Some of the specific terminology is critical in order to have a comprehension of the claims that the technology is proposing. A white paper from the Digital Pathology Association reviewed many of the definitions related to AI/ML.[7] A subset of the definitions within that paper is presented in **Table 1**.[7] The initial studies for AI/ML utilized extensive labor and time-intensive work by pathologists to annotate specific features in order to generate supervised machine learning. This method of AI/ML is only as good as the annotations used for the training and contains the same limits as the quality/expertise of the initial annotations (for instance, general pathologist annotation vs subspecialist pathologist annotation). Unsupervised machine learning was a method used to overcome this

"annotation" limitation; however, the features derived during the development process could be nonsensical (ie, not based in a true morphologic feature) such as date of the staining of the slides or size of the tissue section (or other possible inapparent biases in data). Newer "weakly" supervised machine learning attempts to use some expert confirmation of the feature without the need for explicit labeling by expert pathologists—this is both faster for data generation and cheaper from a study setup. When evaluating the application of new tools, it is critical that users understand the methodology for how the tools are developed and the claims made by the developers in order to know how to ideally implement those developed tools.

This review will focus predominantly on image-based AI/ML as this is more relevant and unique to pathology. Image-based AI/ML has been extensively studied within the radiology discipline and can act as a model for how AI/ML will be used within pathology. Of course, radiology has utilized nearly 100% digital material for their interpretations since the mid to late 1990s. Extensive published

Table 1
Definitions related to artificial intelligence/machine learning

Term	Definition
Artificial Intelligence	A branch of computer science dealing with the simulation of intelligent behavior in computers.[7]
Convolutional neural network (CNN)	A type of deep neural network particularly designed for images. It uses a kernel or filter to convolve an image which results in features useful for differentiating images.[7]
Deep learning	The subset of machine learning composed of algorithms that permit software to train itself to perform tasks by exposing multilayered artificial neural networks to vast amounts of data. Data are fed into the input layers and are sequentially processed in a hierarchical manner with increasing complexity at each layer, modeled loosely after the hierarchical organization of the brain. Optimization functions are iteratively trained to shape the processing functions of the layers and the connection between them.[7]
Machine learning	A branch of artificial intelligence in which computer software learns to perform a task by being exposed to representative data.[7]
Supervised machine learning	Supervised learning is used to train a model to predict an outcome or to classify a dataset based on a label associated with a data point (ie, ground truth). An example of supervised machine learning includes the design of classifiers to distinguish benign from malignant regions based on manual annotations.[7]
Unsupervised machine learning	Unsupervised learning seeks to identify natural divisions in a dataset without the need for a ground truth, often using methods such as cluster analysis or pattern matching. Examples of unsupervised machine learning include the identification of images with similar attributes or the clustering of tumors into subtypes.[7]

work within radiology for the use of AI/ML has centered around the determination of lung nodules, but many other clinical issues have been developed in radiology. Pathology is currently within this transition to using digital pathology with a slight push from the coronavirus disease 2019 pandemic.[8–14] There are several excellent review articles that have described clinical deployment of digital pathology systems.[15–17] Some investigators have even suggested that AI/ML applications might drive digital pathology adoption.[18]

APPLICATIONS

The possible uses of AI/ML in lung pathology can affect all areas, but much of the research has concentrated on oncologic applications. Although oncologic applications are the areas that are heavily researched, application of this technology may actually be more fully appreciated within the inflammatory area. Specifically, to date there have been limited descriptions of the inflammatory milieu that characterizes inflammatory conditions because the evaluations are limited to semiquantification. The use AI/ML could present novel features that might be predictive for the clinical management of these patients. AI/ML may be used to replace a task that is currently being done by pathologists using immunostains or special stains (similar to automated image analysis), hematoxylin and eosin (H&E)–stained slides (routine pathologist work), or extracting novel features/biomarkers (novel features that currently do not have any "analog" correlates). The author will briefly present some published examples of these tools.

ARTIFICIAL INTELLIGENCE/MACHINE LEARNING APPLICATIONS IN IMMUNOHISTOCHEMISTRY AND HISTOCHEMISTRY

We developed, together with a technology company, a screening automated algorithm to use as a tool for pathologists when they interpret acid-fast stains.[19] Briefly, we used 297 cases from our institution and 15 cases from Wan Fang Hospital to develop the algorithm. The algorithm was based on a region of interest (ROI)/patch-based approach. The training data used consisted of ROIs/patches identified by experts as either positive or negative. The slides for this were generated using 2 different staining methods for acid-fast organisms (commercial acid-fast bacillus stain kit and manual Kinyoun method) and the slides were scanned on 2 different digital scanning platforms—Leica/Aperio (0.25 µm/pixel resolution; 40

x equivalent) and Hamamatsu (0.23 µm/pixel resolution; 40x equivalent).[19] The final algorithm was then tested against an independent set of 78 cases. Once the algorithm had been trained with satisfactory performance, we implemented it for clinical use through a web portal (Fig. 1). In this figure, the suspicious ROIs are displayed alongside the whole-slide image. Annotations on the whole-slide image will exclude ROIs outside the annotation area—allowing the pathologist to reduce the likelihood of false positives from debris or stain accumulation outside of the tissue section. This deployed workflow did not depend on graphics processing units (GPUs) for performance, and processing takes around 30 minutes per slide. An email with a link to the case in the web portal is sent when the slide has been processed to the attending pathologist facilitating communication about the processing of the slides. The pathologist can use this workflow to aid in identifying suspicious regions on the actual glass slide or use an entire digital workflow for the interpretation of the stain. Given the frequency of acid-fast evaluation within thoracic pathology, our faculty members have found this to be a positive contribution to their interpretation of acid-fast stains.

A recent article described the development of a deep learning computational system for the interpretation of programmed death ligand-1 (PDL-1) staining in non–small-cell lung cancer.[20] This system contained 2 steps—one to detect the tumor area and another to determine the tumor proportion score for 2 clones (22C3 and SP263) of PDL-1 immunostains. The slides were scanned using a single scanning platform Leica/Aperio at 20x magnification.[20] Manual annotations of tumor and stroma regions were performed in the QuPath application by 5 pathologists with disagreements resolved by a consultant pathologist.[20] Once the determination of tumor was made, a cell segmentation algorithm from QuPath that had been optimized for thresholds based on a randomly chosen group of 3 to 5 whole-slides images.[20] 239 slides stained with 22C3 clone (677 regions) were used for the development of the tumor detection algorithm (563 regions for training and 114 regions for testing).[20] 210 slides (110 22C3 clone immunostains and 100 SP263 clone immunostains) were tested to compare with manual interpretation.[20] The investigators then compared their automated workflow with various methods of manual and AI/ML-assisted workflows across the 2 different clones.[20] The investigators found that this workflow improved diagnostic repeatability and efficiency in the evaluation of PDL-1 expression.[20]

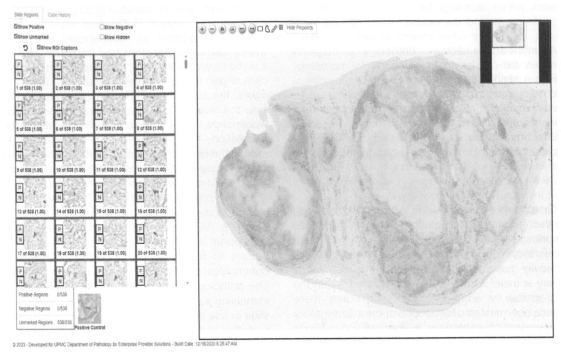

Fig. 1. An example of the web portal for an automated screening tool to assist with the evaluation of acid-fast stains for organisms. An email with a link to the case within the web portal is automatically sent to the attending pathologist for the clinical case. On the right side of the image, there is a slide viewer that can be annotated for specific broad areas that a pathologist has high concern for the presence of organisms (for instance, necrotizing granulomas). On the left side, there are regions of interest for possible organisms. These regions are ranked according the highest likelihood at the top. When the region is selected/clicked, the area within the whole-slide image on the right side is brought up. When the whole slide is annotated, the regions outside the annotated area will be hidden from evaluation. A reference-positive organism in a region is provided at the bottom of the regions panel.

ARTIFICIAL INTELLIGENCE/MACHINE LEARNING APPLICATIONS ON HEMATOXYLIN AND EOSIN STAINS

A recent paper described the development of a deep learning algorithm for diagnosing the histologic patterns of invasive nonmucinous lung adenocarcinoma.[21] This study used 523 H&E-stained slides scanned at 400x magnification (0.15 μm/pixel) and they were categorized by the following 6 patterns—lepidic, acinar, papillary, solid, micropapillary, and cribriform.[21] The labeling of patterns and percentage of each subtype was performed by a single pathologist with subsequent confirmation by a second pathologist. 376 cases were used for training, 27 for validation, and 120 for testing. The investigators found that the algorithm that they developed had various areas under curves for the histologic subtypes—solid = 0.98; cribriform = 0.95; lepidic = 0.85; micropapillary = 0.85; papillary = 0.80; and acinar = 0.75.[21] Interestingly, similar findings were found in examiner-interobserver variability in the manual assessment of histologic subtypes by international experts.[22] Of course, the morphologic assessment is ultimately a reflection of the training data, and the results could be impacted by the data annotation or by limited numbers of specific subtypes. The investigators concluded that the algorithm could be useful for pathologists due to its sensitivity.[21]

Another recent study developed an algorithm for pleural mesothelioma based on 2981 slides.[23] The unsupervised algorithm was based on tiles (small subsets of whole-slide images) from 40x-scanned slides of hematoxylin, eosin, and saffron–stained slides.[23] The developed algorithm, called Meso-Net, provides a continuous risk score for outcomes over the categorization that was traditionally performed by manual assessment.[23] The outcome of the algorithm was then compared to some other assessments of risk for pleural mesothelioma cases—pathologist assessment of the histologic type alone, combination of histologic type and tumor grade, and a naïve machine learning approach.[23] The investigators suggest this algorithm could be used to augment current reporting elements.[23]

NOVEL OUTPUTS FROM ARTIFICIAL INTELLIGENCE/MACHINE LEARNING

A recent article used outcomes from a cohort of non–small-cell lung cancer patients treated with PDL-1 inhibitors to create an algorithm that would predict outcomes of therapy based on H&E-stained images.[24] The dataset consisted of 291 whole-slide images from 198 patients scanned at 20x magnification.[24] The whole-slide images were broken into tiles and each tile for a case was labeled according to the progression-free survival outcome for that case.[24] The developed algorithm was able to properly predict 50 out of 62 cases in an external validation cohort.[24] This algorithm provides a prediction of progression-free survival—an output that pathology reports do not currently report and as such, this represents "novel" functionality that pathologists could provide in their diagnostic reports.

Another recent paper examined murine lung cancer models and tissue microarrays from human lung cancer to develop an algorithm for quantifying the tumor microenvironment.[25] The tumor areas were manually annotated for the 2 cohorts and the slides were scanned at 20x and 40x magnification.[25] Using a commercially available software (HALO AI nuclear phenotyping software), the investigators characterized the 19 human and 33 murine samples.[25] The investigators used conventional immunohistochemistry to verify the results from the software program.[25] In this study, the investigators were able to report the quantity and distribution of inflammatory milieu in association of lung cancers—an example of a "novel" output that is not currently able to be reported reliably in lung pathology.

Another recent study looked at interstitial lung disease in which the investigators used 180 cases (535 whole-slide images) to build a predictive algorithm for usual interstitial pneumonia versus others in interstitial lung disease that they validated on 51 cases (180 whole-slide images).[26] The investigators scanned the slides at 20x magnification and created a novel method to allow for pathologist oversight of the training process that they can "MIXTURE (huMaIn-the-loop eXplainable artificial intelligence Through the Use of REcurrent training)".[26] This combined human-software algorithm performed better than a nonintegrated algorithm.[26] This study highlights how combined human-integrated software can aid in providing a more precise/confident diagnosis in interstitial lung disease.

Several studies have examined nondestructive tissue visualization methods.[27–29] Although not all methods utilize machine learning for visualization, AI/ML is becoming integrated with these orthogonal methods for tissue examination. For example, one study used multispectral imaging combined with principal component analysis (a common unsupervised machine learning method) in order to detect and derive relevant areas within paraffin-embedded pathologic tissue from mice.[28] These techniques could shorten the processing time that has historically been present for pathologic review or create better-quality slides upon initial evaluation, also reducing the time for evaluation. However, these techniques are still immature and whether they reach the pathology mainstream remains to be seen.

REGULATORY

The regulatory framework around AI/ML is evolving. In a fashion similar to automated image analysis, AI/ML regulation may be up to the oversight of the pathologists who use it. In the author's opinion, the application of the AI/ML will determine the level of required oversight—that is, if the AI/ML will be working autonomously to a human or the result can be verified by a human. AI/ML that works independent to human assessment would require a higher safety bar and evaluation before implementation. For radiology where a lot more research with AI/ML applications have been completed, the use of AI/ML has been split into 2 main application methods—software as a medical device and software in a medical device.[30,31] This area of regulation is actively changing within the Food and Drug Administration as it applies for the practice of medicine. Many authors have suggested that developers should make the AI/ML "explainable" in order to facilitate pathologist understanding/acceptance of the technology.[32,33] AI/ML can be deployed in an "open-loop" or a "closed-loop" workflow. The open-loop workflow would include the pathologist within the decision process of the algorithm while the closed loop would be outside the pathologist's opinion. A closed-loop algorithm workflow could be considered a black box and would likely reduce use within the broader pathology discipline.

Pathology has for a long time needed to be flexible with the clinical needs/tests offered within the laboratory and therefore the "laboratory-developed test" pathway was created in order to safely bring tests into the clinical testing environment. Careful evaluation and deployment must be taken when providing tests through this pathway. Although there has recently been some discussion within the federal government of overhauling this regulatory pathway, it is unclear what direction this will take. The use of AI/ML tools within the pathology environment could certainly be deployed within a "laboratory-developed test" pathway. Of course, laboratory-developed tests generally are developed by the local institution rather than being provided from a commercial vendor. As you can see from the prior descriptions of various AI/ML applications they have been developed both within "open-source" environments as well as commercial environments. Similar correlates for laboratory-developed assays can be seen within AI/ML space in regard to institutionally created tools versus commercially available tools.

REIMBURSEMENT

Beginning in January 2023, the American Medical Association introduced "test" codes for the digital scanning of slides.[34] This was for technical work related to using digital pathology and could provide a revenue source that might create a return on investment for using digital pathology and subsequently facilitate AI/ML adoption. Although radiology has more development within the image-based AI/ML environment, reimbursement for the use of AI/ML is still evolving.[35] Of course, reimbursement for the use AI/ML would certainly spur adoption but payors will need to see the clinical benefit for such tools before they will pay for the tools.

DEPLOYMENT

Another aspect of AI/ML is how the algorithm is integrated into the diagnostic workflow. The current development process has been focused on developing tools with less focus on how to integrate the tools into the diagnostic workflow. To some extent, the lack of regulatory guidance has hindered the establishment of pathology workflows. Broadly, these tools can be applied in a "preprocessing" fashion or in an "on-demand" fashion. In the author's opinion from a practical standpoint, most AI/ML should be deployed in a "preprocessing" fashion so that the results are readily available for the sign-out pathologist when desired (ie, at the time of case sign-out). The scenario where a pathologist has the slides and is ready for case sign-out but needs to wait for AI/ML to be performed on the case does not seem likely to be utilized unless the value provided from the AI/ML is so high to justify the delay. As you can see from these different scenarios, a lot of variables feed into the determination of what to do with the AI/ML.

Additionally, the technical resources to run the tools may require higher level of computing function than is available at an institution. This can be overcome with cloud-based computing resources but then the image files need to be transferred from the institution to the cloud environment. This transfer of whole-slide images needs to occur in a secure fashion and security needs to be present with the clinical information within the cloud space. However, it does seem that many software companies are moving toward cloud-based environments, which should facilitate ease of image transfer, in theory. The technical resources needed to run AI/ML tools (ie, high-performance computer clusters or GPUs, and so forth) may not be available on premise at institutions necessitating a cloud environment in order to efficiently support the technical needs of the AI/ML tools.

DISCUSSION

Many research studies have described AI/ML tools that attempt to solve problems within lung pathology. These tools can involve immunostains or special stains, routine H&E slides, or derive novel reporting elements that are not currently reported. Although some institutions have started deploying AI/ML tools, the applications are relatively narrow in scope and are deployed in a very controlled environment to reduce any potential risk for patient safety. There are public image–based challenges that are currently assisting with the development of AI/ML tools for use within pathology.[36] These tools are still early within the adoption phase but do seem to offer beneficial aspects to diagnostic pathology, and so it does seem that at some point AI/ML tools will be available for routine use in lung pathology. As research studies describing AI/ML tools are published, it is important that pathologists become discriminatory about the studies so that the best end product is created for clinical use. Regulatory, workflow, and payment structures around the use AI/ML are still being determined which can either aid or impede further adoption beyond the current status.

CLINICS CARE POINTS

- Artificial intelligence/machine learning tools for lung pathology are being created.

- Deployment and regulatory factors are still evolving which are acting as headwinds to adoption.

- Although most work with artificial intelligence/machine learning has been replicating/augmenting work that can be done manually, future tools will provide information that is currently not reported by pathologists.

DISCLOSURE

The author has no disclosures related to the subject matter of this article.

REFERENCES

1. Zarella MD, McClintock DS, Batra H, et al. Artificial intelligence and digital pathology: clinical promise and deployment considerations. J Med Imaging 2023;10(5):051802.
2. Steiner DF, MacDonald R, Liu Y, et al. Impact of Deep Learning Assistance on the Histopathologic Review of Lymph Nodes for Metastatic Breast Cancer. Am J Surg Pathol 2018;42(12):1636–46.
3. Recht M, Bryan RN. Artificial Intelligence: Threat or Boon to Radiologists? J Am Coll Radiol 2017; 14(11):1476–80.
4. Baxi V, Edwards R, Montalto M, et al. Digital pathology and artificial intelligence in translational medicine and clinical practice. Mod Pathol 2022;35(1):23–32.
5. Do HM, Spear LG, Nikpanah M, et al. Augmented Radiologist Workflow Improves Report Value and Saves Time: A Potential Model for Implementation of Artificial Intelligence. Acad Radiol 2020;27(1): 96–105.
6. Harrison JH, Gilbertson JR, Hanna MG, et al. Introduction to Artificial Intelligence and Machine Learning for Pathology. Arch Pathol Lab Med 2021; 145(10):1228–54.
7. Abels E, Pantanowitz L, Aeffner F, et al. Computational pathology definitions, best practices, and recommendations for regulatory guidance: a white paper from the Digital Pathology Association. J Pathol 2019;249(3):286–94.
8. Hanna MG, Reuter VE, Ardon O, et al. Validation of a digital pathology system including remote review during the COVID-19 pandemic. Mod Pathol 2020; 33(11):2115–27.
9. Ardon O, Reuter VE, Hameed M, et al. Digital Pathology Operations at an NYC Tertiary Cancer Center During the First 4 Months of COVID-19 Pandemic Response. Acad Pathol 2021;8, 23742895211010276.
10. Lujan GM, Savage J, Shana'ah A, et al. Digital Pathology Initiatives and Experience of a Large Academic Institution During the Coronavirus Disease 2019 (COVID-19) Pandemic. Arch Pathol Lab Med 2021;145(9):1051–61.
11. Araujo ALD, do Amaral-Silva GK, Pérez-de-Oliveira ME, et al. Fully digital pathology laboratory routine and remote reporting of oral and maxillofacial diagnosis during the COVID-19 pandemic: a validation study. Virchows Arch 2021;479(3):585–95.
12. Hassell LA, Peterson J, Pantanowitz L. Pushed Across the Digital Divide: COVID-19 Accelerated Pathology Training onto a New Digital Learning Curve. Acad Pathol 2021;8, 2374289521994240.
13. Giaretto S, Renne SL, Rahal D, et al. Digital Pathology During the COVID-19 Outbreak in Italy: Survey Study. J Med Internet Res 2021;23(2):e24266.
14. Cimadamore A, Lopez-Beltran A, Scarpelli M, et al. Digital pathology and COVID-19 and future crises: pathologists can safely diagnose cases from home using a consumer monitor and a mini PC. J Clin Pathol 2020;73(11):695–6.
15. Zarella MD, Bowman D, Aeffner F, et al. A Practical Guide to Whole Slide Imaging: A White Paper From the Digital Pathology Association. Arch Pathol Lab Med 2019;143(2):222–34.
16. Montezuma D, Monteiro A, Fraga J, et al. Digital Pathology Implementation in Private Practice: Specific Challenges and Opportunities. Diagnostics 2022; 12(2).
17. Hanna MG, Reuter VE, Samboy J, et al. Implementation of Digital Pathology Offers Clinical and Operational Increase in Efficiency and Cost Savings. Arch Pathol Lab Med 2019;143(12):1545–55.
18. Cheng JY, Abel JT, Balis UGJ, et al. Challenges in the Development, Deployment, and Regulation of Artificial Intelligence in Anatomic Pathology. Am J Pathol 2021;191(10):1684–92.
19. Pantanowitz L, Wu U, Seigh L, et al. Artificial Intelligence-Based Screening for Mycobacteria in Whole-Slide Images of Tissue Samples. Am J Clin Pathol 2021;156(1):117–28.
20. Wu J, Liu C, Liu X, et al. Artificial intelligence-assisted system for precision diagnosis of PD-L1 expression in non-small cell lung cancer. Mod Pathol 2022;35(3):403–11.
21. Zhao Y, He S, Zhao D, et al. Deep learning-based diagnosis of histopathological patterns for invasive non-mucinous lung adenocarcinoma using semantic segmentation. BMJ Open 2023;13(7):e069181.
22. Thunnissen E, Beasley MB, Borczuk AC, et al. Reproducibility of histopathological subtypes and invasion in pulmonary adenocarcinoma. An international interobserver study. Mod Pathol 2012;25(12): 1574–83.
23. Courtiol P, Maussion C, Moarii M, et al. Deep learning-based classification of mesothelioma improves prediction of patient outcome. Nat Med 2019;25(10):1519–25.
24. Li B, Yang L, Zhang H, et al. Outcome-Supervised Deep Learning on Pathologic Whole Slide Images for Survival Prediction of Immunotherapy in Patients with Non-Small Cell Lung Cancer. Mod Pathol 2023; 36(8):100208.
25. DuCote TJ, Naughton KJ, Skaggs EM, et al. Using Artificial Intelligence to Identify Tumor Microenvironment Heterogeneity in Non-Small Cell Lung Cancers. Lab Invest 2023;103(8):100176.
26. Uegami W, Bychkov A, Ozasa M, et al. MIXTURE of human expertise and deep learning-developing an explainable model for predicting pathological

diagnosis and survival in patients with interstitial lung disease. Mod Pathol 2022;35(8):1083–91.

27. Bishop KW, Barner LAE, Han Q, et al. An end-to-end workflow for non-destructive 3D pathology. bioRxiv 2023. https://doi.org/10.1101/2023.08.03.551845.

28. Sijilmassi O, López Alonso JM, Del Río Sevilla A, et al. Multispectral Imaging Method for Rapid Identification and Analysis of Paraffin-Embedded Pathological Tissues. J Digit Imag 2023;36(4): 1663–74.

29. Borowsky AD, Levenson RM, Gown AM, et al. A Pilot Validation Study Comparing Fluorescence-Imitating Brightfield Imaging, A Slide-Free Imaging Method, With Standard Formalin-Fixed, Paraffin-Embedded Hematoxylin-Eosin-Stained Tissue Section Histology for Primary Surgical Pathology Diagnosis. Arch Pathol Lab Med 2023.

30. Watson A, Chapman R, Shafai G, et al. FDA regulations and prescription digital therapeutics: Evolving with the technologies they regulate. Front Digit Health 2023;5:1086219.

31. Administration, F.a.D.; Available from: https://www.fda.gov/medical-devices/software-medical-device--samd/your-clinical-decision-support-software-it-medical-device.

32. Marchesin S, Giachelle F, Marini N, et al. Empowering digital pathology applications through explainable knowledge extraction tools. J Pathol Inf 2022; 13:100139.

33. Plass M, Kargl M, Kiehl TR, et al. Explainability and causability in digital pathology. J Pathol Clin Res 2023;9(4):251–60.

34. CPT codes for digital pathology. 2023; Available at: https://www.cap.org/advocacy/payments-for-pathology-services/2023-digital-pathology-codes.

35. Lobig F, Subramanian D, Blankenburg M, et al. To pay or not to pay for artificial intelligence applications in radiology. NPJ Digit Med 2023;6(1):117.

36. Hartman DJ, Van Der Laak JAWM, Gurcan MN, et al. Value of public challenges for the development of pathology deep learning algorithms. J Pathol Inf 2020;11:7.

Moving?

Make sure your subscription moves with you!

To notify us of your new address, find your **Clinics Account Number** (located on your mailing label above your name), and contact customer service at:

Email: journalscustomerservice-usa@elsevier.com

800-654-2452 (subscribers in the U.S. & Canada)
314-447-8871 (subscribers outside of the U.S. & Canada)

Fax number: 314-447-8029

Elsevier Health Sciences Division
Subscription Customer Service
3251 Riverport Lane
Maryland Heights, MO 63043

ELSEVIER

Moving?

Make sure your subscription moves with you!

To notify us of your new address, find your Clinics Account Number (located on your mailing label above your name), and contact customer service at:

Email: journalscustomerservice-usa@elsevier.com

800-654-2452 (subscribers in the U.S. & Canada)
314-447-8871 (subscribers outside of the U.S. & Canada)

Fax number: 314-447-8029

Elsevier Health Sciences Division
Subscription Customer Service
3251 Riverport Lane
Maryland Heights, MO 63043

*To ensure uninterrupted delivery of your subscription, please notify us at least 4 weeks in advance of move.

Printed and bound by CPI Group (UK) Ltd, Croydon, CR0 4YY

03/10/2024

01040363-0017